Ethical, Legal and Social Aspects of Child Healthcare

Edited by

Patrick H. T. Cartlidge DM FRCP FRCPCH

Senior Lecturer in Child Health and Honorary Consultant Paediatrician,
Department of Health, Cardiff University, Cardiff, UK

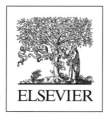

ELSEVIER

EDINBURGH LONDON NEW YORK OXFORD PHILADELPHIA ST LOUIS SYDNEY TORONTO 2007

ELSEVIER

ISBN: 978-0-08-044682-0

British Library Cataloguing in Publication Data
A catalogue record for this book is available from the British Library.

Library of Congress Cataloging in Publication Data
A catalog record for this book is available from the Library of Congress.

Note
Knowledge and best practice in this field are constantly changing. As new
research and experience broaden our knowledge, changes in practice, treatment
and drug therapy may become necessary or appropriate. Readers are advised
to check the most current information provided (i) on procedures featured
or (ii) by the manufacturer of each product to be administered, to verify the
recommended dose or formula, the method and duration of administration,
and contraindications. It is the responsibility of the practitioner, relying on
their own experience and knowledge of the patient, to make diagnoses, to
determine dosages and the best treatment for each individual patient, and
to take all appropriate safety precautions. To the fullest extent of the law,
neither the Publisher nor the Editor assumes any liability for any injury
and/or damage to persons or property arising out of or related to any use
of the material contained in this book.
The Publisher

Working together to grow libraries in developing countries

www.elsevier.com | www.bookaid.org | www.sabre.org

ELSEVIER   **BOOK AID** International   Sabre Foundation

ELSEVIER your source for books, journals and multimedia in the health sciences
www.elsevierhealth.com

The publisher's policy is to use **paper manufactured from sustainable forests**

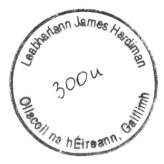

Printed in China

Contents

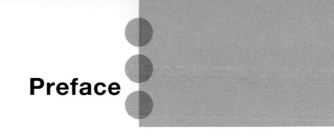

Preface

Many of the problems faced by paediatricians in their professional lives relate to ethical dilemmas and the legal aspects of child health. The scope of potential problems is enormous, including the appropriate use of life-sustaining treatments, child-protection issues, ethics of genetic screening, prioritizing care in a resource-limited health system, etc. Yet, it is difficult to find guidance on how to deal with these issues from standard textbooks.

This book brings together papers written by highly experienced authors, including the Chief Medical Officers for England and Wales, a High Court Judge, paediatricians, psychiatrists and social workers. Insight is provided on how to manage the many ethical dilemmas faced by paediatricians and families. I anticipate the book being a valuable source of guidance for all those involved in promoting the health of children.

Patrick H. T. Cartlidge

Contributors

Mary Y. Anthony MD MRCP FRCPCH
Consultant Neonatologist, Women's Centre, John
Radcliffe Hospital, Oxford, UK

Christopher J. Bacon MA MB BChir MRCP FRCPCH
Retired Consultant Paediatrician, Danby Wiske,
Northallerton, UK

Gillian Baird MD FRCPCH
Honorary Professor in Neurodisability, Newcomen
Centre, Guy's Hospital, London, UK

Michelle A. Barber MA BCh MRCPCH DipPallMed
Consultant Paediatrician, Royal Gwent Hospital,
Newport, UK

Jane Barlow DPhil Hon FPHM
Primary Care Career Scientist, University of Oxford,
Health Services Research Unit, Institute of Health
Sciences, Oxford, UK

Amanda Billson BA MBBS MRCP FRCPCH DipMedEd
Consultant Paediatrician, Royal United Hospital,
Bath, UK

Richard Bowker MA MBBM MRCPCH
Paediatric Specialist Registrar, Nottingham University
Hospital, Nottingham, UK

Anna Boyce MBBS MRCPCH MRCPsych
Specialist Registrar in Child and Adolescent Psychiatry,
Queen Elizabeth Hospital, Gateshead, UK

Rachel Brooks MB ChB DCH MSc PCME
Department of Child Health, University of Wales College
of Medicine, Cardiff, UK

Pamela A. Cairns MB BCh MRCP MRCPCH DH MD
Consultant Neonatologist, Department of Child Health,
St. Michael's Hospital, Bristol, UK

Angus Clarke DM FRCP FRCPCH
Department of Medical Genetics, University of Wales
College of Medicine, Cardiff, UK

Helen Cockerill BSc(Hons) RegMRCSLT
Consultant Speech and Language Therapist, Evelina
Children's Hospital, St. Thomas' Hospital, London, UK

Monica Cockett BA Diploma in Social Administration
Department of Child Health, Peninsula Medical School,
Universities of Exeter and Plymouth, and Director,
Devon Family Mediation Agency, Exeter, UK

David P. Davies BSc MD FRCP DCH DObst FRCPCH
Emeritus Professor of Child Health (Retired), Department
of Child Health, Cardiff University, Cardiff, UK

Sir Liam Donaldson MSc MD FRCS(Ed) FRCP FRCP(Ed)
FRCGP FMedSci FFPHM
Chief Medical Officer, Department of Health, London, UK

Clare Edmonds MBBS BSc MRCP MRCPCH
Specialist Registrar in Paediatrics, Royal United
Hospital, Bath, UK

Martyn Evans BA PhD
Centre for Arts and Humanities in Health and Medicine,
Durham University, Durham, UK

William I. Fraser MD FRCP(Ed) FRCPsych FAcadMedSci
Professor Emeritus, University of Wales College of
Medicine, Cardiff, UK

Stefan J. Friedrichsdorf MD
Medical Director of Pain & Palliative Care, The
Children's Hospitals and Clinics of Minnesota,
Minneapolis, MN, USA

A. Bryan Gill MB MRCP FRCPCH
Consultant Neonatologist and Deputy Medical Director,
Leeds Teaching Hospital NHS Trust, Leeds, UK

Stephen J. Gould MB BS FRCPath
Consultant Paediatric Pathologist, Women's Centre,
John Radcliffe Hospital, Oxford, UK

Sian Griffiths MB BChir FRCP FFPHM FHKCCM
Professor of Public Health Director, School of Public
Health, The Chinese University of Hong, Hong Kong

Richard D. W. Hain MD MSc MRCP FRCPCH DipPallMed
ATCH Senior Lecturer and Honorary Consultant in
Paediatric Palliative Medicine, University Hospital of
Wales, Cardiff, UK

Aidan Halligan MA MD FRCOG FRCP FFPHM MRCPI
Formaer Director of Clinical Governance for the NHS,
Leicester, UK

Tammy Hedderly MRCPCH MBBS BSc(Hons)
Consultant Paediatric Neurologist, King's College
Hospital, London, UK

The Hon Mr Justice Hedley
Family Division of the High Court, Royal Courts of
Justice, London, UK

Michael F. Hird MB BS BSc DCH MRCP(UK) FRCPCH
Consultant Neonatal Paediatrician, The Royal London
Hospital, London, UK

Chris J. Hobbs BSc MB BS DObstRCOG FRCP FRCPCH
Retired Consultant Community Paediatrician, St. James'
University Hospital, Leeds, UK

Tony Jewell FFPH FRCGP
Chief Medical Officer, Welsh Assembly Government,
Cardiff, UK

Alison Kemp MB BCh DCH MRCP FRCPCH FRCP(Edin)
Department of Child Health, Cardiff University,
Cardiff, UK

Victor F. Larcher BA MB BChir FRCPCH MA
Consultant in Paediatrics and Clinical Ethics, Great
Ormond Street Hospital, London, UK

Martine Marshallsay RNLD RGN MSc
Assistant Head of Nursing, Learning Disabilities
Directorate, Bro Morgannwg NHS Trust, Cardiff, UK

Helen McConachie MA MPhil PhD
Professor of Child Clinical Psychology, Newcastle
University, Newcastle upon Tyne, UK

Neil McIntosh DSc(Med) FRCP(Edin) FRCP(Lond) FRCPCH
Professor of Child Life and Health, University of
Edinburgh, Edinburgh, UK

Alex Mellanby MPH MD MRCGP FFPH FRCP
Director, NE & NC London Health Protection Unit,
London, UK

Jaime Morey-Canellas MRCPsych MScPsychiatry
Consultant in Developmental Neuropsychiatry, Learning
Disabilities Directorate, Bro Morgannwg NHS Trust,
Cardiff, UK

Alexandra Murray BSc MBBS MRCP
Consultant Clinical Geneticist, Institute of Medical
Genetics, University Hospital of Wales, Cardiff, UK

David Niven CQSW
Managing Director, David Niven Associates (DNA). Past
Chair of British Association of Social Workers, and past
Chief Executive of the Children's Charity ACHE

Andrea Nussbaumer MD MRCPCH
Specialist Registrar in Paediatrics, Sheffield Children's
Hospital, Sheffield, UK

Heather Payne MB BS FRCPCH DCH ILTM MIHSM
Senior Lecturer in Child Health, Cardiff University,
Cardiff, and Consultant Paediatrician, Ystrad Mynach
Hospital, Caerphilly, UK

Jean Price MD MBBS FRCPCH
Child & Family Services, Central Health Clinic,
Southampton, UK

Annie M. Procter MD MRCP
Consultant and Clinical Director, All Wales Medical
Genetics Service, Institute of Medical Genetics,
Cardiff, UK

John Rees BEd(Hons) CertEd
APAUSE Programme Manager and Honorary Research
Fellow, Peninsula Medical School, Exeter, UK

Robert I. Ross Russell MD FRCPCH
Consultant Paediatrician, Addenbrooke's Hospital,
Cambridge, UK

Peter T. Rudd MD FRCPCH
Consultant Paediatrician, Royal United Hospital, Bath,
and Honorary Senior Lecturer, University of Bath, Bath,
UK

Joanne Saunders BSc MBBCH MRCPCH
Specialist Registrar in General Paediatrics, Royal Gwent
Hospital, Newport, UK

Julian Savulescu BMedSci MB BS MA PhD
Chair in Practical Ethics, University of Oxford,
Director of the Oxford Uehiro Centre for Practical
Ethics, Director of the Programme on Ethics and
the New Biosciences in the 21st Century School,
University of Oxford, Oxford, UK

David J. Scott MA MBA MB BChir FRCP FRCPCH DCH
Medical Director and Consultant Paediatrician, Clinical
Practice Directorate, East Sussex Hospitals NHS Trust,
Conquest Hospital, St. Leonards-on-Sea, UK

Edward P. Sein MBBS FRCPsych
Consultant Child and Adolescent Psychiatrist, Linhope
Unit, Wansbeck Hospital, Ashington, UK

Mike Shooter MA MB BChir FRCPsych CBE
Former Consultant in Child & Adolescent Psychiatry,
The Children's Centre, Nevill Hall Hospital,
Abergavenny, UK, and Past Prersident, Royal College
of Psychiatrists, London, UK

Jo R. Sibert OBE MA MD FRCP FRCPCH DCH
Emeritus Professor of Child Health, Department of Chid
Health, Cardiff University, Cardiff, UK

Justin Simon BSc CQSW
Independent Social Work Consultant, Child Centred
Consultancy, London, UK

Nick J. Spencer MPhil(Nott) FRCPH FRCP(Edin)
Emeritus Professor, School of Health and Social Studies
and Warwick Medical School, University of Warwick,
Coventry, UK

Terence Stephenson BSc BM BCh DM FRCP FRCPCH
Professor of Child Health, Faculty of Medicine
and Health Sciences, University of Nottingham,
Nottingham, UK

Sarah Stewart-Brown BM BCh PhD FFPH FFRCPH FRCP
Professor of Public Health, Warwick Medical School
(LWMS), University of Warwick, Coventry, UK

Elizabeth Towner PhD MA PGCE BSc FFPH
Professor of Child Health, Centre for Child and
Adolescent Health, University of the West of England,
Bristol, UK

John Towner PhD MA BA PGCE
University of Northumbria, Newcastle upon Tyne and
Independent Researcher, UK

John H. Tripp MD FRCR
Senior Clinical Lecturer in Child Health, Peninsula
Medical School, Universities of Exeter and Plymouth, UK

Bryan Vernon MA DipTheol
Lecturer in Ethics of Health Care, The Medical School,
University of Newcastle upon Tyne, Newcastle upon
Tyne, UK

Debbie Wall BEd(Hons) MA
Senior Researcher, NHS Clinical Governance Support
Team, Leicester, UK

Elspeth Webb FRCP FRCPCH MSc DTM&H
Senior Lecturer in Child Health, College of Medicine,
Cardiff University, Cardiff, UK

Jan Welbury MB ChB FRCPCH DRCOG DFMB
Consultant Community Paediatrician, The Children's
Centre, Sunderland, UK

Richard Wilson MB FRCP FRCPCH DCH
Honorary Consultant Paediatrician, Department of Child
Health, Kingston upon Thames, UK

Jane M. Wynne D(of Univ) MB ChB FRCP FRCPCH
Retired Consultant Community Paediatrician, Leeds, UK

Chapter One

Clinical governance: improving the child's experience of healthcare

1

Sir Liam Donaldson • Aidan Halligan • Debbie Wall

SUMMARY

The concept of clinical governance, and the philosophy of quality-centred care is being implemented throughout the National Health Service, not least in the cross-government 'Change for Children' programme. Clinical governance integrates the systems, processes and mechanisms necessary to ensure high-quality and safe care for children. It also demands standards, robust assessment, local innovation and patient empowerment. The clinical governance agenda in child healthcare builds on the lessons of the Bristol Royal Infirmary and Climbié inquiries, with an emphasis on supporting the delivery of child-centred, safe and high-quality care, underpinned by effective multidisciplinary teams, integrated across organizations and whole-systems.

INTRODUCTION

Twelve-year-old Claire* stayed on the children's ward for a week, receiving treatment for cancer. Jenny, the Trust's patient liaison manager, asked Claire to keep a diary during her time in hospital and use a disposable camera to take pictures of anything she felt was really important, or that she would like to see changed.

Claire took pictures of her bed, the room she was in, the toilet, and the food; 'the usual sort of things that you'd expect' according to Jenny. However, a number of photographs were quite different. They showed the bottom half of the faces of hospital staff; just their mouths and their chins. Jenny told Claire that she could not understand why she had taken these pictures. Had she meant to take full-face photos? And Claire said, 'no', the reason she had taken them was because people do not smile enough in hospital. When people smiled at her it made her feel happy; it made her feel confident and good about things.

Claire's response surprised Jenny. It drove home the message that asking patients for their views, whether adults, or children, may elicit responses that do not meet with professional expectations. It also exemplified, in a small way, the unique perspective of the child, and how children's and young people's concepts of hospital care, illness and health risks differ from adults.[1, 2] Their concepts may differ, but children's entitlement to patient-centred, safe and high-quality care, delivered through clinical governance, remains the same as for adults. Children, too, need equitable access to care on their own terms; to people who will listen, who will value what they say, who will respond to their specific needs, and who they can trust implicitly.

By taking their sick child to a doctor, a parent trusts that the treatment and care they will receive will be safe and delivered by a competent professional with the up-to-date knowledge and skills required to meet their child's needs. Clinical governance reflects this privileged relationship: it unifies the activities necessary to ensure the clinician's duty of trust to patients by providing a framework through which National Health Service (NHS) organizations are accountable for continually improving the quality of their services and safeguarding high standards of clinical practice.[3] Clinical governance is also the framework through which organizations influence the informal psychological and social functioning of their staff. It resides more in behaviour than structure. Both the law and clinical governance need structure, but, ultimately, depend upon individuals choosing to behave in an accountable fashion.

In 1998 the consultation document *A First Class Service*[4] set out this quality framework for the NHS, introducing clinical governance as a responsibility of all local NHS organizations. This became a statutory duty of quality under the 1999 Health Act,[5] requiring corporate accountability for clinical and organizational performance.

THE BRISTOL AND CLIMBIÉ INQUIRIES

Despite the enthusiasm and commitment to quality improvement by health services and health professionals over the past decade, public confidence and trust is still very susceptible to media coverage of problems in delivery of health services. The factors which led to poor standards of care for some children treated by the Bristol children's heart surgery service, and identified in the subsequent wide-ranging public inquiry,[6] were intimately related to the components of clinical governance. The Inquiry Report, published in 2001, was a chilling indictment of an NHS culture that failed to embrace quality. The report pointed to issues such as:

- a lack of child-centredness
- a dysfunctional clinical team
- the absence of truly reflective practice
- a failure to place patient safety above other service considerations

---

*Claire and Jenny are pseudonyms; names have been changed to protect anonymity.

- no tradition of using and acting on good performance data
- lack of organizational systems to ensure responsibility for children's healthcare.

The coincidence of the above, combined with an adverse culture, led inevitably to a failing service, with attendant risks for patients and for clinical reputation. The national clinical governance agenda has, in part, been driven by the lessons from Bristol and by other organizational, service and individual failures of the 1990s, which damaged public confidence in the quality and standards of services available to patients.[7, 8]

Similar themes, however, recurred in the 2003 report into the death of Victoria Climbié.[9] Successful clinical governance relies on proper arrangements for accountability, including the accountability of staff to take appropriate action to safeguard the welfare of children in their care.[10] The Climbié report cites 'gross failure' in the organization, management and leadership of the key public services which were designed to protect Victoria Climbié from deliberate harm. Senior staff failed to accept responsibility for the quality of children's services: teams had overlapping remits, staff were poorly trained and information was not exchanged among 'those in the know'.

The combined recommendations of the Bristol and Climbié inquiries and the Government's responses[11, 12] provided the backdrop to radical reforms in the health and social care agenda for children and young people. The objective shared across Government departments, agencies and key public services is to improve measures to protect the health and well-being of children and vulnerable groups through more effective, joined-up working, utilizing the principles of clinical governance.[13] The 2004 Children Act[14] is the legislative basis for reforms introduced through the *Every Child Matters: Change for Children* green paper[15] and the resulting programme being implemented across children's services.[16] In addition, *Choosing Health: Making Healthy Choices Easier*, The Public Health White Paper, identifies children's and young people's health as a key governmental priority for the future.[2]

MULTIDISCIPLINARY AND MULTI-AGENCY TEAMS

The programme for clinical governance within the NHS is about transforming teams and the local organizations in which they operate so that quality assurance and improvement are inherent within everyday routines and practices – 'everyday', rather than being part of an occasional discussion, or an agenda item raised at the next clinical team meeting.

It is only in recent years that working in multidisciplinary teams has become more common, and there is growing evidence that they make a critical contribution to the delivery of effective and innovative healthcare in the NHS:[17, 18]

I am in no doubt that effective support for children and families cannot be achieved by a single agency acting alone. It depends on a number of agencies working well together. It is a multi-disciplinary task. (Lord Laming, 2003: 6)[9]

However, developing teams, let alone those that collaborate across public sector agencies, has been difficult in the NHS. Only 43% of staff participating in the 2004 NHS national staff survey reported working in teams that met regularly to discuss their effectiveness, and had clear objectives to achieve with other team members.[19] Yet 91% reported working in a 'team'.

To implement the quality agenda, teams need to become truly multidisciplinary and, increasingly, multi-agency, with an understanding of team members' roles, the effective sharing of information and knowledge across organizational and professional boundaries,[20, 21] and ways of working that constantly revisit assumptions about the quality and safety of care being provided. This is crucial in an area as diverse as child health, where varied stages of physical and emotional development require different approaches to care, and where specific groups of children need safeguarding from harm.

In addition, an increasing number of children are being treated for long-term, complex illnesses. These children, too, are reliant on a wide range of highly specialized services. Professionals with complementary skills from health, education and social services will need to cross existing boundaries of understanding and form multi-agency teams, agreements on integrated services for children will need be brokered, and different working cultures come together to focus on common outcomes for children.[12, 22] The National Service Framework for Children, for example, recommends that healthcare professionals know social services staff at a personal level, so professional trust builds up over time. Case Illustration 1.1 demonstrates how this may occur.

Case illustration 1.1

Health and social care professionals met to process-map a patient's journey through children's services, so they could see where improvements could be made. They discussed the input of social services into the journey. At lunchtime, a paediatrician, who had worked at the same hospital for 15 years, walked over to a social worker, shook his hand, and introduced himself. Snapshots of conversation were heard by the meeting facilitator:

Nice to meet you. We've never met have we?

I hate to tell you this, but I didn't really know what you did either.

They shared the same patients, but this was the first time they had met face to face to share information about their respective roles in the process of care.

ORGANIZATIONS

Effective leadership is required at all levels of an organization if joined-up working, with cross-sector communication and collaborative working practices, is to become a reality. Organizations need to put in place systems and local arrangements to support individuals and teams and ensure the quality of care provided. Leadership from the NHS Trust Board is crucial for this to occur and to demonstrate, by example, that change for the better really is possible. A children's lead should also be appointed within every Trust Board to oversee clinical governance arrangements, including the introduction of national quality standards.[10] The organizational ethos needs to be one where frontline staff, who have the most contact with children and young people, feel valued, supported and empowered to take the clinical governance agenda forward, and to talk openly about mistakes and learn from them.

The cultural change required to 'shift the balance of power'[23] is difficult to implement in organizations that remain hierarchical and where professional boundaries exist that hamper relationships between staff, and between staff and patients. Opportunities for real change and learning often lie in the details of organizational life: in everyday practices, mundane interactions and normal ways of understanding.

In a constantly developing paediatric team, good leadership means influencing people's attitudes and behaviour towards each other, and towards the children in their care. Individuals need to embrace behavioural change by building a modern approach to reflective practice that places patients at the centre of their thinking: they need to show a genuine interest in the concerns of children and young people, answer children's questions about their care truthfully and clearly; and treat all patients as they would want to be treated themselves.[6] For some, the imbalance of power that can exist when adults communicate with children (and, in some cases, with other adults too) will need to be recognized and redressed.

NATIONAL STANDARDS

Integral to the delivery of clinical governance across the NHS is the identification of clear standards and rigorous inspection to ensure quality of services. The framework of core and developmental standards introduced in *Standards for Better Health*[24, 25] reinforces quality and safety at the centre of the NHS agenda. The Standards also apply to private and voluntary providers of NHS care. All NHS organizations are required to comply with the core standards when developing, providing and commissioning healthcare.

Standards are also set and disseminated through the Royal Colleges, National Service Frameworks (NSFs) and guidance from the National Institute for Health and Clinical Excellence (NICE).[26] A rolling programme of NSFs was launched in April 1998 to address unacceptable variations in health services. NSFs set national standards and identify key interventions for particular services or care groups.

The *National Service Framework for Children, Young People and Maternity Services* (2004)[22] sets out a 10-year programme to improve the quality of children's health and social care, whereby local services are to become designed and delivered around the needs of children and families rather than around the needs of organizations: a cultural shift requiring, according to the Children's Commission, 'a fundamental change in the way we think'.[27]

The NSF also addresses the recommendation of the Climbié Inquiry that child protection should come under the framework of clinical governance[9] by setting standards that cover child protection services: evidence suggests that child protection issues have not always been viewed as a responsibility at NHS Trust Board level.[28]

THE HOSPITAL STANDARD FOR CHILDREN

Children and young people should receive appropriate high quality, evidence-based hospital care, developed through clinical governance and delivered by staff who have the right set of skills. (Hospital Standard Part 2)[10]

The first standard to be published in the Children's NSF was the Hospital Standard for Children.[10] Its implementation sits within a Trust's overall clinical governance framework, giving children explicit recognition as a separate and vulnerable group. This arrangement should be clearly identified within the Trust's Clinical Governance Development Plan, and in an action plan that includes an annual report to the Board on children's services in the hospital. Many aspects of the Standard can be summarized under clinical governance themes (Box 1.1).

Patient safety is a specific strand of the clinical governance framework, with mechanisms in place, via the National Patient Safety Agency (NPSA), to deal with poor practitioner performance as well as reporting, analysing and learning from adverse events and 'near misses' involving NHS patients.[29] The NPSA has established a national reporting and learning system (NRLS) that allows NHS organizations to report patient safety incidents. The learning culture advocated through clinical governance is also being promoted through the publication of statistical trends and comparative information to inform safe practice.

THE HEALTHCARE COMMISSION

Besides clear standards, inspection arrangements are also integral to the delivery of clinical governance across the NHS. In England,

BOX 1.1

Clinical governance and the children's NSF

- **Patients first** – clinical governance systems explicitly focused on the different needs of the child and taking account of their views.
- **Teams** – clinical governance approached on a multidisciplinary and, where appropriate, multi-agency basis to include social work staff and other professionals.
- **Education and training** – staff treating and caring for children and young people having the appropriate education, training, knowledge and skills to provide high-quality care.
- **Evidence-based** protocol and guideline development for children and young people linked into programmes of staff education and training.
- **Information systems** to safeguard children: a reliable system of accurate and comprehensive record-keeping to ensure records are always available when children are seen and assessed.
- **Risk management** – risks to children managed and addressed explicitly, as an integral part of the overall clinical governance arrangements.
- **Clinical audit** – clinical governance and multidisciplinary, child-specific clinical audit arrangements in place to ensure the quality of systems, processes and practices to safeguard children.
- **Safety** – use of medicines guided by the best available evidence of clinical effectiveness, cost effectiveness and safety for children (essential in child health, where children may receive medicines that are unlicensed or off-label).

local NHS clinical governance arrangements and specific standards are inspected and reported on by the Commission for Healthcare Audit and Inspection, commonly known as the Healthcare Commission (HCC), which also regulates the independent and voluntary healthcare sectors, and awards an annual performance rating to NHS organizations.[30] In April 2004 the organization replaced the work of the Commission for Health Improvement (CHI), which formerly undertook clinical governance reviews of NHS Trusts and initiated national patient surveys (since 2004, a young patients survey has been included). The HCC's new approach to assessment is based on checks and follow-ups of organizational self-assessments. The HCC is required by statute to take 'Standards for Better Health' into consideration in doing so, to ensure continuous improvement and that basic standards are being met. A single framework for the inspection of children's and young people's services, led by Ofsted, has been created by merging teams from several inspectorates, including the Healthcare Commission and the Commission for Social Care Inspection. Joint area reviews (JARs) of children's services across local authority areas are conducted by integrated, multidisciplinary teams that report on the experiences of children and young people, and the contributions services make to improve the five outcome areas set out in the Children Act 2004,[14] namely: being healthy, staying safe, enjoying and achieving, making a positive contribution and economic well-being.

Improvement reviews are a part of the HCC's new system of assessment, with services for children in hospital identified as a national priority. The Hospital Standard of the Children's NSF is used as a framework for the assessment of children's acute hospital services in England, focusing on access to local child-specific services provided by staff who are experienced and appropriately trained in the care of children.[31]

CONCLUSIONS

After organizations fail we look with 20:20 vision and see, with remarkable clarity, why it was always an accident waiting to happen. Why can we not anticipate such disasters? Partly, because our peripheral vision is limited by overwhelming and oppressive cultural factions and constraints. Partly, also, because we still rely on outdated, unfit for purpose, retrospective audit methodologies. Clinical governance, properly implemented, offers a readily applicable dynamic diagnostic tool that will anticipate dysfunction and its consequences.

Clinical governance, when appropriately applied in children's healthcare, is a way of working, and a way of rethinking professionalism and partnership with children, young people and their families. It places patients at the centre of delivery of care rather than professional groups or organizations. In this it is inextricably linked to the current transformation in services for children across and beyond the NHS. The *Change for Children* agenda focuses on improving the quality and safety of services for the health and well-being of the whole child. This means acknowledging that health is not the exclusive preserve of the NHS: it requires a whole-system approach that integrates key public services across the community.[12] The fundamental challenge for clinical governance is to align behaviour and attitudes, processes and systems at the level of local NHS and these partner organizations. Its delivery needs to be underpinned by good communication systems, strong leadership and multidisciplinary working practices that are seen to be effective by patients and their families.

Despite the major challenges of implementing clinical governance, integrated teams are identifying new ways of delivering care which make their services more accountable and responsive to the particular needs of children. These services prioritize children's rights and place them firmly at the centre of their care.

Chapter Two

Child safeguarding and UK law: what paediatricians need to know

2

Heather Payne

SUMMARY

The Children Act 1989 was a radical piece of legislation that brought together for the first time numerous private and public laws affecting children into a single Act, which was focused on the well-being of the child. For the first time in legislation regarding children, the welfare of the child was made the paramount consideration. The law removed the concept of 'parental rights' and substituted 'parental responsibility' towards the child. It reflects an approach based implicitly on the rights of the child and explicitly on the belief that children are generally best looked after within the family, with both parents playing a full part and without resort to legal proceedings unless there is significant harm to the child.

BOX 2.1

The Children Act 1989: Statutory Welfare Checklist

Under Section 1(3) of the Children Act 1989 the court must have regard in particular to:

1. the ascertainable wishes and feelings of the child concerned (considered in the light of his age and understanding)
2. his physical, emotional and educational needs
3. the likely effect of any change in his circumstances
4. his age, sex, background and any characteristics of his which the court considers relevant
5. any harm which he has suffered or is at risk of suffering
6. how capable each of his parents, and any other person in relation to whom the court considers the question to be relevant, is of meeting his needs
7. the range of powers available to the court under this Act in the proceedings in question.

INTRODUCTION

The Children Act 1989 (CA89)[1] came into force in England and Wales in 1991 and (with some differences) in Northern Ireland in 1996, and in Jersey as the Children (Jersey) Law 2002.[2] Due to the different legal system in Scotland, it does not apply under Scottish Law.

The CA89 not only reformed the law relating to children, it also made provision for local authority services for children in need, and amended the law regarding children's homes, foster homes, voluntary organizations, looked-after children, day care and adoption.

The 'no order' presumption states that courts will only make orders regarding children if to do so would be better for the child than not doing so. Parents who may be in dispute (e.g. over residence following divorce) are encouraged to seek agreement wherever possible. Where the child is considered to be at risk and a Care Order is being sought, the court will grant the order if the threshold conditions for significant harm are met and the protection of the child cannot be achieved in any other way.

The 'no delay' principle states that legal issues must be determined as soon as possible so that minimum disruption is caused to the child's life. To minimize delay the court must draw up a timetable at a preliminary hearing in respect of subsequent proceedings. The court must have regard to a prescribed Statutory Checklist (see the welfare checklist in Box 2.1) of the factors to be taken into account in deciding the future of children.

The CA89 established the concept of 'significant harm' to a child, this being the threshold for intervention into family life. This is not precisely defined in the Act, as it is a potentially wide ranging definition that may be very specific to an individual child's circumstances. Section 47 of the Act places a duty on the local authority to make enquiries when it has 'reasonable cause to suspect that a child who lives, or is found, in their area is suffering, or is likely to suffer, significant harm'.

Sometimes, significant harm[3] can be indicated by a single traumatic event (e.g. a violent assault, suffocation, shaking or poisoning). However, significant harm may be due to an accumulation of significant events that damage a child's physical or psychological development, such as neglect or long-term minor physical abuse, or involvement in inappropriate sexual activity. Harm is defined in Section 31 of the Act as 'ill-treatment or the impairment of health and development'.

PARENTAL RESPONSIBILITY

Parental responsibility[4] is a legal concept introduced by the CA89 consisting of 'the rights, duties, powers, responsibilities and authority that parents have regarding their children'. It includes the right to give consent to medical treatment and to apply for access to the health records of their child.

Further legislation in the Adoption and Children Act 2002 (see below) has modified who has parental responsibility. In relation to children born on or after 1 December 2003 (England and Wales), 15 April 2002 (Northern Ireland)[5] or 4 May 2006 (Scotland),[6] both of a child's biological parents have parental responsibility if they are registered on the child's birth certificate (whether or not the parents are married). For children born prior to these dates, both biological parents automatically acquired parental responsibility if they were married at the time of the child's conception or at any time thereafter. If the parents were never married, only the mother automatically has parental responsibility, the father needing to acquire it via a parental responsibility agreement (witnessed by a lawyer), or through a parental responsibility court order.

Where the child has been born as a result of assisted reproduction, there are rules under the Human Fertilisation and Embryology Act 1990 that determine the child's legal parentage.

Parental responsibility is not lost following divorce or if a child is accommodated by the local authority or in police custody. It can, however, be restricted by a range of Court Orders (a local authority shares parental responsibility with the parents while the child is the subject of a Care Order).

Parental responsibility is extinguished permanently from birth parents only when a child is adopted; the adoptive parents become the child's legal parents and acquire parental responsibility. Another person can acquire parental responsibility by being appointed as the child's guardian (usually taking effect on the death of the parents) or via a residence order (parental responsibility lasts for the duration of the order).

In England, Wales and Northern Ireland, parental responsibility may be exercised until a young person reaches 18 years of age. In Scotland, parental responsibility is lost when the young person reaches 16, but the ability to give 'guidance' endures until the age of 18 years.

CONSENT

Competent children (legally, minors) can consent to accept diagnosis and treatment on their own behalf if they understand the implications of what is proposed ('Gillick competent'),[7] although they cannot decline treatment[8] (which may be needed in life-saving situations). The competent minor's consent is sufficient in law, although it is always desirable to involve parents, with the child's agreement.[9]

The slightly different legal situation regarding the legal capacity of young people in Scotland led to the Law Lord, Lord Fraser, offering a set of criteria that must apply when medical practitioners are offering contraceptive services to those aged under 16 years without parental knowledge or permission. These are known as the 'Fraser Guidelines'.[10, 11]

The consent of one person with parental responsibility is sufficient to proceed with diagnosis or treatment. If there is parental disagreement, the onus is on the dissenting parent to take steps to reverse the doctor's decision. If the dispute is over a controversial and elective procedure (e.g. male infant circumcision for religious purposes), doctors must not proceed without the authority of a court. In Scotland,[12] there is an obligation on any person exercising parental responsibility to have regard to the views of any other person with the same rights and responsibilities.

CHILD MALTREATMENT

The definition of 'child abuse and neglect' or 'child maltreatment' varies in different cultures and at different times. The CA89 introduced the concept of 'significant harm', which is effectively the working definition of whether a child needs protection. The types of abuse generally recognized[13] are physical abuse, sexual abuse, neglect, emotional abuse, factitious and induced illness (previously called Munchausen syndrome by proxy). NSPCC research shows that a significant minority of children suffer serious abuse or neglect at some time during childhood:

- 7% of children experienced serious physical abuse at the hands of their parents or carers during childhood
- 1% of children experienced sexual abuse by a parent or carer and another 3% by another relative during childhood; 11% of children experienced sexual abuse by people known but unrelated to them; 5% of children experienced sexual abuse by an adult stranger or someone they had just met
- 6% of children experienced serious absence of care at home during childhood
- 6% of children experienced frequent and severe emotional maltreatment during childhood.

All forms of inflicted abuse involve some emotional distress to the child: emotional abuse occurs in the absence of other physical effects (e.g. when the child is excluded, scapegoated, verbally abused, bullied, racially abused or involved in inappropriate activities). The adverse physical and emotional effects on children of being exposed to domestic violence are also increasingly recognized as abusive.

THE PROCESS OF CHILD PROTECTION

Anyone who suspects that a child may be suffering harm has a duty to take appropriate action. Given that a child may come into contact with a wide range of statutory and voluntary agencies, all of which may possess some, but not all, information about the child, the underlying principle is that agencies must work cooperatively in order to protect children. The *Working Together* document[14] sets out how all agencies and professionals (health, education, police, social services, probation, and others working with children) should work together to promote children's welfare and protect them from abuse and neglect. The guidance applies to the statutory, voluntary and independent sectors.

Local authority social services departments are the lead agency in child protection, and have the role of coordinating the child-protection process. Any report of a child-protection concern will be investigated according to the process laid out in *Working Together*. Under Section 47 of the CA89, health (and other) agencies are under a duty to help a local authority with its enquiries in cases 'where there is reasonable cause to suspect that a child is suffering, or is likely to suffer, significant harm'. This requirement means that a medical examination conducted as part of a Section 47 investigation has a different status from an ordinary consultation in terms of confidentiality and sharing of findings, and medical reports may be sent to social services without explicit parental consent, although it is good practice to attempt to engage parents' as well as children's consent to the whole process.

THE CHILD PROTECTION CONFERENCE

This is the interagency forum where concerns about children can be shared, a decision made as to whether further protective action is required, and a child-protection plan formulated. At present, if there is a need for a child-protection plan, the child's name is placed on the Child Protection Register. The local authority is required (by *Working Together* 1999[14]) to maintain this register, identifying children in its area who are thought to be at continuing risk of significant harm and therefore in need of protection by the authority. There are four categories of abuse for recording the type of significant harm from which a child is thought to be at continuing risk. These are neglect, physical abuse, sexual abuse and emotional abuse. Children can be registered under more than one category. The decision to register a child's name is taken at an initial child-protection conference.

An interagency child-protection plan is drawn up for each child on the register; this describes in detail how the child will be protected and how their health and development will be promoted. The progress of the plan will be monitored and reported to the child-protection review conference, at which a child may be deregistered if there is no longer a need for a child-protection plan.

The move to Local Safeguarding Boards specified in the Children Act 2004 (see page 9) will change the regulations around child-protection registers, and changes are being implemented throughout the UK.

EMERGENCY PROTECTION OF CHILDREN

In an emergency situation the police have powers to remove a child to a place of safety on the grounds of reasonable cause to suspect the child may be suffering, or is likely to suffer, significant harm. Under Section 46 of the CA89 the police have the power to remove a child from their home or elsewhere, or prevent the child being removed from a safe place such as a hospital, for up to 72 hours. The police must inform social services as soon as is practically possible, and this service must provide accommodation. The police must inform parents of the action taken, but not necessarily where the child is, and may restrict contact between the child and his or her parents.

An emergency protection order[15] may be requested from the court under Section 44 of the CA89 if a child is in immediate danger[16] from the risks of returning home, but the parents will not agree to the child being accommodated by the local authority under Section 17 of the CA89 as a child in need.

Any individual may apply to a magistrate for an Emergency Protection Order (EPO), but the application is usually made by social services. EPOs may be granted on the application of:

- Any person, where there is reasonable chance a child will suffer significant harm if not removed to a safe place or kept in a safe place.
- Local authorities, where enquiries are being made as to whether a child is suffering or at risk of harm, and where these enquiries are being frustrated or access to the child is unreasonably refused.

- The NSPCC, where there is reasonable cause to suspect a child will suffer significant harm or where enquiries into a child's welfare are being frustrated or access to the child is unreasonably refused.

An EPO may last for up to 8 days and may be extended for another 7 days. The child may be protected for a longer period if the local authority starts care proceedings (see below). Parental responsibility is shared by the local authority during the time an EPO is in force. Parents are entitled to have contact, although this may be supervised by the local authority.

Rather than the child having to leave home during an EPO, an 'exclusion requirement' can be made as part of the EPO, requiring an adult who is considered to be a danger to the child to leave the home. This can only be done with parental agreement, as the parent has to ensure its enforcement

SECTION 8 ORDERS UNDER THE CHILDREN ACT 1989

These are Court Orders that may be granted in respect to children involved in family proceedings.[17] They are:

- Contact Order – an order requiring the person with whom a child lives, or is to live, to allow the child to visit or stay with the person named in the order, or for that person and the child otherwise to have contact with each other
- Prohibited Steps Order – an order that no step which could be taken by a parent in meeting his or her parental responsibility for a child, and which is of a kind specified in the order, shall be taken by any person without the consent of the court
- Residence Order – an order settling the arrangements to be made regarding the person with whom a child is to live; this order confers parental responsibility
- Specific Issue Order – an order giving directions for the purpose of determining a specific question that has arisen, or which may arise, in connection with any aspect of parental responsibility for a child.

If a Care Order is in force, no other Section 8 order, except a Residence Order, may be granted.

SECTION 17 AND SECTION 27 SUPPORT REQUIREMENTS OF THE CHILDREN ACT 1989

Section 17 imposes a general duty on social services departments to safeguard and promote the welfare of children 'in need' living in the area, and to ensure that appropriate services are provided for those children.[18] The local authority is obliged to provide accommodation for children who cannot live at home due to child-protection concerns or other reasons. These accommodated children fall under the Looked After Children regulations. Social services do not have any right to opt out of this requirement or any other part of the Act on the grounds that they do not have resources. The term 'in need' is not tightly defined in the legislation, but is left open to reinforce preventive services and support for families.

A child is defined as being 'a child in need' under the Act if:

- he or she is unlikely to achieve or maintain, or have the opportunity of achieving or maintaining, a reasonable standard of health and development without the provision of services by a local authority under this part of the Act
- his or her health or development is likely to be significantly impaired or further impaired, without the provision of such services
- he or she is disabled.

Section 27 of the CA89 imposes an obligation on health and other agencies to cooperate with local authorities in providing support and services to children in need. If social services do not have the resources available to respond under the terms of the Act, they should call on other statutory agencies for assistance.

SECTIONS 20 AND 21 OF THE CHILDREN ACT 1989

Sections 20 and 21 impose a duty and a power on social services to provide accommodation for:

- Any child in need who is lost, abandoned, or without a carer or person with parental responsibility. This includes any child whose carer is prevented from caring for him or her either permanently or temporarily.
- Any child aged 16 years or over whose welfare may be seriously prejudiced without accommodation. If a 16–17 year old is intentionally homeless, sleeping rough, or at risk of custody or reoffending, their welfare is likely to be seriously prejudiced without the provision of accommodation and, as such, social services should be called upon to provide accommodation under this Section and challenged if they provide a negative response.
- Any child in the area where to provide accommodation will safeguard that child's welfare. This clause is applicable regardless of whether there is anyone with parental responsibility. An example of this may be if a young person is at risk of violence in the family home and his or her welfare will be safeguarded by a move elsewhere.
- Any child subject to police protection, detention or remand under the terms of the Police and Criminal Evidence Act 1984 and the Children and Young Persons Act 1969.

Under Section 20, social services have a duty to ascertain and consider the child's wishes in respect of any accommodation that is offered.

CARE AND SUPERVISION PROCEEDINGS[19]

If a child is considered to be suffering 'significant harm' attributable to the care given (or not given, as in neglect) by the parents, or if the child is out of parental control, the court has the power to grant an Interim Care Order or a full Care Order[20] in favour of a local authority. This gives the local authority a share of parental responsibility and allows them to determine where the child lives. A child may be placed at home with parents, or removed from home and placed in foster care or a children's home.

All these arrangements must be covered in a written care plan for the child, detailing where the child should live, their carers, and any special professional help or support the child may need to maintain their health, education or general functioning. The plan must also lay out contingency plans, in case the care plan for the child is not achievable within a reasonable timescale.

Parents do not lose parental responsibility when a Care Order is in force, but their ability to exercise it (i.e. make decisions about the child) is limited by the local authority. Parents have a right to contact with their child (unless the court makes a No Contact Order), but the frequency, site and level of supervision is determined by the local authority. Parents may apply to have a Care Order discharged.

A Supervision Order allows the local authority social services department to help and advise the parents or carers regarding the care of the child, who may live with their mother or father, or both, or another person. The local authority does not acquire parental responsibility. A Supervision Order lasts for 12 months but can be extended up to a maximum of 3 years.

COURT PROCESSES IN CARE PROCEEDINGS

When a local authority applies for a Care Order, the court must hear the application within 6 days. The court must decide whether to make an Interim Care Order (ICO) or some other interim order (supervision, residence or contact). An ICO lasts for up to 8 weeks in the first instance, and can be renewed for 4-week periods thereafter.

Once an ICO has been granted, there is usually a series of interim hearings, where the court will decide the child's residence, contact and how the case will proceed. Orders and directions may be renewed or changed.

The court may hold a Case Management Conference, to decide what evidence it will need for the final hearing. This may result in directions about:

- any statements, reports and assessments needed from professionals – likely to include social workers, teachers, doctors, health visitors and any other professionals working with the child or his or her family
- when these should be filed (given to the court), so that there is enough time for everyone involved to respond to them before the final hearing
- which experts can see the child (if any are needed) and when their reports must be filed at court
- whether the case should be transferred to a higher court
- any other procedures that need to be followed before the final hearing.

At the final hearing, the court may make any order that it considers to be in the child's best interests (even if it was not the order applied for by the local authority). This may be a Care Order, providing the criteria for significant harm are met, and the local authority's care plan is suitable and achievable. The Care Order lasts until the child is 18 years old, or marries, or is revoked by the court or another order substituted.

Other orders that may be granted are:

- *Residence Order* – this is an order to a specific person, often a grandparent or other family member. This confers parental

responsibility and lasts until the child is 18 years old, marries, or the order is revoked by the court on application by the parent.
- *Supervision Order* – this gives the local authority power to 'supervise' the child's care, but no share in parental responsibility. A supervision order lasts up to 1 year and can be extended for a maximum of 2 years more. If a Supervision Order is made, the local authority will generally agree a 'contract' or supervision plan.
- *Special Guardianship Order* – this is a new order available under the Adoption and Children Act 2002. It allows a court to place a child long term with someone who is not their parent, and to confer parental responsibility. It is more permanent than a Residence Order because a parent cannot apply to revoke the order without the court's permission. Special guardianship is like a 'halfway house' to adoption, as it is intended to be long term, but does not break the legal relationship between a birth parent and child. However, the special guardian has the right to override birth parents' wishes if agreement cannot be reached.

LOOKED-AFTER CHILDREN

A child is 'looked after by the local authority' if they are accommodated by the local authority as a 'child in need' under Section 17 of the CA89, or if subject to a Care Order (full or interim).

The local authority is obliged formally to review the child's well-being (health, education and social care) every 6 months under the Looked After Children regulations using an Independent Reviewing Officer. As part of this process, a health or medical assessment is required.[21] This assessment should not only identify any illness or significant medical condition, but also offer health promotion and ensure health protection via routine surveillance and immunization programmes. A healthcare plan should always be produced, and shared with the child, their carers, social worker and their primary healthcare team (GP and health visitor).

ADOPTION AND CHILDREN ACT 2002

This Act replaced the Adoption Act 1976. It was implemented in stages and became fully operational in December 2005. The main provisions of the act are:[22]

- To overhaul and modernize the legal framework for domestic and intercountry adoption, and in particular to replace provisions of the outdated Adoption Act 1976.
- To put adoption law in line with the existing provisions of the CA89 to ensure that the child's welfare is the paramount consideration in all decisions relating to adoption.
- To place a duty on local authorities to maintain an adoption service and provide adoption support services.
- To provide for adoption orders to be made in favour of single people, married couples and unmarried couples.
- To introduce a new independent review mechanism for prospective adopters who feel they have been turned down unfairly.
- To provide a new system for access to information held in adoption agency records and by the Register General about adoptions which took place after the Act came into force.

- To provide additional restrictions on bringing a child into the UK for adoption.
- To provide restrictions on arranging adoptions and advertising children for adoption.
- To cut delays in the adoption process by establishing an Adoption and Children Act Register to suggest links between children and approved adopters.
- To bring in new court rules governing the making of adoption orders and measures requiring the courts to draw up timetables for adoption cases to be heard. Freeing Orders were replaced by Placement Orders.
- To introduce a new special guardianship order for children for whom adoption is not a suitable option but who cannot return to their birth families.
- To provide that an unmarried father can acquire parental responsibility for his birth child where he and the child's mother register the birth of their child together.
- To introduce arrangements for step-fathers to acquire parental responsibility.

Since the implementation of this legislation, a child can only be placed for adoption: with parental consent; or if the child is subject to a Care Order and the parents consent; or if the child is subject to a Care Order and a Placement Order is granted.

The medical role in adoption continues to be an important part of the multiprofessional task in achieving new families for children who cannot be brought up in their birth family. The role of the Medical Adviser in Fostering and Adoption[23] is described in publications from the UK umbrella organization the British Association for Adoption and Fostering (BAAF).[24]

THE CHILDREN ACT 2004

This legislation provides the legal framework for implementing the *Every Child Matters*[25] governmental programme aimed at ensuring that children's services are effective and children are safeguarded. The Act places an obligation on statutory agencies to cooperate with each other via Local Safeguarding Children Boards[26] (LSCBs) in England to achieve the 'well-being' of children. Well-being is described in the Act using five desired outcomes – that every child should:

- be healthy
- stay safe
- enjoy and achieve
- make a positive contribution
- achieve economic well-being.

LSCBs replaced the former Area Child Protection Committees (ACPCs) in England, and placed their functions on a statutory footing, their objective being to coordinate and to ensure the effectiveness of their member agencies in safeguarding and promoting the welfare of children. The core membership of LSCBs is set out in the Children Act 2004, and includes local authorities, health bodies, the police and others. These regulations came into force on 1 April 2006. These do not apply in Wales, Scotland or Northern Ireland at present, as their devolved governments are preparing their own legislation and guidance documents. Until new legislation is issued by the Scottish Parliament, Welsh Assembly Government or Northern Ireland Assembly, all existing legislation and guidance applies.

ORGANIZATIONAL RESPONSES TO CHILD SAFEGUARDING

Legislation has been enacted to ensure that systems are made safe for children. Police checks are now mandatory for individuals who may have contact with children in the course of professional or voluntary work, in order to establish a coherent cross-sector scheme for identifying those people considered to be unsuitable to work with children.

The Protection of Children Act 1999 (POCA),[27] modified by the Care Standards Act 2000, introduced the Protection of Children Act (PoCA) List in which the Secretary of State has a duty to record the names of individuals who are considered unsuitable to work with children.

The POCA places a statutory obligation[28] on all regulated child-care organizations (as defined in the Act) to refer the names of those individuals who are unsuitable to work with children (due to convictions, cautions or other concerns) for possible inclusion in the PoCA List. The Act also permits other organizations, such as voluntary organizations, sports clubs and Scout associations, to refer names for possible inclusion in the PoCA List.

Child-care organizations (including health, education and care) are now obliged to check names of prospective employees against the list (through the Criminal Records Bureau) before offering employment, and must not employ individuals whose names are included on the PoCA List, its equivalent in Scotland, or List 99 held by the Department for Education and Skills, on the grounds that they are unsuitable to work with children. Employers must also cease to employ such individuals in child-care positions if they subsequently discover that they are included on these lists.

The Criminal Justice and Court Services Act 2000[29] made it an offence knowingly to offer work to or to employ in a so-called 'regulated' position (including child-care positions) an individual who is disqualified from working with children. Individuals who apply or offer to work, accept work, or continue to work with children in such positions are committing a criminal offence. The definition of 'employment' is wide so that a child-care position refers to work with children in all sectors (statutory, voluntary and independent), irrespective of whether the work is paid or unpaid, and whether or not it is under a contract.

Chapter Three

Influence of deprivation on emotional development

3

Nick J. Spencer

SUMMARY

Emotional and mental health problems in childhood are among the most important causes of childhood morbidity and disability, with increasingly recognized adverse effects into adulthood. Although the social patterning of child mental health problems has been widely recognized, attention has focused mainly on family and parental level factors correlating with adverse outcomes. This chapter considers the background or distal socio-economic factors influencing child mental health. The extent and consistency of the social gradient in adverse child mental health outcomes is demonstrated using UK and Canadian data. An explanation of the social gradient based on the cumulative and additive effects of risk and protective factors, which are themselves socially patterned, is discussed. The implications of the social gradient for prevention and intervention are considered, with particular reference to practical measures that can be taken by paediatricians to modify the adverse effects of material deprivation on the mental health of children.

PRACTICE POINTS

- Child mental health problems show marked social gradients, with increasing problems associated with increasing material deprivation.
- Proximal risk factors, such as parenting, maternal depression and parental psychopathology, show similar gradients.
- Paediatricians need to acknowledge and be sensitive to the role of material deprivation in the aetiology of child mental health problems.
- Advocacy at national and local level is likely to be the most effective paediatric preventive intervention.

INTRODUCTION

Emotional and mental health problems in childhood are recognized as major causes of morbidity and disability in childhood, extending their effects into adult life. A minimum annual incidence of 5–10% of children living in relatively stable semi-rural communities, and 10–20% for those in inner cities was reported in the 1970s, and more recent reports suggest an overall national incidence of 10%.[1] Based on a random sample of parents and young people in one of the most deprived areas of London, Davis et al.[2] report a much higher incidence; 76.9% of the whole sample had at least one psychosocial problem, with 40.5% having three or more problems. There is some evidence of a rise in incidence of some disorders in the past 40 years.[1] Associated adverse outcomes are wide ranging, encompassing suicide, school failure, behaviour problems, criminality, and adult mental and physical health problems.

Although the association of emotional and mental health problems with socio-economic status and material disadvantage has been recognized for some time, the importance of distal or background social factors has tended to be minimized, and proximal factors such as parenting and maternal mental health have been the main focus of practice and research interest. This chapter examines the influence of deprivation and material disadvantage on the emotional and mental development of children, and the implications for paediatric practice, research and health policy.

The chapter briefly reviews the association between social factors and emotional development, drawing particular attention to the social gradients in adverse emotional and mental health outcomes. The possible factors mediating the relationship, and possible explanations for the observed gradients, are then discussed. Finally, the chapter considers the implications for paediatric practice, research and health policy.

SOCIAL FACTORS AND EMOTIONAL HEALTH OF CHILDREN

Evidence for the influence of social factors on the emotional health of children arises from a number of sources. These are briefly considered below.

Social gradients in adverse child mental health

Conditions reflecting adverse emotional health among children demonstrate consistent social gradients, with increasing burden of disease associated with increasing material and social disadvantage. The social gradient of mental health problems among UK children measured by income (Fig. 3.1)[3] is similar to that for behaviour problems, the most common form of mental health disorder, among Canadian children (Fig. 3.2).[4] Emotional disorders in UK children show the same pattern (Fig. 3.3).[3] Suicide rates among adolescent boys in the UK are finely graded by social group, with a clear trend

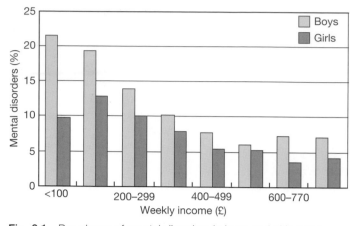

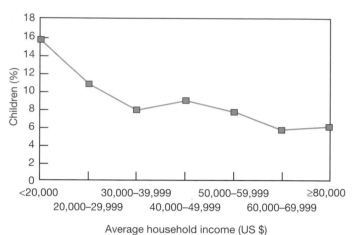

Fig. 3.1 Prevalence of mental disorders in boys and girls aged 5–15 years in Great Britain by weekly family income. (Data from Meltzer et al.[3])

Fig. 3.2 Percentage of children engaging in frequent delinquent behaviours compared with average household incomes. Two-parent families with children aged 4–11 years. (Data from Ross et al.[4])

over the last 20 years towards an increasing social gradient.[5] Attention-deficit hyperactivity disorder (ADHD), often characterized as a biological disorder of the developing brain, is positively correlated with adverse socio-economic circumstances.[3, 6]

Work from the USA confirms the importance of looking beyond the simple contrast of poor and non-poor; children who have experienced permanent and severe poverty have a higher risk of behavioural problems and intellectual impairment than those experiencing transient, less severe poverty who, in turn, have a higher risk than non-poor children.[7] Many children present more than one mental health problem. The number of problems presented by children significantly increases with declining family income.[2]

Social influences on risk and mediating factors

Known risk factors for impaired emotional development also demonstrate a similar gradient, and empirical evidence suggests a direct influence of socio-economic factors on parenting, educational attainment, maternal mental health and other variables with known effects on the emotional development of children.

Parenting is the focus of much current interest, and the UK government has committed considerable resources to parenting programmes as part of the Sure Start[8] initiative. Parenting is often presented as an attribute of individual families divorced from their social and economic context. Historically, it was described as 'maternal inefficiency' and 'maternal incompetence'. Although the terminology has changed, the focus on individual attributes of mothers, almost to the exclusion of fathers, continues to dominate. A more detailed account of the effects of social, economic and political factors on parenting can be found elsewhere.[9] Here the evidence for the direct and indirect effects of social factors on parenting is briefly summarized.

Economic hardship and heavy income loss has been directly associated with more punitive, arbitrary and rejecting parenting by fathers, a decrease in parental nurturing and an increase in inconsistent discipline by both parents. Unemployed fathers display fewer nurturing behaviours than other fathers. Low income, in combination with low levels of perceived social support, has been associated with a higher probability of punitive behaviour by the parent

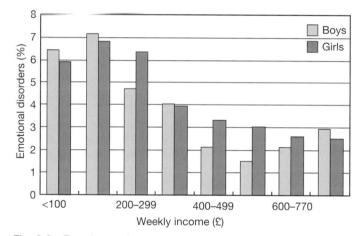

Fig. 3.3 Prevalence of emotional disorders in boys and girls aged 5–15 years in Great Britain by weekly household income. (Data from Meltzer et al.[3])

towards the child. The socio-emotional functioning of children living in poor families seems to be mediated by the psychological functioning of parents and the level of distress in family interaction patterns. The effects of economic hardship and material disadvantage on parenting are partially mediated by marital stresses. The psychological well-being of adults in the household is affected by economic hardship, as is the marital relationship. Stress-related changes in parent–child interactions lead to increasingly coercive parenting, with a resultant increase in childhood behaviour problems and future delinquency. Marital happiness and life satisfaction have been reported to be significantly lower in families with no earner, and these families also tended to show more aggressive parenting strategies. A higher level of parental education seems to protect children against emotional problems. Educational attainment in the UK is socially patterned,[10] so poor children are more likely to have parents with low educational levels. Childhood poverty is a major determinant of poor achievement in adult life, having its main effect as a handicap to good education. Mental health of young adults is also linked to family background and childhood socio-economic circumstances, working through to success and failure in the education system; in the 1958 and 1970 UK national cohort studies, those with no qualifications were three times more likely to be classed as depression-prone than were graduates.[11]

Parental mental ill health is a potent risk factor for childhood emotional problems.[2] Maternal depression has a well-established relationship with adverse social conditions. In Davis et al.'s random sample of children in a deprived London borough,[2] 33.9% of the mothers and 18.9% of the fathers/partners had mental health problems. Parental psychopathology seems to show the same social gradient as childhood mental health problems.

Similar social gradients are observed in risk factors such as marital problems, divorce, inadequate housing conditions and adverse life events. It is also likely that protective factors, which have been reported to protect some children from emotional damage in adverse social circumstances, are themselves socially patterned.

EXPLAINING THE SOCIAL GRADIENT IN CHILDREN'S EMOTIONAL HEALTH

As the evidence presented above suggests, the links between children's emotional well-being and their social circumstances are strong. Behavioural problems are finely graded by socio-economic status, indicating that the causal pathways do not simply work through severe poverty but at different levels of material well-being. This dose–response relationship is further supporting evidence for the causal role of socio-economic factors in childhood emotional health. Further understanding of the influence of social factors on emotional development can be gained by considering the mechanisms by which the social gradient develops. Much research focuses on single risk or protective factors. However, these risk and protective factors are likely to be additive and cumulative over time. The lower the income of the family, the more likely the child is to be exposed to inadequate housing, family unemployment and marginalization. A similar graded, cumulative exposure to poor parenting skills, negative life events, marital conflict, lone-parent status, parental psychopathology and academic failure is likely. Equally, the child is less likely to encounter protective factors as the level of family disadvantage increases. Davis et al.'s findings support this explanation, showing that the number of risk factors rises in inverse proportion to income.[2]

The additive and cumulative effects of risk factors, which are themselves socially patterned, is likely to explain why childhood mental health problems, such as behaviour problems, demonstrate a fine social gradient. These observations provide strong confirmation of the key role played by social factors in childhood emotional health.

IMPLICATIONS FOR POLICY, PRACTICE AND RESEARCH

The public health consequences of impaired childhood emotional health are huge, not only for the current and future mental health of individuals but also for society. Poor emotional health in childhood is associated with poor adult mental health, antisocial behaviour, educational and career underachievement, and later physical ill health. Preventive and curative approaches based on modifying single risk factors, such as parenting programmes, home visiting and early childhood education on the High Scope model, have been shown to have some effect among individual children. However, in the light of the cumulative and additive effects of multiple risk factors considered above, the effects of these single-factor interventions are likely to be small compared with the overall effects of adverse social, economic and environmental conditions. Such interventions are often targeted at the highest risk groups on the basis that the efficacy is likely to be highest in those most 'at risk'. On good theoretical grounds, it can be argued that risk-based interventions are less effective than interventions aimed at changing the risk profile of the whole population.[12] There is a real danger that well-meaning government initiatives such as Sure Start, targeted to very deprived areas, will have only a marginal effect on the risk profile of the whole population.

Undoubtedly, the elimination of poverty in childhood would have the most profound effect on the emotional health of children. In a country such as the UK, where almost one-third of children live in households with incomes below 50% of the national average, this may seem a daunting task. However, other countries, such as Sweden, Finland and France, have achieved much lower levels of child poverty by tax and credit transfer.[13] For example, Sweden reduces so-called 'market child poverty' (the level before tax and credit transfer) by 20% among households with children compared with nearer 5% in the UK. UNICEF estimate that it would take only 0.48% of the UK Gross National Product to eliminate child poverty.

Paediatricians may view social and economic policy issues as beyond their remit. There is a long and honourable tradition of medical intervention on behalf of population groups to promote health. If mental and emotional health are powerfully linked with social and economic conditions, as the evidence suggests, it is legitimate for paediatricians to enter the policy arena on behalf of poor children. The Royal College of Paediatrics and Child Health, although slow to adopt an advocacy role, has now taken positive steps towards influencing government policy on a range of issues.

Can paediatricians do anything to assist children whose emotional health is compromised by their social conditions? The main requirement is sensitivity to the realities of life for families experiencing social and material disadvantage. While this should not prevent the practitioner from acting on the principle that the child's welfare is paramount, it will allow the practitioner to provide sympathetic and realistic advice that takes account of the social context in which parenting is taking place. Paediatricians should be familiar with the benefit entitlement of families, or at least know where families can obtain advice. Many families in financial difficulties fail to claim their full benefit entitlement, pushing them further into poverty. Experiments with introducing the Citizen's Advice Bureau (CAB) into health service settings have proved effective in increasing household incomes. Group- and community-wide approaches to reducing emotional damage to children may allow practitioners to access hidden resources within families, and overcome some of the social isolation of families suffering multiple social disadvantage. There are now many government-funded initiatives, such as Sure Start, developing early educational and parenting interventions to attenuate the effects of material and social deprivation on the health and development of children. Paediatricians can play an active role in these initiatives, providing advice and support in relation to the emotional health needs of children.

Further research into the social influences on the emotional health of children should focus on pathways to various outcomes. Longitudinal studies are the best way to explore these pathways, which are likely to be complex. A better understanding of the cumulative and additive effects of risk and protective factors requires methods that can account for complex relationships exerting their effects over time. Properly conducted, methodologically sound studies are required to test interventions designed to modify risk factors and influence the pathways to adverse outcomes. Such studies need to account fully for the effects of social disadvantage, preferably using a randomized, controlled trial design.

CONCLUSION

Adverse socio-economic circumstances appear to play an important role in the development of emotional problems in childhood. Interventions at a societal level are likely to be most effective in promoting mental health across the widest number of children, but local initiatives to promote the emotional health of children can be effective if they are sensitive to social context.

Chapter Four

Neglect of neglect

4

Chris J. Hobbs • Jane M. Wynne

SUMMARY

Neglect is the absence of adequate parental care and supervision. It is the most frequently registered form of child maltreatment in the UK. Prevalence studies reveal that 6% of adults say they experienced serious absence of care as children. Therefore, many cases escape detection and intervention. Neglect is insidious, chronic, and often neglected or ignored by professionals. Neglect is linked to poverty, and both may have a negative, depressing effect on families and professionals alike. Important indicators of neglect can be found in the child, the parents, family function and especially in the quality of interaction between parent and child. Neglect is associated with significant mortality and with long-lasting morbidity. Victoria Climbié died from the effects of malnutrition and hypothermia, which were the result of neglect. She was also physically abused and had numerous marks of violence on her body when she died. Effective intervention requires a determined coordinated team response in which the paediatrician's role is central to the progress and effectiveness of any treatment programme, through assessment of the child's growth and developmental progress.

PRACTICE POINTS

- Neglect is the most commonly recognized form of child maltreatment, and is increasingly diagnosed and child protection plans developed.
- Neglect may occasionally present as a crisis but more typically is an insidious and pervasive process, which slowly erodes the child's developmental potential.
- There is a strong association with poverty, and families who neglect their children frequently experience a wide range of adverse circumstances.
- Parents who are unable to meet their child's needs, socially, emotionally, intellectually and physically, may also struggle in a wide range of other areas in their own lives.
- Intervention must be planned, following careful assessment, with specific goals, have realistic time limits and always centre on the parents. Progress is usually slow, but significant improvements in care can be achieved for many children, although there are some where alternative care will be required.

INTRODUCTION

The terms 'child abuse' and 'neglect' are inextricably linked. One receives massive attention in the media and professional literature, while the other rarely surfaces. At the time of writing an unusual court case is being reported in the media where parents have been prosecuted for neglect. Their unsupervised children died when a train struck them on a railway line the family had chosen for a picnic spot. Public opinion was divided over whether there should be a prosecution. One view held that the parents had surely suffered enough. Neglect is now the most frequently reported form of maltreatment in the UK. There can be no doubt about its potentially harmful effects, including its significant contribution to childhood mortality. So why is it that it receives so much less attention and remains frequently unreported? One reason may be that we understand it less. Stone[1] wrote:

Neglect appeared to be poorly understood in terms of theory. This was reflected in the shortage of literature specifically about child neglect, the small number of research studies investigating neglect and the absence of professional training for practitioners in this area.[1]

These and other powerful reasons mean that there is much truth in the term 'neglect of neglect'.

Professionals may fail to act because:

- They feel uncertainty regarding the thresholds of harm and may experience a lack of agreement on what is neglect.
- There are legal difficulties and few prosecutions. The term 'wilful neglect' may confuse the issue. The criminal justice system may shift the focus onto the parents' culpability and deflect attention from issues that are better viewed from the child's perspective.
- The outcomes are more difficult to measure and may not become apparent immediately.
- There is denial – terms such as 'low-level neglect' and 'faltering growth' may reflect minimization of the child's situation.
- Over-identification with the mother's often overwhelming needs.
- Burnout – parents feel tired and unsupported – 'all like that in this estate'.

DEFINITION

The concept of neglect is complex, and any definition needs to reflect this. The following are definitions that have attempted to capture the complexity.

The child has a right to expect, and the adult caretaker has a duty to provide: food, clothing, shelter, safekeeping, nurturance and teaching. Failure to provide these constitutes neglect.[2]

Child abuse consists of anything which individuals, institutions or processes do or fail to do which directly or indirectly harms children or damages their prospects of safe and healthy development into adulthood.[3]

Neglect refers to the failure to act. The definition used in *Working Together* is:

The persistent or severe neglect of a child, or the failure to protect a child from exposure to any kind of danger, including cold or starvation or, extreme failure to carry out important aspects of care, resulting in the significant impairment of the child's health or development, including non-organic failure to thrive.[4]

Neglectful behaviour is behaviour by a caregiver that constitutes a failure to act in ways that are presumed by the culture of a society to be necessary to meet the developmental needs of a child and which are the responsibility of the caregiver to provide.[5]

This latter definition places the term 'neglect' clearly in the realm of caregiver behaviour, as opposed to the causes of such behaviour (e.g. poverty, mental illness or malevolent motive) or the effects of the behaviour (e.g. physical or psychological harm).

Neglect, therefore, is most commonly thought of as the absence of adequate parental care and supervision. Neglect is not a fixed condition, and what has been termed neglect in one culture or era may be considered adequate child care in another time and place. It is also important to distinguish chronic persistent neglect from episodic neglect.

EPIDEMIOLOGY

There are few prevalence studies of neglect in the general population. The definitions are broad and the boundaries of what constitutes neglect may be unclear. Emotional abuse and neglect are closely linked categories that are less tangible but often very visible to practitioners. There are no simple definitions with which to measure prevalence.

However, what information is available would suggest that neglect is common. It has been estimated that about 3% of children (350,000–400,000) live in a home environment that is consistently low in warmth and high in criticism(emotional neglect).[6] A recent NSPCC study[7] used a large random probability sample of 2,869 18–24 year olds in the UK. The response rate was 67%. Around neglect issues they focused on basic physical nurturing, healthcare and supervision. Of these, 6% experienced serious absence of care as children, which included: frequently going hungry; frequently having to go to school in dirty clothes; not being taken to the doctor when ill (under age of 12 years); regularly having to look after themselves because parents went away or had problems such as with drugs or alcohol; being abandoned or deserted; or living in a home with dangerous physical conditions. The study also found that one or more criteria were experienced by a further 9% of the sample but with less frequency and/or children were often expected to do their own laundry before the age of 12 years. Generally, there were few distinctions by socio-economic grade, although poorer grades more often experienced serious absence of care. Interestingly, fewer subjects assessed themselves as not having been well cared for (4%), and only 2% felt they had been neglected.

Neglect frequently coexists with other forms of abuse. Oliver[8] followed a geographically determined cohort of generational maltreating families over many years. He identified 560 children born over a 20-year period and found that 513 were maltreated. Of these, 499 were neglected, and of which for 285 this was the predominant form of maltreatment.

Department of Health figures for 2003[9] reveal that of 26,000 children on child protection registers, the numbers in each major category were: neglect alone 10,400; physical injury alone 4,160; sexual abuse alone 2,600; and emotional abuse alone 4,940. Therefore, neglect has overtaken physical abuse as the most common reason for child protection registration. What does this represent? Is it a shift in practice away from the 'neglect of neglect', a changing pattern of morbidity, or a retreat from other forms of abuse? Almost certainly there are many more neglected children than those registered. Such children are not involved within the child protection system and are left 'bumping along the bottom until something assessed as a higher risk, such as physical or sexual abuse, stimulates action'.[3]

POVERTY

Over the past 20 years the UK has experienced an overall increase in poverty, although in the year 2000 there was a modest decrease in child poverty. Child health is closely related to poverty. Poverty, material disadvantage and deprivation are all linked to neglect. The association of reported child abuse and neglect with poverty is well established.[10] Poverty is also linked with childhood malnutrition, i.e. failure to thrive (FTT) or obesity. Poverty is the most important single risk factor for FTT because of the close association between poverty and childhood malnutrition. Although FTT may occur in children of all social classes, most clinical cases come from low-income families.[11] The link between poverty and neglect may be one of the reasons for the lack of interest in neglect. The relationship of poverty to neglect is complex. Fewer resources mean it is more difficult to cope with the demands of life, including child rearing. Not all poor families neglect their children, although some material poverty is likely to be present. It is important to distinguish the former, which can be alleviated by financial help, from neglect caused by emotional poverty.[2]

Poverty is related to:

- low income
- unemployment
- single parent
- poor health, diminished life expectancy
- poor housing/homelessness
- black and ethnic minority groups
- mental health problems
- drugs, alcohol and tobacco use.

CLINICAL FEATURES

Features that determine a diagnosis of neglect are given in Table 4.1.

Recognition of neglect[2]

In the absence of a fully explanatory medical cause, the following conditions indicate a diagnosis of neglect:

Table 4.1 The 'jigsaw' in the diagnosis of neglect

Denial of problems by parents (may have learning problems)	History from child – bullied, no friends, aggressive	'Attention seeking'. Concern by nursery school of standard of care
Physical symptoms, e.g. pain from dental caries	Poor physical condition – dirty, thin hair, nappy rash	Growth – stunted/fail to reach potential height
Development delayed, e.g. language, social skills	Poor compliance with treatment, e.g. asthma	Increased risk of accidents: road traffic accident, fire, drowning
Supportive network, i.e. with family and friends – little effect as share similar problems	Poverty with poor housing, diet, parents with poor health (physical and mental), little education	Large number of involved professionals – health visitor, school nurse, social worker, home care, housing, GP, paediatrician, etc.

- A lack of attachment to the parent, or the child is anxiously or avoidantly attached.
- A lack of emotional nurturance for emotional growth.
- The child is left unattended and in unsafe situations.
- The child is placed in situations of unnecessary risk for emotional or physical harm by his or her caretaker's omission or commission.
- The child is not sent to school.
- The child is not stimulated and is developmentally delayed, especially in language and social development. Social development may be aberrant.
- A lack of age-appropriate and consistent limit setting.
- The child is not given needed preventive or curative medical care.

Significant indications of neglect identified by practitioners include:[1]

Child:
- delayed development
- lack of stimulation
- behaviour problems
- aggression
- physical injury/abuse
- sexual abuse/disinhibited sexuality
- poor hygiene, inappropriate clothing and grooming
- hunger/feeding problems/inadequate diet
- FTT
- health problems, inappropriate medical requests.

Other features are child not wanted, not planned, fetal abuse with physical abuse, alcohol and substance abuse, and poor antenatal care, including malnutrition.

Parents/caregivers:
- poor parenting of caregivers
- history of neglect/abuse in caregivers
- caregivers experienced care system/prison
- substance abuse
- mental illness/learning disability
- inability to nurture/lack of bonding

Case illustration 4.1

Case history from a Part 8 Review under Working Together Regulations

A 5-year-old girl was admitted to hospital suffering from severe anaemia (haemoglobin 2.4 g/dl) and gross head lice infestation. She had signs of cardiac failure and 'looked in a dreadful state'. Any further delay in treatment would have made it likely that she would have died. Following treatment with a blood transfusion and hospital care she was quickly restored to reasonable health. She also had infection with giardia and entamoeba, severe dental caries and there was a history of sexual abuse. Neither she nor any of her six siblings were on the Child Protection Register at time of her admission, although there had been a history of involvement with statutory agencies for many years. However, in the past, three older siblings had been on the Child Protection Register under the category 'at risk of Sexual, Physical and Emotional Abuse'. The family had led an unsettled existence, with at least nine changes of address, including hostels and returns to the mother's family home. FTT had been identified in a younger sibling, who had been admitted to hospital and then discharged having gained some weight. Despite concerns, the parents failed to attend outpatient appointments with the child who was failing to thrive, although immunizations were given. Failing to present their children at outpatient appointments was a consistent factor over the entire 12-year period during which professionals were actively involved with the family.

The parents had a volatile and unstable relationship, with episodes of domestic violence inflicted by the father on the mother. There were many occasions when the mother would leave the father and seek alternative accommodation, usually in a hostel or with her own family. The father had a history of substance abuse. There were longstanding concerns about the parenting abilities of both the adults. When the case was reviewed externally, it was noted that in the weeks prior to admission there was liaison between the local social services area office, health and housing personnel, school and the police. However, despite agencies holding information and each having concerns regarding the child, there was both an overall failure to communicate effectively and, more importantly, no coherent strategy to address the children's needs, in a coordinated manner. This contributed in part to the life-threatening crisis that finally precipitated removal of the children into local authority care.

- poor parenting skills
- disorganization/mismanagement.

Family dynamics:
- high stress levels
- family violence
- unrealistic expectations of child
- parents' needs first
- scapegoating
- lack of boundaries.

Supervision:
- lack of supervision
- inappropriate carers (open house).

Compliance:
- family known to social services
- resistant/non-cooperative
- failure to keep appointments
- poor school attendance.

Social factors:
- poverty/deprivation
- debts, financial problems
- unemployment/reliance on benefits
- poor housing
- social isolation (exclusion).

Physical examination findings include:

- cold, dirty (toenails in infants), inappropriately dressed, infestation, inattention to grooming, chronic nappy and other rashes (e.g. untreated cradle cap)
- excessive decayed, unfilled or missing teeth
- FTT, stunted height
- anaemia, nutritional deficiencies (including vitamin D deficient rickets)
- delay in development, especially language and social, but less often motor
- excessive accidents, including ingestion, scars from old injury
- lack of protection/signs of abuse, physical or sexual
- untreated conditions (e.g. squints, disfiguring minor untreated conditions)
- untreated infection (e.g. otitis media with discharge), unusual severe presentation of illness, repeated infection (e.g. gastroenteritis)
- behaviour may include attention seeking, indiscriminate seeking of contact, angry/aggressive, living in own world/cut off, chaotic
- lack of understanding of others.

Child death related to neglect

Neglect can be a major factor in a child's death linked to:

- malnutrition/poor care – lowering of resistance to infection
- lack of supervision – accidents (e.g. leaving child alone – house fires)
- failure to respond to illness in child – sudden infant death
- failure to use preventive healthcare (e.g. immunization)
- parental use of drugs – intoxicated adult/lack of supervision, accidental ingestion.

Underreporting and lack of recognition of neglect in child death are both common.

Nutrition and emotional neglect

Emotional neglect can be manifested as:

- FTT
- inappropriate diet
- obesity.

Case illustration 4.2

A 4-year-old boy was referred with the complaint that he would only eat tubes of chocolate toffees and chocolate mousses. He drank milky tea. Other food was refused. He was failing to thrive and had iron-deficiency anaemia (haemoglobin 4.0 g/dl). In addition, his development was considerably delayed – he pointed to indicate needs, with very few words, and was still in nappies day and night. He attended only with his father, as his mother stayed at home to look after a number of other children, some of whom also had problems related to inadequate care.

'Failure to thrive' refers to children who are growth retarded secondary to malnutrition.[12] Non-organic FTT is a form of nutritional neglect, where the infant or child is fed inadequate calories for normal growth. Children who fail to thrive show long-term deficits in physical growth, cognitive functioning, and emotional and social development. The problem is largely reversible if treated early by feeding additional calories over the expected requirements for the age of the child to induce catch-up growth.

Important body measurements include weight, head circumference and mid-upper-arm circumference (Table 4.2). Height is usually affected but to a lesser extent than weight.

Abnormal growth patterns

Abnormal growth patterns in FTT include:[12]

- Falling centiles: crossing one or two major centiles downwards should be a cause for concern.
- Parallel poor centiles: after the weight centile has fallen, many children occupy a position on the growth chart where they continue to gain weight and height but below and parallel to the

Table 4.2 Mid-upper-arm circumference (MUAC) for children aged 12–60 months

MUAC	Action
< 14 cm in a child > 12 months old	Likely to be significantly malnourished – warrants referral to a paediatrician
14–15 cm	If older (i.e. 4–5 years), likely to be malnourished – refer to a paediatrician
	Younger child – monitor carefully and assess in detail
> 15 cm	Nutrition is likely to be adequate
16–17 cm in a child at school entry (5–6 years old)	Likely to be adequately nourished

lowest centiles. This must not be interpreted optimistically, as these children are not achieving their potential and suffer significant harm.

- Markedly discrepant height and weight centiles: some children appear to grow better in height than weight. A discrepancy of two or more major centiles is likely to be significant. However, many children who fail to thrive are both underweight and stunted. Growth hormone secretion is likely to be suppressed.
- Discrepant family pattern: calculations of mid-parent-height are, in theory, of value but caution is needed if there is any evidence that one or both parents may themselves have failed to thrive. Observing parents' heights and weights may give useful information in assessing the child's problems.
- Retrospective pattern: obvious improvement of a child's growth may occur following changes in their life situation, including a change of carer. Catch-up growth provides sure evidence of earlier nutritional neglect and more accurate appraisal of the child's true growth potential.
- Dipping or sawtooth patterns: this pattern of weight gain is common in FTT and reflects the fluctuating nutritional intake.

Although weight is the primary measurement in diagnosing and assessing progress in FTT, mid-upper-arm circumference is a useful additional measurement. It assesses thinness and is sensitive to improvements in nutritional status. Guidelines for the use of the mid-upper-arm circumference in clinical practice are given in Table 4.2.

Psychological dimension in FTT

Major aetiological factors considered in FTT include:[13]

- maternal psychopathology
- family functioning
- inadequate nurturing.

Mothers often:

- show depression, anger, low self-esteem
- have eating difficulties
- neglect themselves as well as their children
- have poor health
- have distorted or unrealistic expectations of the child
- have unresolved issues of loss or bereavement
- abuse drugs or alcohol
- are in poverty and unemployed.

Not all mothers of children who fail to thrive show such overt psychopathology as suggested here. More striking in careful research studies are the findings relating to the interaction of the mothers with their children.[14] Mothers showed less frequent verbal and physical contact, less positive reinforcement and warmth. They talked to, played with and cuddled these children less often than mothers of children who were thriving. Where mothers had both children who were growing normally and those who were failing to thrive, they said that they got on better with the thriving ones. Some mothers described feelings of helplessness and despair when attempting to feed their children. Others reported little or no pleasure from their baby, or a disturbance in their sense of the child belonging to them.

The infants and children show a wide range of emotional signs, ranging from the active, irritable, restless, aggressive, poor sleepers, to quiet, lethargic, sad, undemanding children who appear to withdraw.

Attachment behaviour of mothers of FTT children has been studied. In one study, which used adult attachment assessment tools, 96% of FTT mothers showed an insecure pattern of attachment as compared with 60% of controls.[15]

Assessment of FTT in the clinical setting

A multidisciplinary team approach is valuable.[16] Paediatrics, dietetics, health visiting, clinical psychology and social work each have important roles.

Dietary assessment can be done in the clinic or home using:

- a 3-day diet diary
- dietary recall
- mealtime observation
- biscuit test.

In the biscuit test, biscuits are offered to the child (after seeking parent's consent) in the clinic. The child's responses are carefully noted. Children who are not catching up may be observed to consume several biscuits in a 30-minute clinic consultation, although previously described as not eating. The parent's responses can reveal attitudes to food and feeding.

Medical assessment in FTT

The clinician's task is to assess growth, development and health, and to identify the likely cause of the inadequate nutrition. One study found that FTT occurred in 5% of infants born to mothers in inner city areas, and of these only 6% had an organic disorder.[17] The presence of an organic disorder may mean that the parent finds the child more difficult to care for and FTT may result.

Laboratory and radiological investigations are reserved for cases where the history or physical examination suggests an organic component. Many children will show an improvement in growth after a discussion about feeding, and this will be proof enough of the cause of the FTT. The risk of missing an organic condition should be balanced against the dangers of overemphasis of a 'medical' solution. The child needs extra food.

Denial is frequently encountered in FTT. This affects both family and professionals. Denial may relate to the cause, consequences or need for treatment of the FTT. Examples of statements that indicate denial include:

- He's just small.
- Everyone in our family was like this at this age. (Rarely true.)
- He'll catch up when he is older.
- He eats like a horse, and more than his parents.
- He must have a medical problem – can't you do more tests?
- I'm not having you thinking that I don't feed him.
- This clinic is a waste of time – we don't need to come.
- Its all your [the doctor's] fault for putting pressure on the mother/family.

Managing neglect

A balance needs to be struck between informal and formal interventions and treatment. While FTT and neglect are clearly child-protection issues, Taylor and Daniel[18] noted that there were differences in the way that health and social care providers responded to and intervened in children who failed to thrive. FTT has been subsumed in the English child-protection system within the category of neglect, and such children, even those not showing the more characteristic features of physical neglect, can be registered if it is felt appropriate. There is evidence that professionals are less willing to use the formal child-protection system with FTT, reserving its use for cases where there are multiple social and family problems. Taylor and Daniel feel it is important to know whether outcomes are better if FTT is treated as a child-protection issue.

Working with neglect

Neglected children receive help as 'child protection' or 'child in need'. Whichever system is followed, there is need for:

- *Assessment* – key questions to be asked:
  - Why are parents failing?
  - Are parents motivated to change?
  - How can parents and child be supported?
  - Is the extended family able to support?
- *Intervention* – this should be planned, focused and systematic. Separate interventions may be required for the parents and the child. There are numerous different approaches.
- *Coordinated team working* – this is an effective use of resources, and supports professionals in not feeling defeated. The paediatrician's role includes careful monitoring of the child and family for progress towards an acceptable level of growth and development.

- *Time scale* – this may be longer than for other forms of maltreatment. A realistic framework is required for when to call it a day and remove the child (see Case Illustration 4.1).
- *Prevention programmes* – programmes, e.g. health visiting, Sure Start,[19] parenting programmes and adult literacy, need ongoing assessment. Professionals must be well supported. They may offer the best prospect of limiting the effects of multiple deprivation and neglect.

Outcomes for neglected children

Neglect is insidious and chronic and affects children in many ways. Signs of cognitive and socio-emotional delays appear early in the child's life. Left unattended, poor outcomes are more likely. Failure is manifested in all walks of life, including education, job prospects, and social and intellectual functioning. Links between neglect and mental illness, substance abuse, offending behaviour and general adjustment have been established. The outlook is not uniformly gloomy, and much can be done to improve it. The presence of an attentive person taking genuine interest in the child at some time is important. This person needs to be identified and supported. It is vital, therefore, to recognize neglectful patterns of parenting, and to seek, with the help of others, appropriate resources for the child and family.

Chapter Five

Subdural haemorrhage in infants: when is it not accidental?

5

Alison Kemp

SUMMARY

The most common cause of subdural haemorrhage in children under the age of 2 years is non-accidental head injury. Paediatricians are often challenged to make this diagnosis with confidence. A clinician must approach this problem from a thorough understanding of the epidemiology, clinical and pathological features of the condition. The paediatrician must work with a team of specialists in the field of child protection, and perform a baseline set of investigations to identify all associated features. Once the full clinical picture is evident, the team must make a decision based on the balance of probability as to whether child abuse has taken place. This decision is made in the context of the explanations given, and the type, site and severity of injuries the child has received. This chapter sets out recommendations for this process, and discusses the pitfalls encountered along the way.

INTRODUCTION

In 1946, and again in 1972, John Caffey, an American radiologist, described infants who presented to the clinician with subdural haemorrhage (SDH) and long bone fractures as a consequence of severe child abuse.[1,2] It is widely accepted that the most common cause of this clinical and radiological presentation is a whiplash acceleration–deceleration mechanism. This condition has previously been referred to as the 'shaken baby syndrome', but is perhaps best described as non-accidental head injury (NAHI), a term that is less implicit in terms of cause. There are, however, other causes of SDH in infants, and considerable gaps in our knowledge about the detailed mechanism and pathophysiology of injury. This deficit continues to present major challenges to doctors, social workers and lawyers in the diagnosis and management of this condition. The key question for any paediatrician presented with a small child with an SDH is whether or not the child has suffered from physical child abuse. This chapter attempts to outline the epidemiology and clinical and pathological features of this condition, and to address the current dilemmas in diagnosis and their consequences.

EPIDEMIOLOGY

SDH in infants is a relatively common and serious condition. A population-based study in Wales and south-west England[3]

PRACTICE POINTS

Guidelines for the investigations in an infant or young child with an unexplained subdural haemorrhage (SDH)
- Joint investigation by acute hospital paediatrician and paediatrician with expertise in child protection.
- Detailed history of cause and preceding events.
- Early involvement of social services to detail social history and previous child-protection concern within the family.
- Early involvement of the police to explore forensic investigation.
- Examination and photography of associated injuries.
- Investigations: initial computed tomography (CT) scan with early cranial magnetic resonance imaging (MRI) and follow-up imaging at 6 months; skeletal survey with bone scan or repeat skeletal survey at 14 days; indirect ophthalmoscopy by ophthalmologist; and full blood count and coagulation screen.
- Strategy meeting of agencies and all clinicians involved to make the diagnosis and plan management.
- Clear and accurate documentation in case notes.

What we know about the causes of SDH
- SDH is seen after significant whiplash injury, which is often sustained in a road traffic accident.
- SDH is seen after shaking and shaking with impact.
- There is often clinical evidence of other injuries to support a shaking/shaking with impact event.
- SDH rarely follows a simple household fall from a low height.
- SDH is seen after significant accidental injury (e.g. a fall from a first-storey window).
- An infant with severe intracranial and severe retinal injury has suffered a significant level of head trauma.
- In non-accidental SDH, the description of trauma given frequently does not fit the extent of injury seen.
- The majority of babies who have been shaken have coexisting haemorrhagic retinopathy; however, they may present with SDHs without haemorrhagic retinopathy and no other external injury.
- SDH has been recorded in bleeding disorders, metabolic disorders (e.g. galactosaemia, glutaric aciduria type 1), following brain surgery and in meningitis.

calculated an incidence of SDH arising from intentional injury of 12.8/100,000 children per year in children under 2 years old (one per 7,800). In children under 1 year of age the incidence was 21.0/100,000 children per year (one per 4,700), rising to 37/100,000 (one in 2,700) in children under 6 months old. These high figures in infants have been confirmed by Barlow et al.[4] in Scotland, who concluded that NAHI may still be underrecognized. The mortality rate varies from 12% to 30% in various case series described.[3] The morbidity is serious; 60–70% of survivors suffer from significant neurological handicap[3, 5] and the remaining children are prone to behavioural and learning difficulties at long-term follow-up.[6]

CLINICAL PRESENTATION

The diagnosis of NAHI is usually made as a consequence of the investigation of a sick infant who has been admitted to a ward with symptoms of unknown cause or at post mortem. The presenting symptoms, signs and severity of illness vary from a baby with general malaise and lethargy to a shocked infant who is comatose and fitting. The majority of these children do not present to the child-protection team in the first instance. The history is frequently unclear, and may only include a description of the onset of symptoms, with little or no reference to any traumatic event. SDH is often not the first diagnosis considered, and is only confirmed after cranial imaging. The probability of physical child abuse then needs to be excluded on the basis of associated features and careful review of the history.

There are a number of features that raise the probability of abuse.[3] In line with many cases of physical abuse, several explanations may be proposed, which do not fit the pattern of injury and vary in detail on retelling. Relatively little is known about the characteristics of the perpetrators of this injury; however, a survey of 14 cases that were heard in the criminal court showed that 11 of the alleged perpetrators were male carers (five male cohabitees and six natural fathers) and the remainder were mothers.[3]

Subdural bleeding in NAHI has a characteristic pattern. Injuries arise from the acceleration–deceleration as well as impact force. The haemorrhages are small and of low volume; they are frequently multiple and frequently occur in the interhemispheric space and posterior fossa. The subdural bleeding itself is rarely responsible for the poor outcome in these children, who may have associated hypoxic ischaemia, shearing injuries, contusions and infarctions within the brain itself.

Clinical features associated with the SDH include haemorrhagic retinopathy in 65–90%,[3, 7–9] other injuries (such as rib, skull and long-bone fractures and bruises) in 70%,[3, 10] and a previous history of abuse in the family in 44% of cases.[3] If these features are present, the diagnosis of NAHI becomes more probable. Although there is a high rate of associated trauma in shaken baby syndrome, an infant who has been shaken can present with SDHs alone.

ESSENTIAL INVESTIGATIONS

It is important to investigate fully every infant who has an SDH of unknown origin, in order to identify any of the associated findings that, if present, increase the probability that child abuse has occurred. It is equally important to exclude the associated findings in children where child abuse has not taken place, and to consider other causes.

NAHI should be considered as a possible diagnosis in any infant admitted to the ward with unexplained neurological symptoms. Cranial imaging should be considered as part of the investigation of any child under the age of 2 years who is being investigated for physical abuse. If the infant is younger than 6 months old, has haemorrhagic retinopathy, bone fracture, or neurological symptoms or other abusive injuries, a computed tomography (CT) scan should be a mandatory part of the child-protection medical work-up.

Radiological exploration should include an initial CT scan. This is the best means of identifying acute bleeds and is still the most widely available neuroimaging option. Magnetic resonance imaging (MRI) may identify further subdural bleeds and delineate the extent of associated intracranial injury. A follow-up MRI scan at 3–6 months can monitor the cranial pathology, and give an idea of prognosis. If subdural bleeding is diagnosed, the infant must have a skeletal survey with bone scan or repeat skeletal survey at 14 days. In this way, any coexisting fractures can be identified with confidence, and any information relevant to the age of bony injury determined. All children should have their eyes examined by an ophthalmologist who has the expertise in using indirect ophthalmoscopy to identify haemorrhagic retinopathy, which manifests at the periphery of the retina. All children should have a coagulation screen.

The full clinical picture needs to be assessed in the context of a thorough general examination that documents and photographs the site and number of any coexisting bruises, lacerations, burns or bites. Paediatricians with experience in the field of child protection and a social worker need to be involved in the early stages of investigation to assess the likelihood of child abuse, and implement the child-protection procedure as necessary.

DIFFERENTIAL DIAGNOSIS OF SDH

The differential diagnoses in the 20–30% of infants who present with SDH that is not due to shaking or shaking and impact include serious accidental trauma, disease-related conditions (e.g. leukaemia and disseminated intravascular coagulation) as well as other coagulation disorders (e.g. haemophilia, Von Willebrand's disease, haemorrhagic disease of the newborn and Henoch–Scholein purpura).[7]

Spontaneous bleeding from arteriovenous malformations or aneurysms, complications of traumatic labour, instrumental delivery or neurosurgery can cause an SDH in infants. There are a handful of cases described in the literature where SDH was found in association with hypernatraemia from dehydration or salt poisoning.[11]

Subdural effusions, collections of fluid in the subdural space, can be seen following an episode of meningitis or encephalitis, as well as in congenital metabolic abnormalities such as glutaric aciduria type 1,[12] galactosaemia and Menkes disease. These fluid collections, which are not necessarily haemorrhagic, may be of low attenuation and therefore appear similar to chronic subdural haematomas on CT.

Each of these conditions has its own specific physical signs or diagnostic investigations. Glutaric aciduria type 1, for example, is often diagnosed at around the same age that NAHI prevails, and can present with similar neurological symptoms. Infants with this condition have bilateral front temporal atrophy, with a widened extra-axial subdural space that renders them prone to SDH.[12]

The approach to diagnosis should be to implement the investigation protocol to exclude the most likely diagnosis of physical child abuse in all cases, with full consideration of the different possibilities that exist. In reality, there is a hierarchy of clinical presentation. The 4-month-old baby who presents with subdural haemorrhages, haemorrhagic retinopathy, haemorrhages with finger-tip bruising around the upper trunk and rib fractures has, in all probability, been a victim of physical abuse. The decision to implement the child-protection procedure is relatively straightforward. A child of similar age who presents with an isolated SDH, however, presents a far greater diagnostic dilemma, and justifies a more extensive diagnostic work-up to exclude other causes. The whole picture must be interpreted with clinical rigour and in the context of the differential diagnosis.

DIAGNOSTIC DILEMMAS

From the minute subdural bleeding is identified, there is pressure on the clinical team to decide whether or not the infant has been abused. The consequences of making the wrong diagnosis are serious; a child who has been violently abused may go unprotected, and there can be devastating consequences for a family wrongly accused of child abuse. Decisions can only be made after a thorough and complete clinical investigation, and even then questions remain surrounding the severity and timing of the traumatic event and its relationship to the injuries sustained.

Mechanism of injury

The scientific evidence used to identify the mechanism and forces required to induce an SDH is inconclusive. Much of the theory is based on experimental models, old animal studies and small case series where the perpetrator admitted shaking the child.

In the 1960s, work was published showing that monkeys shaken to the point of concussion developed SDH.[13] This was extrapolated to estimate forces that would be required to injure a human in the same way. This limit was easily exceeded in modelled experimental work undertaken by Duhaime et al.[14] in shaken impact injury, but could not be replicated by violent shaking alone. This experimental model lacks the dynamic components of raised thoracic pressure, leading to high central venous pressure and blood flow through fragile blood vessels that are likely contributory variables in vivo.

It is now widely accepted that shaking a baby or small infant generates the acceleration–deceleration forces that are necessary to generate an SDH. Babies are small and easy to pick up and shake in a way that would be impossible in heavier children. A baby has a large head and weak neck muscles. They have no defence resources to protect themselves from the whiplash mechanism, which sets up shearing forces within the cranium sufficient to tear the blood vessels that cross the relatively wide subdural space, resulting in bleeding.[2, 15] There is evidence that some infants suffer from shaking with impact against a firm or hard surface, and have subdural bleeding with a skull fracture or bruising. However, it is widely accepted that shaking alone can cause the cerebral and ocular injuries; small case series have been published where parents have admitted holding a child around the chest and shaking so that the head flips backwards and forwards forcefully. Clinically, bruising to the torso and rib fractures would support this mechanism.

The generation of subdura bleeding requires these acceleration–deceleration forces on bridging veins and, consequently, SDH is rarely seen in an impact head injury of accidental origin, with the exception of a road traffic accident, where similar whiplash mechanisms are elicited. Minor household injuries, such as a fall off a sofa or bed, rarely cause a skull fracture and are not associated with intracranial injury. If a more serious household fall causes a skull fracture, it is most likely to be a linear fracture; any coexisting intracranial bleed is likely to be in the extradural space underlying the fracture.

There is evidence to support a direct relationship between the severity of eye injury and the severity of intracranial injury.[7] The mechanisms that cause haemorrhagic retinopathy are thought to include significant rotational acceleration–deceleration forces that are sufficient to cause vitreous traction on the retina, and hence tearing of retinal blood vessels and consequential bleeding.[7]

Timing of injury

The medical expert in court is often asked for his or her opinion about the timing of injury, and to supply supporting evidence. In concrete terms, there is still little to offer to pinpoint the time of injury in terms of clinical investigations.

Although it has been stated previously that cranial imaging can differentiate between an acute SDH and a resolving chronic SDH on the basis of the variation in signal density, this is now thought to be less obvious, but adult MRI studies may offer more promise in this field. Cases may present with multiple SDHs of different density, which are not necessarily of different ages. Ageing of fractures, haemorrhagic retinopathy and bruises is also an inexact science.

Bruises vary in appearance due to the extent, site and depth of injury. In a similar way, the colour and appearance of retinal haemorrhages varies according to the size of the bleed and its age. Brown-yellow haemorrhages may be at least 1 month old, and haemorrhages of different colours are likely to be of different ages. Mild retinal bleeds probably clear rapidly (within days) in a similar way to birth-related retinal haemorrhages, moderate bleeds may resolve after a number of weeks, and severe ones may take months.[7]

Sometimes the extent of brain repair at autopsy can contribute to timing the injury. Forensic pathological studies indicate that the presence of haemosiderin in a retinal haemorrhage suggest that it is more than 3 days old.[7]

A lumbar puncture will become blood stained within 6 hours of a bleed and contains oxyhaemoglobin on spectrophotometry. The cerebrospinal fluid becomes xanthochromic after 12–24 hours, which may persist for 3 weeks after an acute bleed but for months in chronic SDH.[16]

Discussion of the timing of the onset of clinical features and the chronology of events, identified in the police and social assessments, often makes the picture clearer and builds a more accurate forensic picture. However, accurate timing of the injury is rarely possible.

CONCLUSIONS

Correct management of infants with subdural bleeding depends on accurate diagnosis, which is challenging but improved when the child has been investigated fully, and the clinician can be confident that they have identified or excluded associated features of child abuse. As in any clinical situation, the clinician is beholden to exclude the most likely diagnosis, which in a baby, infant or small toddler is undoubtedly child abuse. The clinician must work with the child-protection team to weigh up the probability that abuse has or has not taken place, and present the facts that inform this decision coherently to the case conference, civil and criminal courts as necessary.

Unanswered questions remain, and these need to be researched further. We need to clarify the least force necessary to cause subdural bleeding, and evaluate neuroradiological features in the context of cases that have an explained mechanism to clarify their relevance to the severity, timing and mechanism of trauma.

There is no evidence to suggest that the number of infants who are shaken is falling. Indeed, as the threshold for considering this diagnosis falls and our understanding and the availability of cranial imaging increases, it is likely that more infants with SDH will be identified.

Every NAHI caused by shaking or shaking impact is inherently preventable. We need to know more about the characteristics of the perpetrators of this injury to help us to design successful preventive strategies and direct these at the right target population. There is evidence that the majority of perpetrators are male and that many members of the public do not recognize the dangers of shaking.[17] However, there is little evidence that public-awareness campaigns reach the target population or that 'Never Shake a Baby' campaigns reduce the problem.

Chapter Six

Current debates in child sexual abuse

Jean Price

SUMMARY

This chapter debates some of the topics around sexual abuse that appear to be causing some difficulties to practitioners. The incidence is mentioned and the importance of the history from the child is emphasized. Reasons why a child should receive a medical examination, together with when the examination takes place, who should carry this out, and whether this should be one or two practitioners are discussed. The consent to the examination and timing of the examination are also debated, as is the nature of the examination, and the need for good and appropriate documentation, and photography of one sort or another. The examination positions are discussed, as are the clinical findings and sexually transmitted diseases.

INTRODUCTION

Child sexual abuse continues to play a significant role in the daily work of health professionals working with children within the community setting, particularly GPs, community paediatricians and psychiatrists. The diagnosis of child sexual abuse can be difficult, and frequently agencies such as the police and social services look to health professionals to provide evidence. This is not easy, given the numerous configurations of the normal hymen, and the changes in the hymen that occur after injury with rapid healing. Little is known about the healing process, or the end result following a single episode of abuse or following chronic abuse over a period of time. Clearly the effects of this would be different in a prepubertal compared with a postpubertal child. This would imply that there is still considerable work to be done in order to establish more effective and definitive ways of assessing children who allege abuse.

The true incidence of child sexual abuse is impossible to assess. It is estimated, however, that up to 100,000 children each year have a potentially harmful sexual experience,[1] and the recording of sexual abuse on child-protection registers has increased markedly from 5% of all registrations in 1983 to 23% in 1995.

Suspicions that sexual abuse may be occurring can arise from the child's behaviour. This may be sexualized and provocative, or withdrawn, isolated and regressed, with sleep and feeding difficulties. As victims get older, it may present with self-destructive behaviours, such as drug and alcohol misuse, as well as prostitution and running away. All victims may present with psychosomatic symptoms or clinical symptoms pertaining to the genitalia or the anus. Most frequently, however, children are brought to our attention because of a disclosure by them, which may be recent or historical. This usually triggers a child-protection response from all the agencies (health and social services, and the police) under the Child Protection Procedures.[2]

It has been said in the past, and remains so today, that the child's story is the single most important piece of evidence:

> ... the child's story of what happened, together with the child's demeanour and emotional response whilst describing what took place, is the single most important feature in coming to a diagnosis.[3]

In all aspects of medicine, we are trained to take a history before examining, investigating and making a diagnosis. This is also true of sexual abuse, and most physicians would expect some history from the child or the presenting agency prior to clinical examination. It has been shown, however, that the history may alter the interpretation of the clinical findings. This is more likely to be the case for inexperienced practitioners.[4]

WHY IS A MEDICAL EXAMINATION NECESSARY?

Forensic evidence

The presence or absence of injury or the presence or absence of semen is usually the reason for referral for examination. The clinical information can assist the investigation of the allegation, but also provides considerable reassurance to both the victims and their families.

Treatment

The identification and treatment of any infection is necessary. The therapeutic aspect of the medical examination is often not appreciated. It can be the beginning of a healing process. The fact that any damage heals dramatically quickly can be a source of considerable reassurance to both the child and his or her carers.

Baseline

The clinical findings, if carefully recorded, can form the basis for future examinations. It is well known that a number of these children live in a vulnerable environment and may be further abused in the future, hence this baseline examination could be invaluable for future evidence. Frothingham et al.[5] found at 8-year follow-up that further abuse had occurred in 35% of children. There were also other aspects of their functioning that caused concern.

There continues to be debate regarding the need for a medical examination, and there are still some misconceptions by the social services and police as to what the examination involves. They sometimes do not appear to accept that, unless there are acute forensic specimens to be obtained, for example when an offence has taken place within the previous 2–3 days, the examination is primarily one of inspection.

WHO SHOULD BE RESPONSIBLE FOR THE MEDICAL EXAMINATION?

There is ongoing debate as to whether medical examinations should be the remit of the forensic medical examiner or the paediatrician. There is growing support for a holistic examination of the child and, if necessary, remedial intervention, which would more clearly put the examination in the remit of the paediatrician. This is primarily because of the ongoing difficulties that these children display, and the vulnerable environments within which they often find themselves. In a study that investigated the adverse effects 8 years after abuse, Frothingham et al.[5] found a higher occurrence of problems in abused children compared with a control group:

- adverse behaviours 60% versus 16%
- educational problems 24% versus 5%
- chronic health problems 54% versus 36%
- involvement of mental health services 32% versus 1%.

The remit of the forensic medical examiner is to carry out a one-off examination and provide a report. Whoever carries out such examinations should have a comprehensive understanding of childhood development, educational and social medicine, as well as forensic skills. It is, therefore, beholden to paediatricians to become familiar with the needs of the forensic examination.

SHOULD THE EXAMINATION BE CARRIED OUT BY ONE OR TWO DOCTORS?

There are occasions when a two-doctor examination may be necessary. This is usually when the paediatrician has no forensic experience and requires a forensic medical examiner to assist in the collection of forensic exhibits. If the examiner is inexperienced, it would be wise to request a more experienced examiner to assist. A two-doctor examination could provide essential supportive evidence within a court setting, and prevent the child requiring a second medical examination. Nevertheless, good clear documentation of clinical findings, together with photography, could avoid the need for a second examiner to be present, yet still allowing for a second opinion to be provided, either for the prosecution or the defence. There is, therefore, growing support for photographs, and the use of a colposcope for such examinations, particularly where unusual findings or clinical damage is present.

CONSENT TO EXAMINATION

Consent is essential in the current climate. Children over 16 years of age and those less than 16 years but 'Gillick competent' can give their own permission for the medical examination to take place. Those on care orders would require the permission of the court, but otherwise permission can be sought from the parents of the child. It is, however, always good practice to explain clearly to the child and the carer what the examination consists of and to request their permission. A running commentary of how you are progressing through the examination may be of assistance in reassuring the child and the parent, but can also reassure the examiner that the child is giving permission at every stage.

TIMING OF EXAMINATIONS

Most disclosures about child sexual abuse are old, and the examination can therefore be planned to occur at an appropriate time and place to suit both the child and the examiner. Increasingly, practitioners are running a routine clinic for such examinations. This allows appropriate venues, nurse support and equipment, etc. to be made available.

Those alleging sexual interference/rape within 72 hours of the incident require an urgent examination. As time passes, vital forensic evidence may be lost. Christian et al.[6] found forensic evidence present in approximately one-quarter of his cohort of 273 prepubertal children. All were examined within 44 hours and 90% were seen within 24 hours. The majority of forensic evidence (64%) was found on clothing and bed linens. Twenty-three per cent of this cohort had genital injuries and a history of injury, plus ejaculation increased the chance of finding evidence, but in some children there was evidence that was not suspected from the history. The American Academy of Paediatrics states that there should be collection of forensic evidence under the following circumstances:

- when the last event was within 72 hours
- when there is a history of bleeding
- when there is acute injury present.

WHAT THE EXAMINATION INVOLVES

The examination is primarily one of inspection, with labial separation and gentle traction to visualize the hymenal margin more effectively. A moistened swab may be used to either tease the hymen open or to inspect the folds of an oestrogenized hymen looking for damage within the folds. Some examiners used glaistner rods, and in the USA Foley catheters are sometimes used. In adolescents it may be necessary to assess the hymenal ring, particularly in single episodes of rape. The only time it is necessary to pass a speculum is for the collection of high vaginal swabs for forensic evidence in adolescents alleging sexual intercourse within the preceding 72 hours. Equally, on examination of the anus, a proctoscope or internal examination would only be necessary if there were clinical findings or there was an allegation of buggery with ejaculation.

EXAMINATION POSITION

The child's emotional needs should always be considered when positioning the child. Very young children may prefer to be examined on the mother's lap. More commonly, however, children are examined in the supine frog-leg position, with the legs abducted and the knees flexed. An alternative examination position is the prone knee/chest position. The Royal College of Physicians' handbook[3] states this position is not generally used in the UK, although it is used quite extensively in the USA. It requires patience to get the child correctly positioned, with the head and shoulders resting on a pillow, the knees flexed under the abdomen, and the bottom raised in the air. This is an extremely useful examination position when there are suspected abnormalities in the posterior margin of the hymen, as this position allows relaxation of the pelvic floor muscles. Any suspected abnormality in the posterior margin seen in the supine position would smooth out in the prone position if it were a normal artefact, whereas concavities in both positions would be supportive of damage to the hymen.

EXAMINATION FINDINGS

Terminology

There still remains considerable confusion around terminology, particularly that pertaining to damage to the hymen. Despite the request following the Cleveland enquiry that clinicians should use common terminology, this has not happened. Nevertheless, most of the terms used can be found in the Royal College of Physicians' handbook[3] or the *Colour Atlas of Sexual Assault*.[7] A number of colleagues and I have jointly felt that the following terminology is useful.

Transection This may be acute with raw edges or healed. It is a full-thickness tear from the edge to the base of the hymen. This loss of tissue is not replaced by healing and, once present, should remain until the hymen is worn away by regular sexual intercourse.

Partial transection This is a tear from the edge of the hymen that does not reach the hymenal attachment. This again may be acute (fresh) or healed. It will heal leaving some loss of hymenal tissue, and may present as a concavity or a notch on the edge of the hymen. This may be associated with an increase or mounding of tissue to one side of the notch or concavity. This may be described as a bump.

Concavities or notches in the anterior half of the hymen (9 o'clock through 12 o'clock to 3 o'clock) are usually now considered as potentially normal,[3] whereas those in the posterior half of the hymen (3 o'clock through 6 o'clock to 9 o'clock) may be more consistent with damage and therefore indicative of pressure against or through the hymen. It is very useful to follow some acute clinical cases, as some fresh injuries to the posterior margin of the hymen do heal, leaving minimal damage in the form of a minor concavity on the surface of the edge of the hymen, and if they were viewed at a later second examination by an inexperienced examiner, may be considered to be normal clinical findings.

Attenuation Thinning in the depth of the hymen, from its edge to the point of fixation, may appear as a concavity or a notch on the edge of the hymen.

Bumps Bumps are frequently a normal finding and are usually associated with an intravaginal ridge.

Tags Tags are not infrequently found and are usually extensions of the hymen. They may be the end result of a septae hymen that has broken down at one end. Some tags may be quite large and can cause parental anxiety.

Inflammation

Inflammation of the external genitalia or the inner labial margins, fourchette and tissues of the vestibule could be indicative of friction, rubbing and pressure in these areas, as can occur in sexual intercourse. It is important, however, to appreciate that this could also be the consequence of children rubbing themselves as a result of irritation due to skin condition or infection of the genitalia. It is, therefore, important to rule out the possibility of these conditions. It may, therefore, be advisable to screen for infections in such situations (see later). Threadworm may also be a source of irritation to both the anus and the genitalia, and should be looked for and treated if there is inflammation and minor abrasions to the genitalia. A second examination should be done after a course of treatment to ascertain whether there are still abnormalities on the genitalia (e.g. inflammation and oedema), which may mask other clinical abnormalities or may simply be due to threadworm or infection and may be misinterpreted as abnormal findings following an allegation of abuse. After resolution of oedema, it is possible to visualize any underlying damage. Should the child's allegation result in a criminal prosecution, it will be necessary to demonstrate that alternative diagnoses have been considered and eliminated.

Hymenal diameter

The hymenal diameter was considered in the past to be a useful diagnostic clinical finding, but then fell into disrepute.[3] A more recent piece of work by Pugno[8] suggested that the transhymenal diameter between 9 and 3 o'clock is a useful screening parameter for evaluating children in potential sexual abuse cases. In a cohort of 1058 prepubertal girls aged between 6 months and 10 years, examined because of alleged sexual molestation, girls with no definite signs of genital trauma exhibited a mean transhymenal diameter of 2.3 mm and, in general, showed an increase of approximately 1 mm per year of age. In contrast, those with definite signs of genital trauma exhibited a mean transhymenal diameter of 9.0 mm and no significant variants with age. He claimed that the transhymenal measurement is 99% specific and 79% sensitive as a screening tool. This area requires further research.

Anus

There is little new research on anal clinical findings. Anal sphincter dilatation greater than 20 mm is common when stool is in the rectum, but occurs in only 1% of children if stool is not present. Abrasions, lacerations and haematomas have not been observed in the absence of abuse.[9, 10]

No clinical findings

It is acknowledged that, despite an allegation of some form of child sexual abuse, there may be no or minimal clinical findings. The Royal College of Physicians' handbook[3] and Muram[11] reported that, in four prepubertal children, no or minimal clinical findings were found by examination performed 72 hours after an admitted episode of penile penetration.

Sexually transmitted diseases

Sexually transmitted disease (STD) may be transmitted during a sexual assault and the isolation of an STD may be the first indication that abuse has occurred, particularly if this is beyond the neonatal period. Most research on this subject has been carried out on adults, but studies involving children suggest that swabs should only be taken if there are symptoms of infection or there is a clear history of contact with the offender's genitalia.[12]

- *Chlamydia trachomatis* may be the result of perinatal acquired infection, which may persist for as long as 3 years. Thereafter, it is highly likely to be sexually transmitted. It is important from a medico-legal point of view to prove that this is present via culture. This is the gold standard.
- Gonorrhoea is the most frequent STD found in abused children. It can be asymptomatic, particularly in the rectum and the pharynx, and when swabbing for suspected gonococcus of the genitalia, swabs should also be taken from the rectum and the pharynx.[12]
- Bacterial vaginosis has been identified in both abused and non-abused children, but the methods for diagnosing bacterial vaginosis in adults have not been evaluated in children.
- Human papilloma virus has been detected at various sites in children who have not been abused, and the relationship between abuse and the development of clinically apparent genital warts is unclear.
- Human immunodeficiency virus (HIV) can be acquired through sexual contact. The exact risk to children and which children should be screened is controversial.[13]

FUTURE RESEARCH

There is still a need for increased knowledge about the range of normal anatomy of the genitalia and the anus, and how this changes with age. There is also a need to look at the healing process following a single episode of a sexual assault versus multiple chronic episodes. These areas need to be researched in both the prepubertal and the pubertal age groups.

CONCLUSIONS

There are still many areas of knowledge about child sexual abuse that need to be expanded. We still do not have adequate knowledge of the range of normal anogenital anatomy and how it changes with age. Nor do we have information about healing following a single episode of damage or multiple chronic abuse, and we still do not have consistent terminology. There is still an urgent need for further research, which probably needs to be multicentre in order to obtain adequate sample sizes to make evaluation meaningful. It is clear, however, that examinations for suspected sexual abuse must be performed by people with experience and with appropriate facilities and equipment. There must be close support and cooperation between all clinicians working in this field.

Chapter Seven

Recognition and management of fabricated and induced illness

7

Richard Wilson

SUMMARY

Clinical skills include eliciting a clear history and assessing, by examination, investigation and intervention, the reasons for the child being brought for an opinion. We can be misled by reports that are incomplete, exaggerated or untrue. Whatever the motivation, this can lead to inappropriate and harmful acts upon the child by tests or treatments. Improved awareness and clinical skill should be supplemented by early collaboration with colleagues in paediatrics and child protection when there is uncertainty or persisting suspicions.

PRACTICE POINTS

- In every consultation, consider whether the carer's account and views are compatible with the child's condition, and note how much depends on uncorroborated statements.
- Certain factors may trigger a more critical view of whether an illness is fabricated or induced, even though they are not proof.
- Early information gathering from other professionals who have contact with the child is essential.
- If suspicions cannot be allayed, consult early with colleagues in child protection.
- If this issue worries you, get some training.[1]

INTRODUCTION

The understanding of how children can be harmed by carers who fabricate or induce illness has developed since the early reports in the 1960s and the confusing era of the 1980s and 1990s.[2] We have increased our knowledge of the old dramatic problems, which still exist. We are beginning to extend our understanding of the huge area of emotional and psychological harm. We recognize that doctors deliver some physically traumatic and intrusive harm through inappropriate medical and surgical investigation or treatment. This chapter cannot replace reading and consulting the important sources quoted in the Royal College of Paediatrics and Child Health's guidance on fabrication or illness induction (FII),[3] and can only highlight a few areas.

Two issues have changed significantly. First, the terminology 'fabrication or illness induction by carers with parenting responsibilities' is absolutely clear and requires no definition.[4] This is a behaviour to be identified, not a medical or psychiatric diagnosis. It is, of course, linked to the separate consideration of whether a child has suffered or is likely to suffer harm, and whether that harm is significant. The term 'Munchausen syndrome by proxy' should be discarded. Second, covert video surveillance is no longer controversial. It has been shown to have a valid role, but one that is probably diminishing. Such surveillance is now legally the sole responsibility of the police, who follow guidance in line with the law, and it will more often be carried out locally.[5]

PROBLEMS IN RECOGNITION

FII can occur in any setting and with any symptomatology. Although there are well-described clinical situations, the recognition of FII depends on our clinical acumen, both in the medical evaluation of a particular suspected pathology, and in the awareness of triggers that should alert our concerns.[3] It is, however, wrong to use an alerting factor as evidence of proof.

Clinical situations that may be more frequent in leading to physical harm classically include intermittent disorders such as epilepsy, asthma, choking, headache, vomiting and abdominal pain, where the diagnosis rests solely on the history. In other cases there may be fabricated or induced bleeding, or situations such as collapse, drowsiness or diarrhoea associated with hypernatraemia, or hypoglycaemia or poisoning. Unexpected or recurrent deaths in the family emphasize the need for all children's deaths to receive comprehensive investigation.

Other alerting factors are the doctor's inability to correlate reported symptoms or signs with a disease that the child is known to have, or even with any other recognizable disease. Repeated presentation, sometimes to many doctors or with a variety of problems, should suggest the need for a wider view of the child and family where there may be a history of unexplained illnesses or multiple operations, or even deaths. When investigations produce results that do not correlate with symptoms or signs, one must suspect both of being misleading. When treatment fails to produce the desired effect, there may be fabrication of illness, or when treatment is not given, a denial of illness and a fabrication of health. Twenty-five per cent of abusing carers have a history of being victims of child abuse, which is higher than the incidence in the general population. However, that a carer has such a history is no proof of anything except the need to look more closely. Only 20% of abusing carers have previous paramedical training, so such a history is not typical, but it may, like access to drugs or insulin, make certain behaviour a possibility. Previous mental health difficulties, particularly somatizing disorders or deliberate self-harm, are major alerting factors which may be known to family doctors, but do not prove that FII has occurred, or that it has been perpetrated by that person. Understanding the possibility of how harmful parental behaviour may have arisen does not justify it or prove it has occurred. Even a past history of puzzling illness or death in siblings is not proof. There is no psychiatric disorder that inevitably leads to child abuse, and sometimes the perpetrator is another person in the family. There is no easy shortcut.

MEDICAL EVALUATION

Each case needs a scrupulous medical investigation and evaluation. This is well illustrated in a paper comparing two children with hypernatraemia.[6] One, who had a diagnosis of colitis, was found to have been given purgatives and then poisoned with salt. Another, who had a suspicious family history of deaths and unusual illnesses in siblings, was shown to have hypernatraemia due to disproportionate dehydration. The details of investigations required careful scrutiny and comparison with clinical findings to elucidate the aetiologies.

DEATHS

Death from FII occurred in 6% of cases in the UK series reported by McClure et al.[7] The frequency of death in series based on the case loads of experienced practitioners varies with the features that led to their inclusion, and due to inadequate investigation. Retrospective allegations that a series of unexplained infant deaths in a family were inevitably due to homicide cannot be sustained. The subsequent siblings of an infant who dies suddenly and unexpectedly have 25% of genes in common and a similar environment. The risk of a second cot death is six times the risk of the first.[8]

Home Office records show there are around 30 infant homicides each year, compared with over 300 natural unexplained deaths. There have been serial murderers among carers and professionals, but these are rare and the behaviour different from that in FII.

The investigation of individual infant deaths is improving due to local multidisciplinary initiatives and to the Foundation for the Study of Infant Deaths campaign *Responding When a Baby Dies*.[9] This culminated in the joint report form the Royal College of Pathologists and Royal College of Paediatrics and Child Health, *Sudden Unexpected Death in Infancy*, chaired by Baroness Helena Kennedy,[10] which gives clear guidelines. The Association of Chief Police Officers have also given specific instructions on infant deaths in the *Police Murder Manual*. The Department for Education and Skills has proposed that all unexpected child deaths are investigated by the Local Child Safeguarding Boards as part of new Child Death Screening procedures. The uncertainty about infant deaths should diminish.

APPARENT LIFE-THREATENING EPISODES

Frightening episodes that alarm parents and lead to summoning of medical aid or admission to hospital have become known as

'apparent life-threatening episodes'.[11] They have been described in some infants who later died as a result of sudden infant death syndrome (SIDS). In the Confidential Enquiry into Stillbirths and Deaths in Infancy (CESDI), 12% of subsequent SIDS were reported as having such attacks before death, compared with 3% of controls.[5] The SIDS babies had more severe or prolonged attacks, and half went to hospital compared with one-third of the controls. The detailed corroborated history of the events, the child and the whole family needs to be complete enough to direct a filmed reconstruction. The child needs observation at least overnight. Further investigations have been suggested. The hospital paediatric social worker should see the family to support them through their anxieties and assess any needs they may have.[12] In Eminson and Postlethwaite's series,[13] the death rate in infants identified as being subjected to FII through induced apnoea was 20%. One might hope that identification would have reduced some of the mortality. In Southall et al.'s series,[14] no index cases died, but the infants were under investigation for recurrent episodes of apnoea. The death rate among siblings was 26%, compared with 5% in the study by McClure et al.,[7] but the previous death of a sibling was one of the factors which prompted the referral. It is known that some infants die after episodes of smothering intended to quieten the baby, and that death was unintended. Although such deaths are accidental, and therefore manslaughter, if the underlying situation had been understood, the harm might have been prevented and the baby may have survived.

SURGERY

The frequency of induced surgery is highest when signs are induced without smothering or administering poisons of high toxicity, but it also occurs in one-quarter of fabricated cases. When surgery has been performed, there will also have been extensive investigation.

Table 7.1 Analysis of 308 cases not reported in large series[13]

	Cases	Deaths	Surgery	Sibling ALTE/death
Fabrication of history, records or tests	67	0	18	3
Withholding nutrients	14	0	0	2
Producing signs (not poison or smothering)	62	3	37	7
Poisons of low toxicity	41	5	26	6
Poisons of high toxicity	89	22	12	32
ALTE	35	5	7	17
Total	308	35	100	67*

*31 deaths and 36 ALTEs.
ALTE, apparent life-threatening episode.

Operations for symptoms such as vomiting, which depend mainly on history, are a particular risk (Table 7.1).

COMMUNITY PAEDIATRICS

Community paediatricians have specific opportunities for detecting FII.[13] The awareness of children who are frequently absent from school, or who seem to be repeatedly referred to one specialist or another, or where parents insist the child has specific learning difficulties that teachers do not detect, or demands for financial assistance that seem disproportionate, or insistence on unusual dietary or exercise routines, all need to be looked into. The long-term effects of illness exaggeration, overprotection, overtreatment, and teaching the child to view themselves as disabled or different are not fully understood. Sometimes, mild fabrication becomes consolidated into a chronic situation, which later becomes collusion. The child becomes an invalid and the illness is self-induced and perpetuated, by which time the child is too old to be protected. FII can affect children with chronic illness, whose carers are intensely involved with their child and their professionals. These children too may undergo unnecessary and harmful treatments.

REVIEW OF THE MEDICAL ROLE

Failure to identify the fabricating carer is the gateway to harm delivered by doctors. This recognition makes the consultation a jungle with new dangers. We know that we harm children every day by altering their lives, or sticking needles into them, giving them potentially dangerous drugs or scheduling them for surgery. Of course we have the best motivation in the world but, like the carer, motivation is not the issue. Rather the issue is whether the harm is based on a correct assessment and whether the risks are justifiable. In FII the doctor is an intrinsic part of the triangular dynamics, not just an observer of possible parental abuse of the child. We may feel uncertain of what is really happening. Uncertainty empowers the abuser, and disempowers the doctor.[13] However, we can:

- Review our day-to-day clinical acumen. Have you ever seen a video of yourself in a consultation and evaluated your performance? Would you let somebody else see it and, if so, who?
- Be intellectually honest. How much were you presuming or concluding without justification? Did the child you just saw benefit from seeing you?
- Find out what the child knows or feels.
- Record everything in detail.
- Not organize investigations or make referrals before a reliable (corroborated) account of what is really happening is available.
- Answer the question: 'Why has this person brought this child to see me at this time?'

PERSISTING CONCERNS

We need help when we have anxieties. It may be that the figure for FII seems low. From 1992 to 1994, 0.4/100,000 children per annum were recognized by a case conference to be suffering this form of abuse.[7] However, we know that there are many more children whose parents overtreat (or undertreat) them, who exaggerate, who have theories that involve unnecessary regimens, or who believe in ill-defined diseases or unevaluated treatments.[13] Most of these children will never be considered by a case conference. It may help to:

- corroborate the stories by speaking to the GP, health visitor, teacher or grandma
- ask some families to make a video record of what happened to the child in reported episodes
- ask a colleague or the named doctor to review the puzzling situation
- spend time with parents who demand escalation of investigation or treatment in company with another colleague such as a social worker or psychologist, who may be able to help us to decide whether the case should be taken further and, if so, how.

Mostly we need help to develop trust in colleagues in other disciplines so that we can telephone them or call on their help.

THE PROCESS OF IDENTIFICATION[13]

Collaboration is an issue of trust. Initially, we are reliant on our own clinical skills and on verifying some of our suspicions. This can be difficult, particularly when there are inpatients who develop close relationships with other staff with whom we would not wish to share our concerns at that point in time. However, we need to exchange information with colleagues who know the family, and with colleagues in child protection, whether they are paediatricians, police, child psychiatrists or social workers. Sadly, the relationships even between acute and community paediatricians are not always composed of respect, trust and friendship. This is not just a shame, it is shameful. Lack of trust that others would do things as well as we might is not unique to doctors. We need to work to create a team rather than a corps of prima donnas. We need time and opportunity to meet with colleagues in other disciplines to understand the origins of their different perceptions, to work out how the boundaries of our territories can be outlined and how to cross them, and how to develop personal relationships. Those who manage services must give us time for study and multiagency training, joint work and informal meetings in order to build this team. With commitment from the top, we can find shared values, agree thresholds and look at how we use finite resources. We may also need to plan to get this commitment from the top. While such a team may take time to set up, when it is working it will undoubtedly be more efficient and benefit children as well as provide cost benefits.

There are, of course, times when we all fail to listen, fail to answer, fail to attend meetings, fail to let people know what has happened, think it is not our job, think we do not have the resources or think we cannot summon up the courage to do what we know we should. Knowing someone who can help and whom you can phone is essential, but should not lead to cosy exclusive relationships or hierarchies. Being 'along the corridor' is very important, particularly in relation to child psychiatry and social-work staff. To have a social worker based in every paediatric and child health department would lead to major improvements in care for children.

A CAVEAT

Having started along the path of ascertaining FII abuse, it can be difficult to remember that a suspicion or a belief is not proof.

Sometimes there will be other explanations. How do we cope with that? How is the family coping? What will the other agencies think? Care for children and clinical acumen and protocols propel us along the path. The routes are clearly signed when significant harm has occurred, but the paths peter out for both families and professionals when there is no proof, or the child is found to have an unrecognized medical problem, or this is a child and family in need but not at risk of harm. One of the challenges is to make it clear that innocence remains a live option. We should be seeking support for the family and their needs from the outset. Failure to do so is one of the reasons for complaints.

THE LAW

The law is also clarifying its position. Recent cases have determined that doctors do not have a duty of care to the other members of the family. Consequently, if an investigation into possible child abuse has been conducted properly, parents cannot sue for the distress it will have caused them. We would, of course, wish to reduce that in any case.

It is also clear that information about family members can be requested from family doctors if it is needed to prevent harm or the risk of harm to a child. It is also clear that there are situations where one can refuse parents access to their children's notes. It is always sensible in these difficult situations to use risk management and legal advice.

CONCLUSIONS

The focus is now firmly on the child and whether the child has been directly harmed physically or psychologically by the carer, or indirectly using doctors to deliver the harm. Parental motivation is not relevant in identifying whether harm has occurred. Understanding parents neither proves harm nor justifies it. It is, however, important as an alerting sign, in assessing whether rehabilitation is possible, and perhaps in developing strategies for prevention.[15]

'Harm' itself must be considered as the effect on the child rather than the action of the carers. Whether the harm is 'significant' can be one of the most difficult decisions.[16] Physical harm will always cause psychological harm too. The effects of illness induction are a cause of both. Fabrication is more common; it can lead to physical harm delivered by professionals as devastating as direct illness induction. However, when the harm is psychological, we have less information on the outcome, which will depend not only on the perpetrator's activity, but also on the resilience of the child and other positive or therapeutic experiences. We know relatively little about the long-term effects, and this is a priority for research. We need to bear in mind the effects of abuse on the whole being of the child physically, psychologically, mentally and socially, and the effect this may later have on their own children.

Doctors and other professionals know that some carers abuse children, and in the majority of cases this is a straight interaction between the parents and the child. FII is different, because doctors are an intrinsic part of the process. Our assessment of the picture given by a carer is part of every consultation, and his or her account (and even our view) may be wide of the truth. We must be more critical of our consultations if we wish to improve our skills. We must collaborate with others to gain both the comprehensive and corroborated view and mutual trust.[17] Our aim must be to detect and prevent abuse or the risk of harm, and help children and their families earlier. We may then, in some cases, be able to reduce the problems that lead carers to induce illness or deceive us into harming children, and in other cases remove the child from danger as soon as possible.

Chapter Eight

Physical child abuse: responding to the evidence

8

Michelle A. Barber • Joanne Saunders • Jo R. Sibert

SUMMARY

The challenges and pitfalls that present to clinicians when confronted with injuries to a child suspected of suffering physical abuse are many. They have been heightened by a number of high-profile court cases in the UK. It is vital that the diagnosis of abuse is based on the evidence collected in a systematic way. A series of systematic reviews is currently underway which should help. So far reviews have been completed on bruises, fractures, dental Injuries and thermal injuries. A review on non-accidental head injury is ongoing, and one on abdominal injury is planned. Children commonly present with a number of different injuries and a holistic, integrated approach to the assessment and investigation of injuries should be employed.

INTRODUCTION

The UN Convention on the Rights of the Child emphasizes the right of the child to freedom from abuse. Child abuse is a serious public health problem, with the potential for major physical and psychological consequences for affected children, who may carry the legacy of abuse with them into their adult life.[1, 2] The misdiagnosis of abuse, however, can have similarly devastating consequences for the child and the family. The accurate identification of abuse is, therefore, of great importance and should always be our aim. The clinician's task is made more difficult because of the paucity of research evidence and the fact that so little work has been done in putting together the evidence in a systematic way. A group of us in Wales (the Welsh Child Protection Systematic Review Group, led by Dr Alison Kemp and Dr Sabine Maguire) has started a review of the evidence on physical abuse. So far we have completed reviews on bruises, fractures, dental injuries and thermal injuries. We are in the process of reviewing non-accidental head injury, and a review of abdominal injury is panned. These reviews have contributed greatly to this chapter and the latest versions can be found at the Review Group Core Info website.[3]

THE CLINICAL ASSESSMENT

Careful examination and detailed notes that are signed and dated on each page are essential to the assessment, since these may be required in preparation of evidence for court. The purpose of the examination is to make a diagnosis of definite or probable abuse, to exclude medical conditions and to screen the child for other health problems. It should be remembered that child abuse is a symptom of disordered parenting and the affected child may be suffering neglect of other important aspects of their care. The history and examination should be conducted in a non-judgemental manner and in a child-friendly environment. Injuries should be measured accurately and documented on topographical charts wherever possible.

Many paediatric units will have a proforma designed for the purpose, commencing with a page to record signed and witnessed consent from the parent and, if appropriate, the child/adolescent. A photographic record should be obtained where possible, also with consent.

COMBINATION OF PROBABILITIES

At present the diagnosis of physical abuse rests on an informally computed probability of the injuries presented being caused by abuse. This takes into account what we know from available research and also the compatibility of the injuries with the history given. However, each clinical presentation is unique, with a unique constellation of injuries and context. It would be invaluable if we were able to give accurate probabilities of individual injuries being due to abuse or accident and were able to combine them. However, there are many obstacles to this research.

For the purposes of this chapter, child physical abuse is discussed under headings denoting the various types of injury. We explore what is known from existing research at this time and some of the common pitfalls in the diagnosis. Although we have made every effort to give accurate information available in late 2006,[3] we strongly advise that clinicians make decisions on the basis of their reading of the literature, in particular any systematic reviews.

BRUISING

This has been the subject of systematic review, both for patterns of bruising[4] and ageing of bruising.[5] Bruising is both the most common presenting feature in physical abuse and the most frequent reason for referral to the child-protection team.[6, 7] The attending paediatrician must consider several factors in determining the likelihood of bruising being non-accidental. A bruise cannot be interpreted in isolation, but only in the context of other injuries, the medical and social history, developmental stage, the explanation provided, examination and investigations.

Patterns of bruising

This has been the subject of a recent systematic review.[4] The review concluded that the patterns of bruising suggestive of physical child abuse are:

- bruising in children who are not independently mobile
- bruising in babies
- bruising that is away from bony prominences
- bruises on the face, back, abdomen, arms, buttocks, ears and hands
- multiple bruises in clusters
- multiple bruises of uniform shape
- bruises that carry the imprint of implement used.

There is a strong correlation between bruising and motor developmental stage. Bruising in a baby who is not yet independently mobile is uncommon in the absence of disease (in particular coagulation disorder).[8, 9]

In the systematic review, accidental bruises were most commonly seen on the front of the body, particularly the shins and forehead. In abused children bruising to the ear, face, head and neck, trunk, buttocks, arms and hands was seen significantly more frequently than in controls; with the head, and particularly the face, being the commonest site in all eligible studies.[3, 10–13] Abusive bruises were larger and often multiple.[10–12] Clustering of bruising was observed and may arise from defensive injuries; this is typically seen on the upper arm, outer thigh, trunk and adjacent extremity. It should be noted, however, that most of the studies included in the systematic review were retrospective and observational studies. A common criticism of many of the studies was that reverse causality contributed to the definition of the abused population.

Characteristics of the bruise itself may allow a diagnosis of abuse to be made. The bruise pattern commonly mimics the object of injury. When a child is struck with an object or a hand, there may be either an imprint or negative image, with a surrounding rim of petechial bruising where capillary rupture has occurred, or a positive image where vessels are ruptured directly.[13–15] Clues to the shape of the object involved can be derived from the pattern of the bruise and may be highly specific. Common objects of injury include sticks, chains, cords, belts, slippers and hands, and the diagnosis will be less problematic where an older child has disclosed such abuse. Slap marks usually result in a negative image of the fingers with a series of linear petechiae outlining the finger edges, and overlapping linear bruising where there have been repeated blows. Vertical gluteal cleft bruises have been reported, as has bruising to the pinna of the ear, where the profile of the bruise assumes the line of anatomical stress rather than the shape of the injuring object.[11]

Ageing bruises

Paediatricians involved in child-protection cases are frequently asked to give an opinion as to the age of bruises, thus timing the injury and potentially identifying the perpetrator. Classically these estimates were made on the basis of bruise colour and appearance, and utilized textbook classification, which was not evidence based. Many factors will determine the colour of bruises seen, including the depth of injury, location, force employed, vascularity of the tissues involved, skin colour and ambient lighting, in addition to the time since injury. Maguire et al.[5] recently published a systematic

review, which concluded that a bruise cannot be accurately aged from clinical assessment in vivo or on a photograph. Since the practice of ageing by colour has no scientific basis, it should be avoided.

Medical causes of bruising

On occasion there will be a medical explanation for bruising – a coagulation disorder, leukaemia, or a connective tissue disease such as Ehlers–Danlos syndrome. Clues to these conditions should be sought within the history, examination or family history.

Investigation

In all cases a full blood count and a coagulation screen should be arranged at the time of the examination. More detailed investigation of coagulation may be needed, particularly in babies. Advice should be obtained from a paediatric haematologist if there is any doubt. Bruising may coexist with other injuries that are sometimes more specific for abuse than the presenting concern, and hence are commonly used rationales for investigating younger children with unexplained injury. Children under 2 years of age with evidence of abuse should have fracture excluded.

FRACTURES

Fractures are a serious manifestation of abuse in children, being identified in up to 55% of children who have been physically abused, and it is important that they be identified.[16, 17] A number of aspects of abusive fractures have been reviewed systematically.

Ageing fractures

The recent systematic review concluded that dating of fractures is an inexact science.[18] Most radiologists date fractures on the basis of their personal clinical experience, and the literature provides few consistent data to act as a resource. Like bruising, it is unwise to rely on evidence from x-rays to date injuries, particularly in the court situation.

Investigation of fractures in suspected child abuse

In children under 2 years old, where physical abuse is suspected, diagnostic imaging of the skeleton should be mandatory. The recent systematic review[19] suggests that either a skeletal survey or a radionuclide bone scanning alone may miss bony injury and may not identify all fractures. A study has shown that identification of rib fracture is improved by oblique views of the ribs,[19] and Kemp et al.[20] have looked at which radiological investigations should be performed to identify fractures in suspected child abuse.

Generally, both a skeletal survey and a radionuclide bone scan should be performed when screening for occult fractures. An alternative is to x-ray children again after 2 weeks, when healing might be visible. There are considerable logistical difficulties in getting the children back for further x-ray examination, and the child-protection process may be delayed. The British Society of Paediatric Radiology has produced guidelines for the standards for skeletal surveys.[21]

Patterns of fractures in abuse

This was the subject of a recent systematic review.[3] Sixty studies were included. Meta-analysis was possible for rib, humeral, femoral and skull fractures. However, considerable heterogeneity was present. The fracture-specific probabilities are useful guidelines, although caution must be exercised in their application in the clinical and legal contexts. A fracture in a child must be assessed in the context of the history given, the child's developmental level, the number of fractures present, and detailed evaluation of the proposed mechanism of injury. Abusive fractures are more frequent in younger children. Worlock et al.[22] observed that 80% of abusive fractures occurred in infants less than 18 months old, whereas 85% of accidental fractures occurred in those over 5 years old. Abusive fractures are frequently multiple. It is important to note that there may not be external signs of bruising in association with non-accidental fracture.[23, 24]

Rib fractures had the highest probability of being the result of abuse in the systematic review (41%), this probability of abuse rising to 84% if major trauma, bone disease or birth injury were excluded. Rib fractures are particularly associated with abuse in babies, where they are thought to be due to squeezing. Classically abusive rib fractures are multiple and posterior, although they may also be anterior or lateral.[25, 26] Rib fractures rarely present in isolation, and are often found during investigation of other injuries.

In the systematic review for skull fractures, the probability of abuse was 23%, increasing to 37% for complex fractures. Skull fracture with intracranial injury in babies is highly suggestive of abuse.[27, 28] Fracture characteristics indicative of abuse include multiple or complex fractures, depressed, wide or growing fractures, those crossing suture lines and non-parietal fractures.[22, 28] A history of a fall from a cot, bed or sofa as a cause of a skull fracture should be questioned.[29] Linear fractures are the most common abusive and non-abusive skull fracture.

Probabilities of abuse for femoral (12%) and humeral fractures (1%) were low in the systematic review. The low figure for humeral fractures was due to the large number of supracondylar fractures in the accident group. The pre-mobile developmental stage is a discriminator for abuse in femoral fractures. Non-supracondylar fractures of the humerus in very young children are much more likely to be the result of abuse.[22] There were inadequate data on metaphyseal fractures for meta-analysis. Abusive vertebral and pelvic fractures have been described.

In older children, a spiral fracture of the mid or lower tibia known as a typical 'toddler's fracture' or 'childhood accidental spiral tibial (CAST) fracture', is unlikely to be due to abuse and may occur when the toddler stumbles while running.[30] The fall may be trivial, with the child developing a limp and minimal swelling; thus there is often a delay in presentation, which is usually considered to be significantly associated with abuse.

Fractures to the spine in children are uncommon, comprising less than 5% of all reported spinal injuries. Typically they result from high-energy trauma or falls from significant heights, and often coexist with other major injuries. They can occur in abuse and are mostly fracture–dislocations or compression fractures. Classically they may result from hyperflexion–hyperextension injury, either from shaking or direct blows. Fractures may be stable or unstable, and can be associated with injury to the spinal cord. Spinal cord injury may also arise in the absence of a vertebral fracture.[31–33]

Rib fractures and cardiopulmonary resuscitation

This has been the subject of the systematic review.[3, 34] Six studies were included: they represented data on 923 children who had undergone cardiopulmonary resuscitation (CPR). Three children sustained rib fractures as a result of CPR, and in all these three the fractures were anterior (two midclavicular and one costochondral). We did not find any child in the literature that had a posterior rib fracture due to CPR. Medical and non-medical personnel performed resuscitation variably. Rib fractures after CPR are rare, and when they do occur they are anterior and may be multiple.

Differential diagnosis

Systemic disease should always be excluded when a diagnosis of child abuse is being considered for fractures in children. Of the conditions to be considered the most important is osteogenesis imperfecta. In all cases of fractures, which are thought to be due to abuse, a family history of fractures should be taken and the colour of the sclerae should be noted. The skeletal survey should be examined for bone density and the presence of wormian bones. In the future there may well be biochemical tests that will help diagnose osteogenesis imperfecta, but at present these have not been established. Metabolic bone disease in neonates, rickets, osteopetrosis, copper deficiency, osteomyelitis, leukaemia and disseminated neuroblastoma may all cause fracture that can be confused with abuse.

NON-ACCIDENTAL HEAD INJURY

Non-accidental head injury (NAHI) is a significant cause of death and disability in babies. We are unaware of any systematic review on this subject. The triad of encephalopathy, subdural haemorrhages and retinal haemorrhages has been traditionally regarded as diagnostic of shaken baby syndrome, and indeed the majority of medical opinion concurs with this, particularly epidemiological studies.[35] More recently, Geddes et al.[36, 37] have analysed the pathology of NAHI due to abuse. They concluded, probably rightly, that apnoea may be a major factor in the pathological mechanism of death in some subdural haemorrhages in infants. There has been an interpretation of their conclusion (more strongly stated in the lay presentation in *New Scientist* than in the definitive publications in *Brain*) that the apnoea could be caused by relatively little force. Kemp et al.[38] have analysed a series of cases, and in particular cases with apnoea. They found that apnoea, far from being associated with more minor trauma, is associated with features of severity such as fractures. Detailed discussion about this is beyond the scope of this chapter.[39]

However, many subdural haematomas arising in the first 2 years of life are thought to result from abuse. All cases should therefore be investigated for possible abuse, and investigations should include the following:[40]

- a multidisciplinary social assessment
- an ophthalmology assessment
- skeletal imaging
- a coagulation screen
- a brain computed tomography (CT) scan and, later, magnetic resonance imaging (MRI).

The radiology of subdural haemorrhages in infants has recently been reviewed by Datta et al.[41] They concluded that an MRI scan adds information and should be performed in all cases. They also suggest that interhemispheric haemorrhages and subdural haemorrhages in multiple sites suggest NAHI.

Glutaric aciduria may cause subdural haematoma in childhood; however, this is associated also with frontal lobe hypoplasia and developmental delay, and not with fractures.[42] Biochemical investigation of this condition may be problematic, as glutaric aciduria may not be present.

BURNS AND SCALDS

Burns and scalds may be the result of accident, neglect or deliberate abuse. The compatibility of the history with the physical findings has to be assessed, together with any clues in the history, such as late presentation, changing story, vague details or inappropriate level of concern in a carer, indeed as for any other injury. The evidence base from research for thermal injuries has been appraised by the Welsh Child Protection Systematic Review Group.[3] Contact or dry burns in abuse can arise from a wide range of household appliances: irons, curling tongs, heated metal utensils, light bulbs, radiators and, relatively commonly, cigarettes. These items result in a positive image or brand mark, and the object used may in some circumstances be readily identifiable.[43, 44]

Cigarette burns are a common diagnostic problem. Staphylococcal bullous impetigo is an important differential diagnosis. Secondary infection can also occur with thermal injuries such as cigarette burns, so that the diagnosis may not be certain.

Bath scalds arising from abuse present difficult problems for the clinician, and in particular when giving evidence for court. Features that are suggestive of forced immersion include a clear tidemark, incompatible story, associated injuries and symmetrical scald. On the other hand, irregular, asymmetrical and geographical marks, a history compatible with the story with no associated injuries may be more suggestive of accident.[45]

ABDOMINAL INJURIES DUE TO ABUSE

There has not been a systematic review of this subject. Abdominal injuries are rare, but definite, features of abuse in childhood and the mortality may be high. In a survey published through the British Paediatric Surveillance Unit[46] abdominal injury was found to be a rare condition, predominately affecting children under 5 years old. These injuries are likely to be underdiagnosed, because less severe cases may present with non-specific symptoms and signs, especially in infants. Children have poorly developed abdominal musculature and a relatively small abdominal anteroposterior diameter, placing the abdominal organs at risk of injury from blunt abdominal trauma. Abdominal injuries can involve the rupture of any abdominal organ, including the liver, spleen, pancreas and bowel. Small-bowel injuries can arise accidentally as a result of falls and road-traffic accidents, but they are significantly more common in abused children. Internal abdominal injury should be suspected where there is unexplained abdominal bruising; however, it may not be assumed that both will always coexist in abuse.

DENTAL INJURIES

Bite marks may be inflicted by adults, children or animals. They are a common problem in children presenting for medical assessment of possible abuse. Many bites are easily explainable; however, they may present significant diagnostic challenges for the clinician. A partnership between paediatricians and a forensic dentist has been shown to be an invaluable help in the assessment.[47] The Welsh Child Protection Systematic Review Group is also appraising the evidence for oral and dental injuries in child abuse.[3] The diagnosis of an adult bite is largely based on extrapolation from what is known from anatomy rather than on data from case–control studies. Injuries such as torn labial frenum, often held by experts to be pathognomonic of abuse in infants, may occur accidentally in children at a later stage of development.

CONCLUSION

While there is already considerable evidence from existing research on which to base our clinical decision-making regarding the informal probability of abuse, further quantitative research is urgently needed in this field. It should be noted that children commonly present with a number of different injuries and that a holistic, integrated approach to the assessment and investigation of injuries should be employed. The paediatrician should be careful not to overstate the probability of physical abuse and must be clear about their professional limitations when giving evidence in police investigations and court.

ACKNOWLEDGEMENT

We are grateful for the work of the Welsh Systematic Review Group, and in particular Drs Alison Kemp and Sabine Maguire.

Chapter Nine

The prevention of childhood unintentional injury

9

Elizabeth Towner • John Towner

SUMMARY

Unintentional injury is a major cause of death, ill health and disability in childhood. A steeper social gradient is found for injury than for any other cause of death. Children are particularly vulnerable to injury because of their physical, psychological and behavioural characteristics.

However, injuries can be prevented or reduced in severity by a variety of methods: education and training, provision of safety devices, environmental modification, and legislation and its enforcement. A combination of methods is often important. Paediatricians have an important role to play in the prevention of childhood injuries: in data collection, individual education, and counselling and advocacy.

PRACTICE POINTS

- Unintentional injury in childhood is a significant public health problem.
- A steeper social gradient occurs for injury than for any other cause of death.
- Injuries can be prevented by a variety of educational, environmental and legislative methods, and by combinations of these.
- Paediatricians have a key role in data collection, individual education, and counselling and advocacy.

INTRODUCTION

Unintentional injury is a major cause of death in children in the UK, and for every child who dies many more live with the consequences of injury. Furthermore, although children from all levels of society are vulnerable, the burden is not spread evenly, as injuries disproportionately affect more deprived children. This chapter describes children's vulnerability to injury and documents the scale of the problem of injury. It then summarizes what works in the prevention of injuries, and considers what role those involved in paediatrics can play in preventing childhood injuries.

CHILDREN'S VULNERABILITY TO INJURY

Children are especially vulnerable to injury because they live in a world in which they have little power or control. They find themselves in environments constructed by and for adults, whether in the home or outside on the roads and elsewhere. Their voices are seldom heard, and only rarely are places, even playgrounds, designed in consultation with children.

This 'political' vulnerability is compounded by the physical, psychological and behavioural characteristics of children. The small stature of children increases their risk in the road environment: they are harder to see than adults by car drivers and, if hit by a vehicle, they are more likely to sustain a head or neck injury than an adult. Other physical characteristics make children vulnerable to injuries: children under 4 years old are more likely to suffer head injuries in falls down stairs than are older children, and the skin of babies and toddlers burns more deeply and quickly and at lower temperatures than the thicker skin of adults.[1]

Psychological characteristics include the development of children's skills to negotiate traffic safely. Young children often do not know what they are looking for in the traffic environment, and cannot easily distinguish between visual and auditory features that are relevant or irrelevant to the road crossing tasks.[2] Skills to perceive movement and velocity, source of a sound, distance and depth are well developed in adults, but not in young children. What is required in the road environment is the capacity to integrate this information quickly and efficiently, and to judge gaps between moving traffic coming from two directions. How children behave is also very different from adults. Sinnot[3] provides a vivid illustration in the home environment of how children use this fundamentally adult space:

> ... (they) crawl about the floor, climb onto the window ledge, squeeze through stair balustrades, slide down the stair handrail, swing on the gate, run from room to room and ride bikes inside as well as out, making use of their houses in ways that seem to them reasonable, but have not apparently been foreseen by the designer.

THE SCALE OF THE PROBLEM

The picture of childhood injury deaths shows great variations, which relate to children's age and stage of development, their gender and the social background of their families.[4] Where children spend their time and are exposed to risk is important: preschool children are most likely to die from an injury in the home, whereas school-aged children are most likely to die in the road environment. Different patterns emerge for both fatal and non-fatal injuries. Falls, for example, result in relatively few deaths, but are the major cause of both hospital admissions and accident and emergency attendance of children.[5]

What are the overall numbers of childhood deaths from injury? Broadly, the picture is one of considerable improvement. In England and Wales in 2002 there were 261 deaths, and in 2003 there were 248 deaths of children aged 0–14 years.[6, 7] These numbers contrast markedly with those for the early 1990s, when over 500 deaths per year were reported. Even in the late 1990s figures were considerably higher than in 2002–2003: in 1997 there were 386 deaths and in 1998 there were 338 deaths in children aged 0–14 years.[8] Roberts et al.[9] have traced trends in unintentional injury deaths in children between 1985 and 1992 and compared these with children's exposure to risk as pedestrians and cyclists. In this period, pedestrian injury death rates fell by 37% and the average distance walked by children fell by 20%. Cyclist deaths fell by 38% and the average distance cycled fell by 26%. In addition to changes in lifestyle and travel patterns, there is also some evidence that trauma case fatality rates have declined, this probably being the result of improvements in trauma care.

The leading causes of unintentional injury deaths in childhood are: land transport accidents; threats to breathing from suffocation, strangulation, inhalation and ingestion of objects; accidents caused by smoke, fire and flames; and drowning and submersion.[6, 7] Land transport accidents (ICD 10 codes V01–V89) account for just under half of all unintentional injury deaths in childhood (121 and 102 deaths in 2002 and 2003, respectively), but within this injury type different patterns are apparent for pedestrian, cyclist and car-occupant deaths. In 2002, 27 and in 2003, 29 children died in accidents caused by exposure to smoke, fire and flames;[6, 7] 57% of these children were aged less than 5 years. Very young children are vulnerable in house fires because they depend on adults for assistance with escape. Drowning and submersion resulted in the death of 55 children in the 2-year period 2002–2003. Again, preschool children were particularly vulnerable: 64% of the children were under 5 years old.[6, 7]

Injuries disproportionately affect the most vulnerable children in society: those living in the most deprived environments. The social class gradient is steeper for injuries than for any other cause of death. The gradient is particularly marked for residential fire deaths, where the death rate for children is 15 times greater for children in social class V compared with those in social class I. The ratio for child pedestrian deaths is 5:1.[10]

Deaths represent only the tip of the injury 'iceberg'. 'For every injured child who dies, many more live on with varying degrees and durations of disability and trauma'.[11] Some injury types figure little in mortality tables: scalds, for example, represent only a small proportion of deaths and injuries, but they can result in considerable long-term disfigurement and disability, and can be amongst the most distressing and painful injuries a child can receive.

The Health Survey for England provides evidence of the scale of injury morbidity.[12] Self-reported data on 'major' accidents (where a hospital was visited or a doctor consulted) and 'minor' accidents (other accidents causing pain or discomfort for more than 24 hours) were collected for children aged 0–15 years for the years 2001 and 2002. Annual major accident rates of 24 per 100 were found for boys and 19 per 100 for girls, and annual minor accident rates of 210 per 100 for boys and 159 per 100 for girls were estimated.

Most major and minor accidents in children under 2 years of age occurred as a result of a fall. In older children, the two most common types of major accidents were falls and accidents occurring during sports/exercise/play. The proportion of major accidents that involved victims taking a week or more off school was 6% for boys and 9% for girls.[12] Children living in households with only one adult, had significantly higher major accident rates than those living in households with two or more adults.[12]

WHAT WORKS IN PREVENTING CHILDHOOD INJURIES?

Opportunities to prevent injuries occur through a range of educational, environmental and legislative approaches.

Educational approaches

These include changing individual decision-making by both children and parents, but they can also be directed at professionals and policy-makers, and can include lobbying and advocacy. Indeed, there has been a tendency to take a rather narrow view of education in the health field in general, with its role somehow detached from environmental and legislative approaches, rather than being integral to them.[13] The latter do not take place in a social and political vacuum. Education is very much part of the whole process of change. Examples can include increasing the use of safety devices, such as seat belts in cars, bicycle helmets, and smoke detectors, and pedestrian and bicycle skills training programmes. Awareness raising and understanding about issues such as drinking and driving or speed of traffic can, over a long period of time, help to shape a safety culture among the general public, which creates the imperative to act. Thus, in Australia, there was a concerted 10-year campaign to increase bicycle-helmet wearing, and education was very important in influencing public opinion and policy-makers before legislation was introduced in 1990.[14]

Environmental modification and engineering

This involves designing products or the built environment to reduce the potential for the occurrence of injuries. Urban traffic safety schemes, for example, can include measures to reduce traffic speed, redistribute the flow of traffic and reduce more risky manoeuvres. In playgrounds, impact-absorbing surfaces and suitable equipment height can reduce the severity of injuries. In the home, building-design changes to balconies and windows and doors can reduce falls and lacerations, and child-resistant packaging of medicines can reduce poisonings.

Legislation or regulation

This can be used to reinforce safety practices. Examples of single actions that offer passive protection include the control of nightwear flammability and design changes in banisters. Other legislative approaches require repetitive action, such as the use of car seat belts or bicycle helmets.

Legislative, environmental modification and educational approaches all have a part to play, and their effect in combination is important. Community-based approaches by a range of agencies allow injury-prevention messages to be repeated in different forms and contexts.

Evaluation of interventions

Although the above outlines the broad approaches to intervention in the injury field, only a small number of interventions have been rigorously evaluated, and this has hampered development in this area. Evidence for the effectiveness of interventions for reducing injury (RI) or changing behaviour (CB) has been assessed in three main environments where childhood injuries occur: on the road, at home and at leisure.[15] On the road, there is good evidence for: 20 mph zones (RI and CB), cycle helmet education campaigns (CB), cycle helmet legislation (CB), child restraint loan schemes (CB) and child restraint legislation (CB). There is reasonable evidence for: area-wide safety measures (RI), education aimed at parents about pedestrian injuries (CB), cycle training (CB), cycle helmet legislation (RI), child restraint education (CB) and child restraint legislation (RI).

In the home there is good evidence for: smoke detector programmes (RI and CB) and child-resistant packaging to reduce poisoning (RI). There is reasonable evidence for product design (RI), general safety devices (RI), window bars (CB) and parent education on hazard reduction (CB). There is no good or reasonable evidence of effective interventions in the leisure environment, although there is some evidence for interventions targeted at drowning, and play and leisure injuries. There are some general community prevention initiatives targeting a range of injury types in different groups. Reasonable evidence has been found for both reduction of injuries and changing behaviour.[15]

WHAT ROLE CAN THOSE INVOLVED IN PAEDIATRICS PLAY IN PREVENTING UNINTENTIONAL INJURY?

Three main areas for the involvement of paediatricians in injury are outlined here: the collection and enhancement of routine injury data, individual education or counselling for parents and children, and a wider advocacy role. Case studies illustrating the role of paediatricians are then provided.

Data collection

Good data are essential in the development of effective interventions. Injury surveillance systems can be used to confirm, disprove or refine an analysis of an injury problem, as well as to assist the design, implementation and evaluation of a prevention programme. Local data will help identify local priorities and thus improve targeting. Local data are also valuable in an advocacy role, in demonstrating the scale and nature of the injury problem in their community to local people and authorities. Unfortunately, data-collection systems at local and national levels in Britain have very little compatibility. At a local level, most areas have accurate local data only for mortality, where there are very few cases to use for priority setting. Data on non-fatal injuries and their severity are needed and this is an area where paediatricians can play a major role. The Bath injury surveillance system was set up to address the limitations of other systems and information sources. It is based in the Emergency Department at the Royal United Hospital in Bath, and collects additional data on the circumstances of injuries in children and young people aged 0–16 years, as well as demographic

and consequence data. This system is able to provide useful and relevant information for injury-prevention policy and initiatives, with detailed local information on geographical patterns. For example, in the 4-year period from 1997–2000, the average annual presentation rate for 0–4 year olds in Bath for unintentional injury was 131/1,000. The majority of injuries occurred in the home and the most common mechanism of injury was falls.[16]

Individual education or counselling

A health professional such as a paediatrician, health visitor or school nurse can increase the use of safety devices. This can be seen in encouraging the use of infant car-safety restraints, smoke detectors and bicycle helmets.[17] If the health-education message is of short duration and is age paced (i.e. directly relevant to a specific age group or stage of development), it is more likely to be effective than generalized advice. The authority of the advice giver can provide credibility and enhance the effect of the message.

General practitioners and health visitors are in regular contact with the families of preschool children, and are well placed to provide evidence that is directly relevant to them. Routine health checks at child health surveillance clinics and home visits provide the opportunity to point out hazardous practices (e.g. handling of hot beverages near very young children) or dangerous features of the house (e.g. banisters or balconies). Families who are particularly vulnerable to accidents through stress or family illness could be highlighted in parent-held personal child health records. Training materials have been developed for health visitors, which explore a range of ways of tackling the problem of unintentional injuries at a local level.

Although it may be seen as a partial failure of injury prevention, contacts with families of children who have suffered an injury can help to reduce further exposure. These meetings can provide the opportunity for individual counselling or first aid advice. Safety displays within hospitals can raise awareness. The safety of the hospital's own environment for child patients and visitors can also be included. For example, are there improvements that can be made in design or in how people interact in the space provided?

Advocacy

Advocacy takes place at a number of levels, ranging from membership of local multiagency injury-prevention groups to campaigns for safety measures at a national or international level. Pioneer examples of multiagency groups come from Sweden. In the small community of Falköping, an extensive network of contacts was built up of people interested in injury prevention.[18] Education of policy-makers and health workers was a high priority, and resources were produced so that district nurses, for example, had home safety checklists to use on home visits to parents of young children. Importance was also placed on the use of local media.

Paediatricians have a role to play in promoting positive messages of safety in local newspapers, radio and television, and countering more sensational reporting of accidents, which are seen as unfortunate occurrences that are impossible to prevent. The Child Accident Prevention Trust's annual Child Safety Week[19] can help to heighten awareness and provide the opportunity to publicise local activities such as the development of safe play areas or a safety equipment loan scheme.

Advocacy will vary in its political depth, from a wish to see specific environmental modifications, such as traffic calming or changes in the design of products and legislation, to a more radical approach involving the need to tackle the root causes of inequality in society. Spencer[20] has called for health professionals to take political action on behalf of poor children and their families, and has outlined a number of areas where paediatricians can play a key role in injury prevention. These include lobbying national and local government to modify children's environments using traffic-calming strategies, and strategies to reduce reliance on the motor car and promoting community participation and community diagnosis locally, which can identify the main sources of danger to children.

In the UK, the lobbying and commitment of a paediatrician (Dr Hugh Jackson) resulted in the introduction of regulations for Child Resistant Closures for all children's aspirin and paracetamol preparations in 1976. In the year following the 1976 Act, a highly significant fall in admissions for accidental aspirin poisoning was recorded.[21] The creation of the Child Accident Prevention Trust[22] in the late 1970s also resulted from extensive advocacy and lobbying. Maconachie[23] believes that the Royal College of Paediatrics and Child Health can be more active in supporting injury prevention by establishing trauma fellowships, showing more overt support for the activities of the Child Accident Prevention Trust, providing a database of injury-prevention activities that members are involved in, and collecting information on different types of injuries.

CASE STUDIES

The three case studies described include advocacy, data collection, and individual education or counselling.

Case illustration 9.1

Example of paediatric nurse

An example of a health education campaign initiated by a specialist paediatric nurse with first-hand experience of caring for head-injured children is the Helmet your Head campaign, based in Reading. This aimed to increase bicycle-helmet wearing among children aged 5–15 years. It consisted of school-based talks containing age-specific information, true-case scenarios, videos of head-injured children, and information on how to wear a helmet properly. Local media and celebrities raised the profile of the campaign, and a low-cost helmet purchase scheme was established. One person led the campaign and fostered close relationships with the local media and schools. The importance of local data on cycle-related head injuries was also significant in defining the problem locally and in evaluating the campaign.[24]

CONCLUSION

Unintentional injury is a major cause of death in children in the UK and is responsible for considerable morbidity. All children are vulnerable to injury because their physical, psychological and behavioural characteristics place them at risk in a largely adult world. Furthermore, the social construction of that adult world makes the children of the poor even more vulnerable to injury.

This chapter has highlighted proven strategies for preventing many types of injuries in childhood. However, effective interventions and approaches need to be implemented in a far more widespread and comprehensive manner. This is a process in which the active involvement of all those concerned with paediatrics is to be urged.

Case illustration 9.2

Example of hospital involvement

The Injury Minimization Programme for Schools (IMPS) has been developed in Oxford by a group of healthcare professionals. It targets 10- to 11-year-old children and is taught in the school and hospital environments. The focus is on road safety, accidents in the home, fire, electricity, poisons and waterways. The school programme explores aspects of risk and safety. This is complemented by a hospital visit, where children visit the accident and emergency department and receive basic life support and cardiopulmonary resuscitation skills training. The effect of the IMPS programme on knowledge, attitudes and reported behaviours has been evaluated.[25]

Case illustration 9.3

Example of health visitor involvement

In a deprived area of Newcastle, health visitors were involved in a home-safety initiative. A mass media campaign (the television Play it Safe campaign) was supplemented by individual health visitor home visits. Of the intervention group, who had received a home visit, 60% made some physical change to their homes, compared with 9% of the control group, who had only been encouraged to watch the television series. The advice offered to the severely disadvantaged families was specific, small in amount and concrete.[26]

Chapter Ten

Parental conflict and children

John H. Tripp • Monica Cockett

SUMMARY

In recent decades there has been a major research interest in the outcomes for children associated with family environment and changes in family structure. Increasingly children can no longer rely on being part of a family where two parents remain together until the children reach independence. This research has highlighted the risk factors – emotional, physical, social and economic – presented to children by such changes. Although these factors can have a cumulative effect on children's outcomes in relation to future life chances, unresolved parental conflict, especially in relation to children's arrangements, presents children with the most persistent negative effect.

While some parents are able over time, with support, to place the needs of their children at the centre of their plans, others struggle to achieve this. Children become 'caught in the middle'. Some parents never resolve their conflict and remain unable to cooperate throughout their children's dependent years.

During the past 20 years professionals working with families have made every effort to support parents to make cooperative arrangements for their children in spite of their own situation. The aim is to minimize distress and ongoing problems for their children in order to allow them to build their own positive future.

There is a general acceptance of the negative influence of interparental conflict on children. Longitudinal studies have found that the quality of family relationships is closely associated with outcomes for children, regardless of family type.

CHILDREN'S AND PARENTAL CONFLICT

Contact disputes are frequently not about the children concerned, they are the continuation of a power struggle between the separated couple.[1]

The house was like a ghost house, it was so quiet, we used to creep around afraid, in case dad would lose his temper, and hit mum.[2]

Children's awareness

Children as young as 2 years are aware of parental conflict. In a recent study, children graphically described their responses to parental conflict. In qualitative data children described sleep patterns being disturbed as they remained alert to the sound of parental arguments. Others described begging parents to stop arguing; some hid in bedrooms with pillows over their heads. Children described running out of the house when their parents argued to seek refuge with their grandparents.[2]

Emery et al.[3] in the USA report that children's awareness of conflict and levels of intervention were more important indicators of difficulties for the child than the levels of conflict alone. This view was supported by a British study, which examined the effects on children of living in 'disharmonious' homes. The causes of parental discord were grouped under overt or covert hostility, and disagreement about child-rearing practices. Overt conflict between parents was found to have the stronger link to children's behavioural and emotional problems.[4] The findings from the Exeter Family Study also showed that most children were aware of domestic rows, even when parents considered that they 'never quarrelled in front of the children'. Domestic violence and some other categories of conflict, including silence, were viewed as very distressing by the child and threatening to the child's security. One-quarter of the children in the reordered family group had previously been part of a family where the mother had been exposed to physical violence. Children in these situations, while expressing their relief at being removed from the associated fear and responsibility, did express concerns about the departing parent and would have liked more information; some resented being 'kept in the dark'.[2]

Protective factors

Grych and Fincham[5] suggested that exposure to successfully resolved conflict may not be damaging:

> *Conflict resolution, that is the good model, how conflict ends, may be as important as or more important than how it started.*

Rutter,[6] in his work about exposure to risk, and children's adaptation to it, emphasized the importance of providing the child with the necessary emotional skills to withstand the kinds of life experiences that will be an inevitable part of the child's transition into adulthood. He stresses that particular hazards, such as interparental conflict and lowered self-esteem, contribute towards vulnerability, while continuity, good supportive relationships and good self-esteem assist the development of resilience.

Wallerstein et al.[7] suggested that success in overcoming the major obstacles created by divorce can assist the development of resilience. Rutter's studies[6] emphasize the contribution that school support offers vulnerable children, and found that children benefited according to need. Children who obtained reinforcement elsewhere were not so dependent on the school environment. A good relationship with siblings was also found to be a protective factor. Other studies, including the Exeter Family Study, confirmed that self-esteem plays an important protective role for children. Good self-esteem scores were associated with better social, educational and health outcomes for children. Low levels of self-esteem were associated with exposure to parental conflict, both before and after separation, and with the quality of contact with the non-resident parent.[2]

Domestic violence and children

During the last part of the 20th century there was an increasing emphasis on, and research interest in, the effects on children of being part of a family where domestic violence was an issue. The NSPCC also funded research into the link between child protection matters and domestic violence.[8] In February 2002 a report by the Lord Chancellor's Department placed an emphasis on assessing family circumstances for the child, taking into account domestic violence issues when considering appropriate safe contact for children in circumstances where they may be at risk.[9]

FAMILY BREAKDOWN

Over the past 30 years research has also amassed abundant evidence that children fare badly in family structures that do not remain stable. When parents separate, children are exposed to a range of risk factors that can make it harder to preserve good family relationships.[10] An overview of this research conducted by Rogers and Pryor[11] confirmed most of the findings of previous studies that parental separation and divorce present a higher range of risk factors to children than other family structures. However, it also emphasizes the fact that parental conflict, which is ongoing, contributes strongly to children's behavioural problems.[12]

Pryor and Rogers[13] also reinforced the findings from the Exeter Family Study that multiple family reordering presented children with the most risk factors.

As a phenomenon

During the last two decades, although the commitment to the ideal of marriage has remained unaltered, when relationships encounter difficulties couples are now much more likely to replace 'till death do us part' with a legal dissolution of the marriage contract. Putting up with a bad marriage, whatever that entails, is, to many, an alien concept. Although separation may appear at the time to be an ideal solution for at least one of the adults involved, it is not so straightforward for children. It is often assumed that conflict is the main cause of couples parting, but not all marriages end because of bitter disaffection. Some simply end in boredom, lack of interest or frequently because one or other partner has fallen 'out of love' and has transferred loyalty to someone else.

Work carried out by the One Plus One research centre[14] has shown that disagreement between couples over the sharing of household tasks and responsibilities often escalates with the advent of children, when the parental role may eclipse the previous couple role. In fact the largest growing evidence, both anecdotal and research based, shows that the arrival of the second child may present difficulties to parents, and the research figures show that an increasing number of marriages end after 5–7 years, whereas 20 or 30 years ago the emphasis was on much longer marriages and marriages ending later when the children were older. There is evidence that over the last two decades an increasing number of children are experiencing parental separation at a younger age and will be more likely to lose contact with their non-resident parent.[15]

During the early years of the 21st century there seems to be little evidence that family structures are becoming more stable. Figures collected from the Office for National Statistics in 2004 show that the number of divorces in the UK had again begun to rise and now total approximately 1,600,000 per annum.[15] Of the 11 million children in this country 5 million children will experience a period of their lives in a lone-parent family. Statistics also tell us that second and subsequent marriages are even more likely to be unstable for children and will present them with a whole range of fresh problems.

A major contributor to the numbers of children experiencing lone parenting is an increase in cohabitation, which research also shows us is even more unsafe for children.[16] Cohabitation is four times more likely to break down than marriage.

Effects on children

This accumulative evidence of the past 30 years into the effects of separation and divorce on children, and particularly the effects of parental conflict, continue to be highlighted by more recent research that pinpoints the main risk factors, including cohabitation, which can be less secure for children, and repartnering of one or both parents.[11] Research also continues to highlight other risk factors for children, such as maternal psychological stress levels, the quality of the father–child relationship[17] and the quality of co-parenting after separation.

Children respond differently according to their age and sex. Fincham and Osborne[18] emphasized the need to evaluate children's responses in the context of their cognitive and emotional development. In a clinically referred population, Wallerstein and Kelly[19] described the varying reactions of children to their parents' divorce at different ages. Young children frequently, but incorrectly, believed that they are responsible for their parents' divorce, and develop problems associated with guilt. In mid-childhood they tended to blame one parent, making it difficult for them to maintain relationships with both parents, and adolescents were often angry with parents for failing to resolve their problems without 'wrecking the family'. Emery[20] has shown that, when exposed to parental conflict, boys are more likely to exhibit aggressive and disruptive behaviour (externalized), whereas girls are more likely to become withdrawn and depressed (internalized), which may be easier to deal with in the short term, but may have an effect on the child's capability to respond to conflict as an adult.

Interaction with conflict

Research into the effects of family conflict has, in some measure, supported the public attitude to divorce over the past two decades, and has given credence to the belief that it is more important to remove children from conflict than to maintain the family structure. The maxim 'better a good divorce than a bad marriage' is accepted by many parents and family lawyers, although it has no established basis.

Amato[21] states that parental divorce 'interferes with the child's ability to utilize parental resources', and that conflict between parents reduces the quality of relationship between parent and child. Parents' energies are deflected away from their children, thus depleting the resources that would be available to the child and introducing an element of, at best, laissez faire and, at worst, chaotic parenting styles.[18, 21]

Once removed from the immediately stressful situation, some children's problems lessen over time.[20] Conversely, the long-term adverse outcomes associated with family breakdown, revealed in birth and cohort population studies, suggest at least some continuing effects.[22] In the Exeter Family Study, it was found that, although the effects of time were important so that some children, after an initial acute reaction, adjusted to their new life circumstances, the cumulative effects of other life events influenced positive or negative adaptation. This raises the question of whether children's best interests are being served when 160,000 couples each year choose to end their marriages, adding a fresh 176,000 dependent children annually to the unestimated total who no longer live with both natural parents. Parental separation exposes children to a whole range of risk factors, including reduced contact, some of which will be triggered by continuing conflict to which children will become vulnerable because of divorce. The risk factors include school changes, house moves, reduced financial resources, poor maternal psychological well-being and coping, and a loss of other family support, especially from grandparents. Some believe that problems experienced by children are largely due to difficulties experienced before the parents separated.[20] Others consider that all these other factors, which are not the result of conflict but are the sequelae of separation, are highly relevant to children's outcomes.[23] Whatever the mechanisms, the fact that there are short- and long-term negative consequences for children when parents separate is not in dispute and is of great concern to both practitioners and policy-makers.[9]

Research by Wallerstein et al.[7] supports the view that parental divorce in general still presents problems for children even in the absence of violence or other parental psychology. A criticism of their research methodology, particularly by Amato,[24] prompted further research into children's experience of their families separations.[20] This research found that children provided with the right support, which is underpinned by parental cooperation, can be made more resilient to risk factors presented to them by parental separation.[24, 25] Jenkins et al.[4] examined the strategies developed by children to cope with parental quarrelling, in a sample drawn almost entirely from intact families. A high proportion of children said that they intervened in their parents' arguments, while some described siblings comforting each other, talking to friends and, in a small number of cases, thinking that quarrels were beneficial.

Both qualitative and quantitative studies in the UK and the USA have found that children who were upset by their parents' divorce were often already aware of serious parental conflict, but nevertheless had not expected separation to occur.[11] Teenagers vividly recall this situation, and express shock and regret at the outcome of conflict that they had come to accept as part of their family life.[2]

Ongoing conflict after divorce or separation

While divorce may sometimes reduce conflict, conflict between parents often begins, and usually continues, following divorce. In the Exeter Family Study,[2] of the 76 families who had separated, 49 sets of parents remained in conflict, although for most of the group, the divorce itself was 5 years or more in the past. Only 60% of the total group said that there had been major conflict between them during the marriage; in some families this had been resolved by divorce, but in others it had been exacerbated. For a proportion of the 40% of parents who had relatively conflict-free marriages, there had been major conflict at the time of separation that had persisted for over half of this group as part of their post-divorce relationship. It was found that the nature of the conflict between the parents had often changed, becoming much more likely to be centred on issues concerning the child, post-divorce parenting and new partners.[13] Children may be called upon to take sides, keep secrets, and carry overt, as well as covert, messages between parents. Continuing parental conflict was a block to the development of the quality and quantity of contact arrangements, and conflictual contact was found to be associated with increased difficulties for children, particularly with self-esteem. Furthermore, exposure to continual post-separation parental conflict not only has an immediate detrimental effect, but has a 'sleeper effect'; maladaptation may only reveal itself at times of critical development transitions, for example, when young people begin to form their own personal relationships.[26]

Separation and divorce can also lead to much reduced, if not total loss of, contact between parent and children. For children, conflict can often precede or be part of a new partnership formed by their parents. This can centre around the parent–child relationship within the family, or embroil the child in the animosity exhibited by one or other natural parent towards the 'infiltrator'. New relationships can interfere with existing extended family relationships, which may also be lost to the child.

Original research by Grych and Fincham[5] suggests that attribution, deciding who was to blame for the failure of their relationship, is a key issue in determining the development and escalation of conflict at this post-divorce stage. They suggest that if each parent accepts some of the blame, this assists post-divorce adaptation; only then are parents capable of change. Conversely, for children, feeling responsible for their parents' separation has a dramatic effect on their self-esteem. Parents' ability to recognize the burden placed on their children in this manner is often impeded by their own concerns at this time; parents are often unable to reassure their children adequately that the blame lies in the marital relationship and that the children's relationship with their parents will remain intact.[2]

Marriage support

There is a view that the government's attempt to support marriage has been viewed as social engineering and paternalistic, and as an attempt to reassert traditional family values.

This movement to support marriage has been based on the ongoing concerns that the continuing rise in the number of relationship and marriage breakdowns, and the subsequent increase in the number of cohabitation relationships that break down, present problems to children. Further discussion about how the socialization of children and the emotional literacy can be passed on if family structures are no longer sound has also presented the government with challenges.

During the last 10 years there has been a marked increase in support for marriage preparation programmes and other services that can support parents at particular times. There has also been a marked emphasis on the availability of parenting programmes to assist parents from the birth of their first baby onwards.[27] This is a preventive programme encouraged by the government and supported and outlined in publications supporting the family. A network of community trusts have been set up around the country. These aim to provide marriage-preparation classes in conjunction with the registrars and churches, to offer parenting programmes to parents, and to offer relationship education and negotiation skills to teenagers in schools. The government supports some of these programmes financially and the programmes are being evaluated.

The view of the child

There has also been an increasing emphasis on the importance of the voice of the child and the need to reduce risk factors for children outside of divorce. Mediation has been able to contribute to the move to allow children to express their own views.[28, 29] A number of agencies now offer appointments to children to give them the opportunity, in a confidential environment, to express their views, which can be fed back into the mediation.

Evidence shows that a conflictual relationship between parents, particularly based on contact arrangements, can have a detrimental effect on children. The courts have endeavoured to keep the needs of the child uppermost when confronted by opposing parental views. Pressure groups have arisen, some of which consider that there is a 'mother-biased' approach in the law. Recent research shows that contact can be so conflictual that it has to be accepted, for the time being at least, that parents go their own separate ways.[30, 31]

THE ROLES OF PROFESSIONALS

The government has become increasingly concerned about the association of lone parenthood with poorer outcomes for children. Therefore, in the last half of the last century and the early years of the 21st century the emphasis has been on developing support systems for parents and children in whatever family circumstances they find themselves.[32]

Doctors – the GP and the paediatrician

Social influences have always presented a challenge to clinicians dealing with children, but there must now be an increased emphasis on the need to view the medical and social factors as interactive, and interdependent. To the child social influences present a range of risk factors, to which some families and children are unable to respond effectively.

Doctors are well aware of the associations between symptoms, illness, and family structure and breakdown. They have the difficult task of giving these appropriate weight in individual clinical situations where variance means that statistical probabilities may be irrelevant. Dealing with the family issues may be necessary before there is progress toward recovery. An immediate attribution of symptoms to many common family situations is very rarely appropriate. After a careful clinical history, examination and, if necessary, limited investigations to confirm that all is well on the organic medicine front, a careful explanation of the possibility of a functional cause will make the latter much more likely to be accepted as important to explore. Without, or even with, extensive analytical psychiatric or psychological input these factors are often difficult to establish unequivocally. A skilled professional may be able to support children and parents in managing family relations in a positively therapeutic way without having to 'prove cause'. Given the right prompts and an understanding of the role of the subconscious in the origin of symptoms, many children can 'recover', and then work through relevant issues.

The Exeter Family Study was set up partly as a response to the local paediatric and child psychiatry concerns about the number of children referred to outpatient clinics with physical symptoms with no obvious organic cause, or with psychiatric or psychological problems that appeared to have an association with family difficulties, especially family breakdown. There has also been a growing concern among practitioners and policy-makers about the association of single parenthood (usually the result of broken relationships) with the increasing involvement of young children in serious crime, and an increased suicide rate among young men. Furthermore, it is known that the most common perpetrator of the sexual and physical abuse of children is a step parent or new partner, perhaps reflecting the confusion of expectations, roles and boundaries that exists in many reordered families.

In the Exeter study the interesting factor about the nature of children's visits to their family doctor was that, instead of always presenting a spectacular symptom, children in reordered families presented more often with mundane or everyday problems, such as minor respiratory infections. These children were exhibiting lower levels of general well-being which, when experienced over a long period of time, can seriously affect children's school attendance and achievement. Adults are likely not to recognize the impact, as it is more insidious than the acute presentations associated with eating disorders, hysterical conversion symptoms and disruptive behaviour.

Any presenting problem, whether physical or psychological, must therefore be seen in the context of the child's family background. The importance of changes in family structure on children's lives, the age of the child in relation to the severity and length of symptoms, who the child lives with, and his or her place in the family may all be of significance. Sometimes, details of family structure alone are not enough to evaluate family environmental influences on the child. Quality of family relationships, an assessment of the child's interaction with both parents, as well as siblings and, if the parents are not living together, some history of the child's contact and involvement with the non-resident parent, will be relevant to the understanding of the symptoms presented. It can be important to involve both parents in any diagnostic process, particularly a non-resident parent who may not even be aware of the referral. In some situations, parents blame each other for the symptoms displayed by the child. Seeing parents together, whenever possible, will not allow one parent to dominate or to use the referral as a weapon. If step parents are prime carers they may also wish to be involved.

Family doctors, as well as consultant paediatricians, are aware of the need to work together to support families by working with other agencies, including the potentially valuable roles of the children's trusts now established in most areas. These trusts are a combination of health, education and social services departments, which work together to provide a unit to provide a response to family problems, whatever their nature.

Psychological services

In a study on the needs of emotionally disturbed adolescents, carried out for the Health Advisory Service, 60% of the sample of over 50 adolescents attending child and adolescent psychiatry had disrupted family backgrounds, representing a seven-fold relative risk.[33] In the Exeter Family Study (matched pairs)[2] there was an eight-fold relative risk of psychiatric referral in reordered families as opposed to intact families. There was a small group of children (5), mostly in separated families, who had been offered a referral but had refused to cooperate. Children in all family groups studied reported higher numbers of psychosomatic health problems than parents seemed to be aware of. Children in reordered families reported more problems than children in intact families. Children in high-conflict, intact families, as shown in other studies, were more likely to have a problem than were children in low-conflict families.

Research has shown that an increasing number of children are presenting with behavioural problems, and levels of depression have increased in children under the age of 14 years.[34] The child and family adolescent psychological services are overburdened with requests to support families and children.

Family lawyers

The consultation prior to the passing and implementation of The Family Law Act, 1996, did not achieve a no-fault divorce but emphasized the importance of mediation and the consideration of consequences by parents for themselves and for their children. This had a fundamental influence on the way in which solicitors now approach family law. It also highlighted the polarized views about family values, the concept of 'the guilty party', the effects of divorce on children and, especially, the effects of parental conflict.[35]

There has been a strong and healthy debate in Britain about the role of family law, family law courts and the kinds of experiences that families go through.[36] During the late 1990s, a vigorous debate followed the passing of The Family Law Act. On one side traditional family values were seen as being challenged, and on the other there was a call for acceptance that family structures were changing and required a different approach. For those working in the field of family law, one of the encouraging outcomes of this debate was the development and support of family mediation agencies, which promoted an alternative way of addressing family breakdown.

Family mediation

The aims of The Family Law Act to reduce the conflict associated with adversarial divorces, encourage attempts at reconciliation and introduce the option of mediation were only partly fulfilled due to a range of factors, including political pressures. However, one of the great successes in terms of setting up these services has been the solid rooting of family mediation services in the practice of family law throughout the country. Family mediation is a process that enables couples to sit down together to discuss their future role as parents, with the aim of keeping both parents responsible for, and involved with, their children as a matter of course. Its objective is to avoid potentially damaging confrontation and exacerbation of conflict. Mediation pilot projects were set up in 1996 and research has shown that not all families are suitable for mediation and not all outcomes are totally 'successful'.[37–39]

Mediation has introduced a new way of dealing with family problems. Couples are screened for their suitability for mediation, addressing in particular domestic violence issues and child-protection matters, and mediation agencies work closely with solicitors in producing positive outcomes for families. The most recent development has been the growing interest among the family courts and judiciary to resolve matters by mediation, and parents who now engage in proceedings in relation to children's arrangements are likely to find themselves referred back to mediation. In some areas there is a pilot scheme in place where original court welfare officers offer an in-court mediation service to assist conflictual parents.

FAINs

Since 1997, following the setting up of The Family Law Act, a new approach has been developed and is supported currently by the Legal Services Commission Family Advice and Information Service (FAINs). This FAINs pilot sees solicitors as being the key workers in advising families in family breakdown, as they are usually, along with the family doctor, the first person approached by families. The pilot project places an emphasis on the solicitor being the 'case worker for the family' in directing the family to the appropriate help, as ascertained following an in-depth interview with the solicitor. The FAINs approach is underpinned by the need to develop a network of support services so that solicitors can offer a range of services to their clients. Lack of funding for these support services severely hampers their development.

Family justice council

The growth of mediation and the importance of support networks for families and hearing the voice of children has had an influence on the family justice system as a whole. The National Family Justice Council emphasizes the importance of multidisciplinary training for all family professionals, including the judiciary. In 2005 the National Family Justice Council set up Regional Family Justice Councils in order to further the multidisciplinary education and training for family professionals, with an emphasis on family dynamics and the needs of children. These councils are proving to be very successful.[40]

The school

There is a real concern that the major changes to the permanence of family structures will seriously undermine the overall social and educational development of children. The family has traditionally fulfilled this role, which has not been seen as an entirely appropriate responsibility for educators during this century in the UK. Young people almost universally respect their parents more than any other adults and, equally universally, hope for successful long-term, permanent and child-bearing relationships for themselves. Increasing family instability presents an irresolvable paradox for adolescents between their parents' experience and behaviour and their own wishes for the future.

Contrary to generally accepted beliefs, the school provides a milieu where children can discuss sensitive and personal issues constructively, and could in theory take on some of the roles of families in the socialization of developing adults. A recently reported sex-education programme demonstrates that a social-learning-based educational initiative not only increases knowledge but is also associated with changes in belief and, most importantly, with lower rates of sexual activity in young teenagers.[41]

Preparation for adult life and parenthood is a key part of the National Curriculum but is barely visible in many schools because of its relegation to a cross-curricular component, which is not examined and for which there is very little space in a crowded timetable. The fact that few teachers receive either undergraduate or extended postgraduate training in this area – possibly even fewer than when childcare was taught to less able girls – further emphasizes the lack of attention to this area of education. Teaching might include the psychology of relationships, negotiation and conflict resolution techniques.

Building self-esteem and self-efficacy might be more important for this country's social and economic future than training for employment. If this is to be achieved, much more attention will need to be paid to the importance of engaging children and adolescents in educational activity designed to develop the appropriate skills for successful negotiation of the social aspects of adult and family living.

CONCLUSIONS

Parental conflict and children remains an important issue, for several reasons. The number of children who experience family change continues to rise, and longitudinal studies emphasize that family structure change presents challenges to children. Outlining risk factors for children can only assist those who wish to provide support services for families and their children at such a time.[42] Parental conflict always presents challenges to both parents and, particularly, children. Ongoing and unresolved conflict presents the most challenges for children. Therefore, practitioners are faced with the challenge to provide parents with the opportunity to develop cooperative strategies for their children's futures and to reduce conflict, rather than allow their child to be open to being vulnerable in their future lives, when in turn they begin to make their own relationships.

Chapter Eleven

Social paediatrics

11

Jo R. Sibert

SUMMARY

Social paediatrics concerns the duty of paediatricians to do their best to ameliorate the effects of poverty and disadvantage in children. Disadvantage has profound effects on children, but the United Nations Convention on the Rights of the Child helps to focus our work not only on treating disease, but also on preventing it. Specific groups of disadvantaged children (looked-after children, children in refuges and refugee children) have particular health needs. We must focus our clinical practice to deal effectively with socially deprived children using a multidisciplinary and problem-orientated approach.

PRACTICE POINTS

Clinicians should:

- use the United Nations Convention on the Rights of the Child as a basis of their work with children
- recognize the special needs of disadvantaged groups
- use a multidisciplinary, problem-orientated approach
- leave enough time to see disadvantaged groups adequately.

WHAT IS SOCIAL PAEDIATRICS?

'Social paediatrics' is a term that has been used in a number of contexts to describe the practice of healthcare in children in which the social dimension has been included. The words are sometimes used synonymously with 'community child health', and indeed the European society that deals with community matters is the European Society for Social Paediatrics. The boundaries between community child health and general paediatrics have become blurred since the Royal College of Paediatrics and Child Health report *Strengthening the Care of Children in the Community: A Review of Community Child Health*.[1] It is increasingly being recognized, therefore, that paediatricians have a duty to do their best to ameliorate the effects of poverty and disadvantage on children. Social paediatrics will thus have an increasingly important part to play as we struggle to deliver effective healthcare to socially deprived groups, not only in the community, but also in the

hospital setting. The basis for all this work is the United Nations (UN) Convention on the Rights of the Child.[2]

This chapter deals with the effects of disadvantage on children, and how the UN Convention helps us to focus our work not only on treating disease, but also on preventing it. It also deals with specific groups of disadvantaged children (e.g. looked-after children, children in refuges and refugee children), and with how we can focus our clinical practice to deal effectively with those who are socially deprived.

THE EFFECTS OF DISADVANTAGE

There is ample evidence of the effect of social deprivation on most aspects of children's health. This starts around birth. An ecological study of all stillbirths, neonatal and postneonatal deaths for the 908 electoral wards in Wales[3] found, for example, that the relative risk of combined stillbirth and infant death was 2.10 (95% CI 1.69–2.61) in the most, compared with the least, deprived fifth of wards. All categories of death, except early neonatal death, were significantly associated with deprivation. Infant mortality fell throughout the 20th century, but the gradient in social class still remains.[4] This is also the case with sudden infant death syndrome, for which a social gradient was established many years ago.[5, 6]

Injuries are the most common cause of death in children over 1 year old. Kendrick and Marsh[7] emphasize that the social class gradient in childhood mortality from injury is steep and increasing. They found that residence in a deprived ward was independently associated with any medically attended injury, with hospital admission and with the number of injuries received. Avery et al.,[8] in an analysis of the death rates from accidents in children aged 0–14 years by health district in England and Wales, found that, during the 5-year periods 1974–1979 and 1980–1984, death rates were generally higher in the north and west of England and lower in the south and east, as well as being higher in urban than rural areas. There was a more than five-fold difference between the highest and lowest rates by district during both periods, and a very strong correlation with social deprivation.

Adverse socio-economic circumstances in childhood may have a specific influence on health and mortality in later life. Mortality from stroke and stomach cancer in adulthood is increased,[9] but not as a result of the continuity of social disadvantage throughout life. Deprivation in childhood influences the risk of mortality from coronary heart disease and respiratory disease in adulthood, although an additive influence of adulthood circumstances is seen in these cases.

UN CONVENTION ON THE RIGHTS OF THE CHILD

The UN Convention forms the basis of work in social paediatrics, with all countries in the world, apart from the USA, being signatories. The issues are covered by the specific Rights of the Child to Health in Article 24 and also in other articles. This UN Convention has great relevance to the practice of paediatrics and child health in the UK.

Article 24.1 states the right of the child to the highest obtainable standard of health possible. This should mean not only providing an adequate treatment service, but also providing adequate prevention. This article of the UN Convention also affirms that the party states (the countries who are signatories to the UN Convention) shall strive to ensure that no child is deprived of his or her right of access to healthcare services. This is particularly important in the UK context in the fields of:

- looked-after children
- homeless children
- refugee children.

Article 24.2(a) states the duty to diminish infant and child mortality, and Article 24.2(d) affirms the duty to provide adequate care for mothers. This is important in the UK context because, although we have made great progress in reducing infant and child mortality, there are still many problems, especially problems related to the social class gradient found in the UK.

Article 24.2(c) states the duty to ensure the provision of adequate nutritious foods and clean drinking water. Although waterborne disease is no longer a major problem in the UK, we still have problems with iron-deficiency anaemia, mainly among poor children.[10] Article 24.2(e) states the duty to ensure that parents and children have information regarding child health and nutrition; far too much health education information is currently put in terms that are impossible for most parents to understand.

Article 24.2(f) states the duty to develop preventive healthcare. We have had successes with:

- a reduction in the incidence of sudden infant death syndrome with the Back to Sleep programme[11]
- *Haemophilus* influenza B immunization[12]
- a reduction in accidental poisoning arising from better safety packaging.[13]

All these improvements followed research, but funding and facilities for much research into preventive medicine for children may be very difficult. The duty to develop preventive healthcare must also ensure that there is an adequate number of staff (health visitors, GPs, school nurses and community paediatricians) to deliver the programme. It also means that there must be partnership projects with local authorities.

Issues related to health obviously include child protection. Article 3.2 of the UN Convention states the right to such protection and care needed for the child's well-being. In a study of severe physical abuse in Wales, we found that one in 880 babies was physically abused each year,[14] so this is obviously a major issue for children in the UK.

Article 23 makes clear the right of disabled children to special care, a major issue in the UK. We are willing to provide the neonatal care that allows babies to survive with cerebral palsy, but appear less willing to provide the equipment for their needs when they are older. Article 27 provides the right to a standard of living adequate to the child's needs. This is obviously essential to the main concern of social paediatrics. In Wales, where I work, one-third of children live in poverty. Much of this is related to the environment in which the child lives, and Article 27.3 of the UN Convention states the duty to provide material assistance, particularly regarding housing. We also have to recognize the right in Article 31 to rest and leisure, and to engage in play. We have shown that playground injuries can be reduced, but some local authorities in Wales have removed play equipment rather than make it safe.

DISADVANTAGED GROUPS

Particular disadvantaged groups present particular problems to the paediatrician in developing adequate healthcare. These include looked-after children, children in refuges, homeless children and refugee children, as well as children in areas where there is inadequate primary care. These are usually the most deprived areas and provide an example of the 'inverse care law'.[15]

Many of these groups have increased health needs. For example, Webb et al.[16] examined children in women's refuges in Cardiff, and found that the uptake of all assessments and immunizations was low. The authors concluded that the children had a high level of need, as well as poor access to services. Similar situations occur with looked-after children[17] and refugee children,[18] who are poorly provided for, despite their increased need for services.

The conventional National Health Service provision does not allow the flexibility for adequate provision for these children, but they still have their right to health. This is particularly the case for looked-after children, who may often change address and are unable to achieve any continuity with health service or educational providers.

Webb et al.[16] concluded that time spent in a refuge provides a window of opportunity to review health and developmental status. They also suggested that the best person to do this might not be a doctor but a nurse: 'specialist health visitors could facilitate and provide support, liaison, and follow up'. This is a principle that is being used not only in refuges, but also with looked-after children. We are moving away from the routine medical examination, as used to happen with the school medical and with looked-after children, towards a much more targeted multidisciplinary approach that must also include health promotion. This is the approach that has had success with the child surveillance programme.

DEALING WITH PROBLEMS

Dealing adequately with deprived children lies at the heart of good social paediatrics, as there is an increasing consensus that this is best done in an integrated way, with the hospital and community working together. There is no doubt that one of the barriers to good paediatric healthcare is the difficulty of deprived families in travelling a long distance to outpatient departments. Clinicians therefore need to develop strategies with commissioners to bring their care nearer to families, by running clinics in either health centres or community hospitals. There may also be certain practices where secondary clinics within primary care are viable: I do a clinic every 6–8 weeks in a general practice in Barry, South Wales, where there are many families with young children.

This work with deprived families obviously needs to be developed in a multidisciplinary way with professionals working within the health service, particularly nurses. The key to good practice is, however, working with social services, local schools and voluntary organizations, not only in terms of child protection, but also in terms of the whole area of children in need. Clinicians, working together with commissioners, need to develop a strategy for health promotion for deprived families. This will clearly involve the child surveillance programme and work with schools, but will also encompass population-based work. An example of this is how healthcare professions worked with the local authority to reduce the number of playground injuries in Cardiff.[19]

When we see deprived families, we need to ensure that we have enough time to deal with them adequately. If we adopt a problem-orientated approach, we can deal with the problems one by one, remembering that social problems may be more important than health ones. Areas such as poor growth, poor development and dental caries must also be addressed. In addition, we need to consider how long we follow-up children who are also being supervised by the local authority. Social services should not be left to follow-up these children alone. Where there are serious legal issues, one should at least follow cases until the legal process is over.

Chapter Twelve

The nature of social work

David Niven

SUMMARY

Social work has been radically changed over the years but still retains the elements of compassion mixed with patronage, and skilled support mixed with social control. The resolution of conflict in individuals and communities underpins the practice. The general public still appears to have difficulty differentiating between social work and the broader social-care tasks in the community. Only 5% of the social services workforce are traditionally qualified social workers. More tasks are being contracted out by local authorities to the voluntary and private sectors, with commissioning, inspection and monitoring remaining the statutory responsibilities.

The image of social work is changing slowly, although the profession seems sluggish in harnessing contemporary marketing and public relations skills to its advantage.

Child protection is still the division of social work that attracts most polarization and debate and, although successive governments have launched many initiatives, the now multidisciplinary approach is still faced with chronic challenges.

INTRODUCTION

When Mary Stewart became the first paid Almoner at the Royal Free Hospital in London in 1895, it could be said to be one of the first attempts to introduce a degree of formality and organization to activity that has been present in society through the ages. This was caring for the community and protecting the vulnerable.

Social work emerged out of the rapidly changing social landscape of 19th century Britain, where traditional care in the community was a mixture of charitable giving (the lady of the manor giving to the poor of the parish), a reliance on extended family support (much more entrenched due to the lack of mobility in traditional communities) and the slow emergence of political recognition of people's right to a better quality of life, including healthcare, housing, employment conditions, relief from poverty, education and social expectation.

DEFINITIONS

Defining social work has always been fraught with difficulties. The current edition of *Collins Dictionary* describes social work as

social services that give help and advice to the poor, the elderly and families with problems.

True – but only a fraction of the picture. The *Educational Dictionary of Social Work*[1] gives the definition of social work as:

the paid professional activity that aims to assist people in overcoming serious difficulties in their lives by offering care, protection or counselling.

Social workers are there to assist vulnerable people at points of crisis or conflict in their lives. In fact, the resolution of conflict underpins the majority of tasks that social workers are engaged in. My own working explanation of the social work task would be that social workers are:

- trained to make accurate, balanced assessments of need
- trained to coordinate and implement these plans
- trained to obtain the resources to meet that need, and then have an ability to move these resources from A to B in as efficient and effective a manner as possible
- trained to form professional relationships with their clients (now more commonly called 'service users').

For the first 60 years of the 20th century social work developed in a variety of different settings: child care, mental health, hospitals, psychiatric institutions, probation settings and general family welfare initiatives. Some degree of organization began to emerge in the early 1960s, and eventually, in 1970, various parent bodies amalgamated and formed the British Association of Social Workers (although probation officers maintained their own association).

TRAINING

Social services departments in England and Wales and social work departments in Scotland are charged with delivering services to the communities that they operate in. Their employers tend to be local authorities, the voluntary sector, charities and a growing private sector. There is, however, still, in the public eye, a great deal of confusion as to the differences between social-work tasks and social-care tasks. Social workers have to obtain a professional qualification. This consists of the Diploma in Social Work, which can be added to with various post-qualifying or advanced awards. The

Diploma course normally takes 3 years, unless added to a first degree, when it can be 2 years. There is often confusion in the public eye between the tasks that qualified social workers perform and the tasks that others in the personal social services are charged with. The majority of workers in the personal social services do not have a social-work qualification, but thankfully their qualifying and training needs are now being much more thoroughly addressed and new qualifying structures and training opportunities are being introduced nationwide. These can be staff who work in residential or daycare settings or those who provide domiciliary services in people's own homes.

The myth that social workers were young idealists with little life experience has largely been exploded. In the mid-1990s a survey was done that showed that practising social workers had an average age in the early 30s and usually had considerable other experience to bring to the profession.

Social work courses are usually a balance of formal, assessed study and rigorously assessed work practice placements. Academic study includes sociology, psychology and social policy, among other subjects

ORGANIZATION

It is still usually the case in the UK that personal social services are organized broadly as services to children and services for adults. Those that work with children and young people do so in areas such as adoption and fostering, disability, child protection, looked-after children, education welfare, young offenders, homelessness, specific initiatives (e.g. drug action programmes), and in a burgeoning voluntary sector across a broad variety of subjects and tasks. This is all in addition to children and families teams who tackle the full range of family vulnerability and dysfunction.

Social work with adults is principally with those who are particularly vulnerable or at a crisis point in their lives. Many are called Care Managers now, whose function involves putting together complex packages of care with individuals who include the frail and elderly, and the mentally or physically ill. Others work with adult offenders and substance abusers. Some work in hospitals, institutions and daycare settings, as well as coordinating help within the individual's own home. Specialization occurs in adult social work too, an example being in mental health where social workers have to obtain the Approved Social Worker qualification (Mental Health Officer status in Scotland).

PRINCIPLES

The British Association of Social Workers (BASW) has adopted and endorsed 12 principles of social work practice. These are upheld by all BASW members and influence their work whatever setting they are in and whatever particular specialization or discipline they adhere to (Box 12.1).

IMAGE

Too often the public's attention is drawn to the 'drama' of social work. In a world of instant communication, rapid delivery of news and the prevalence of soundbites, you would be forgiven for

BOX 12.1

The 12 principles of social work practice

1. Knowledge, skills and experience used positively for the benefit of all sections of the community and individuals.

2. Respect for clients as individuals and safeguarding their dignity and rights.

3. No discrimination exercised nor tolerated in others on grounds of origin, race, status, sex, sexual orientation, age, disability, beliefs, or contribution to society.

4. Empowerment of clients and their participation in decisions in defining services.

5. Sustained concern for clients even when unable to help them or where self-protection is necessary.

6. Professional responsibility takes precedence over personal interest.

7. Responsibility for standards of service and for continuing education and training.

8. Collaboration with others in the interests of clients.

9. Clarity in public as to whether acting in a personal or organizational capacity.

10. Promotion of appropriate ethnic and cultural diversity of services.

11. Confidentiality of information and divulgence only by consent or exceptionally in evidence of serious danger.

12. Pursuit of conditions of employment, which enable these obligations to be respected.

thinking that the only thing that social workers do involves child protection or work with the mentally ill. Bad news always makes the headlines. Melodrama sells in newspapers. When was the last time anyone read a tabloid headline that said 'Social workers do good job'? It just would not sell newspapers. Social work still has a very difficult image problem.

Day in, day out, the vast majority of social workers, up and down the country, are involved in preventive work. Just like all others in the caring professions, the daily task is to improve the quality of people's lives, balancing intervention against the wish to empower people to choose for themselves. They work to prevent families breaking down and children being taken into care; to prevent people with a mental illness reaching breaking point; to prevent the frail elderly feeling as though they have been abandoned by society just because they have not got the means to pay for care; to prevent children and adults with disabilities being isolated and let them live a normal life, included in society, instead of excluded at the margin. All of these and many more are the points of daily conflict in society that involve social workers and bring their skills to bear. Without drama and, like many other professions, with a lot of hard work, social workers just get their heads down and get on with it.

Thankfully, the days when the image of social workers was portrayed as young, long-haired with sandals, stuffed full of quasi-communist ideas, politically correct to an excruciating degree and just hovering at the end of your street to snatch your children away from you, seem to have receded. The fact that a social worker is not legally entitled to set one foot across a threshold without the house owner's express permission (unless there is a Court Order and the worker is accompanied by the police) seemed to escape much of the media in the 1970s and 1980s. The constantly running stories in the press of children's homes in the 1960s, 1970s and 1980s, where some social services workers abused their position of trust (all were called social workers in the media), is a legacy we all have to live with, but still makes the task for today's social workers more difficult. The fact is that the climate for disclosing abuse has considerably improved, and this, coupled with better investigation methods, is part of the reason why victims are coming forward today to talk about what happened in the past. The climate for disclosure is safer and more therapeutic, and less confrontational and frightening than it used to be. Some would argue that the pendulum has swung too far, and regulation, inspection, monitoring and bureaucracy (as a mechanism of control) leave too little 'face-to-face' time with the client.

PARTNERSHIP

One of the measures contributing to the improvement of profess-ional care in the community has been the organization of multi-disciplinary working. In the past, far too often, agencies worked in isolation. There is now an increasing formalization and wish for multiagency working. In all types of service delivery, whether it is pathways for disabled children through the caring systems, child protection, mental health matters, working with offenders or dis-charge arrangements for elderly patients from hospital, and any of the many other settings, cooperation is proving far more effective. Partnerships between social services, health, education and the voluntary sector are now bearing fruit. The concept of integrated care is emerging as one of the most effective ways forward. The need to avoid duplication and miscommunication, and the maximizing of resources seems to have, at last, taken root. Social workers are increasingly now part of multidisciplinary teams and are playing their part in a more holistic approach to personal care.

Child protection is still the most dramatic and talked about area of multidisciplinary working, where cooperation between the agen-cies is not only crucial but sometimes life-saving. The recognition of signs and symptoms cannot be the responsibility of just one agency. Too often in the past one particular professional has taken individual decisions that turned out to be flawed. More and more, collective responsibility has to be the order of the day. The danger, as illustrated by the fallout from the recent 'shaken baby' debate, could be that individual professionals will not put themselves or their experience on the line, and therefore the possibility is increased that someone who is actually abusing a child will not be challenged.

In February 2000 Victoria Climbié died having suffered a catalogue of abuse from those caring for her. A government inquiry, started in April 2001 and chaired by Dr Herbert Laming, high-lighted widespread mistakes. The net result was 108 recommend-ations that all services with any contact with children should be working together to safeguard children. The latest update was published in October 2006.[2]

One key structural change was that the Area Child Protection Committees became 'Local Safeguarding Children Boards'.

THE FUTURE

We are at an interesting moment in history for social services, and social work in particular. There have been great advances in the effectiveness and the delivery of care. There is an argument, however, that social work is increasingly moving from the statutory sector (i.e. local authorities) to the voluntary sector in the role of 'provider'. Legislation dictates that social services are accountable for the provision of many services. It may be that fewer and fewer people will be employed by local government and that their role will concentrate down to one of inspecting and monitoring rather than direct provision. Social work will not disappear. It is just becoming realigned and redefined all the time.

As well as a number of disciplines cooperating more together, other countries and cultures are having an impact on the shape of social work. The International Federation of Social Workers repre-sents over half a million people in 55 countries, and is purposefully pulling together, in definitions and principles of practice, more universal and commonly acceptable regulations and guidance. For a profession that embraces all, from the Ukrainian Association of Social Pedagogues and Specialists in Social Work to the volunteer nature of social work in Sri Lanka, and from the highly organized professionals in many industrialized countries to the emerging identities in many African nations, the challenges are great.

Here in the UK, one of the most significant events and changes in the social work environment has recently come into being. This is the General Social Care Council. At last, argued for over the last 30 years, there will be a visible body that will regulate and register the profession. All professional social workers have to register with the council and, in increasing numbers, as they develop qualifi-cations, those working within the social care sector will also register with the council. The four home countries will each have their own council arrangements and perhaps some difference in emphasis, but the principle will be the same. For social workers whose practice is bad, the withdrawal of registration (being 'struck off') will become a real possibility, and that recognizable public sanction will, I believe, be more reassuring to the wider community, helping to increase trust. Eventually the General Social Care Council will be responsible for around a million people in the workforce.

CONCLUSION

I do not know what Mary Stewart would have made of the last 110 years of social work activity and organization, but I think she would have seen that the need for social workers is as strong as ever. Great paradoxes exist within the profession – an increased amount of cooperative activity with other disciplines, balanced against the starburst that seems to have occurred in specializations. The great weight of legislation and regulation that social workers have to adhere to seems, at times, as much of a burden as a checking system – a not uncommon cry from professionals in health, education and law enforcement. But the fundamental principles of providing a paid, well-trained, safety mechanism for the most vulnerable in our community still exists and, sadly, seems as needed as ever.

Chapter Thirteen

Fostering and adoption: the paediatrician's role for children who require substitute parental care

Heather Payne

13

SUMMARY

The work of providing medical advice for fostering and adoption is a specialized paediatric role, where the paediatrician works as part of a multiagency team with social services departments, and voluntary and other agencies. The aim is to offer support and healthcare services to children who cannot live with their original families for a variety of reasons (looked after by the local authority[1] or referred for adoption[2]). The needs of children and the similarity of the principles involved in caring for children outside their family of origin mean that the spectrum of health services required for children in substitute care can be seen as a continuum. The role of the paediatrician[3] is to identify the current and future health needs of the children, to work as part of a multidisciplinary team to ensure access to and coordination of health services, and to liaise with and advise other professionals, as well as children and young people and their carers, on health matters.

THE ADOPTION OR FOSTERING TRIANGLE

'The triangle' is a term that was first used in adoption,[4] but is a concept that is useful throughout the spectrum of substitute parental care. The triangle comprises the child, the birth family and the substitute carer (foster parent or adoptive parent, or residential key worker). The child's needs will be met in varying combinations by the two other parts of the triangle, with support and help from external agencies (schools, health carers, social services, etc.). The balance will change with time and circumstances, but the three components must always be considered.

THE DEVELOPMENT OF ADOPTION AS A SERVICE FOR CHILDREN

The significance of adoption as a service for children can only be appreciated in a historical context. Although adoption has been described throughout history and in literature in many stories including Moses,[5] Oedipus,[6] *As You like It*,[7] and *Oliver Twist*,[8] the first ever Adoption Act in Britain was not until 1926. This legislation was a response to large numbers of babies born to unmarried women after the First World War in the context of social attitudes of the time towards illegitimacy.[9] Adoption was seen as a neat solution to all these problems, the social engineering required seemingly viewed as purely beneficent, in securing a good home for the child, avoiding stigma for the birth mother and providing a child for the infertile couple. Doctors were often involved in private placements; there was much secrecy, and the main concern was that babies were free of syphilis and 'fit for adoption'.[10] The emotional needs of the 'adoption triangle' (birth mother, adoptive parents and the adopted child in later life) were not considered.

The real revolution in attitude came in the 1970s, when it was articulated that the purpose of adoption was to find parents for children, and not the other way around. Children with disability, previously considered 'unadoptable', were successfully placed with adopters.[11]

Birth mothers were properly enfranchised into the process, following the Adoption Act of 1976 and the Children Act 1989. The latter made the child's welfare paramount but emphasized that professionals must work with families and also consider the wishes and feelings of the child.[12] In addition, the growing understanding from the Post Adoption Centre that adopted people want to know about their origins led professionals to realize that children are better off in terms of identity development and adjustment if they are told the truth about their adoption from the very beginning.

Adoption and fostering in 2005

The numbers of children adopted in Britain climbed steadily with the growing population, reaching a peak in the early 1960s. Numbers of adoptions have declined steadily since then, and the average age at adoption has gone up. Current figures show that around 4,000 domestic and around 350 intercountry adoption orders are made in the UK per year (Table 13.1). The majority of children currently being adopted into a new family (i.e. not a step-parent adoption) are older, as very few babies are now relinquished for adoption.

Around 60,000 children per year in England and Wales are in public care (looked after), and some 5–10% will go on to plans for adoption. Many of these children will have special needs with regard to placement because of the history of abuse or neglect that caused them to be in care, as well as medical or developmental problems, and difficulties with attachment or behaviour.[13] Adoption will not be achieved for all those children for whom it is planned.

Table 13.1 Trends in adoption in Britain 1968–1989

Year	Total adoptions (to nearest 1000)	Proportion by step-parent
1968	24,000	NA
1975	21,000	44%
1980	11,000	35%
1989	7,000	49%
2003	5,000	30%

THE CHILD IN FOSTERING AND ADOPTION

Care needs of the child for fostering or adoption, and legal status

Fostering aims to provide the child with a home, usually for a temporary period, whilst maintaining strong links with the birth family with the aim of reintegration. Adoption aims to offer the child an entirely new family, extinguishing all legal links with the birth family. In reality, this sharp distinction is often blurred by long-term fostering, or adoption with contact arrangements.

The majority of children requiring adoption have been in the care system for a variable period of time, and have experienced neglect or abuse. In order to avoid delays in ensuring a secure and stable life for the child, the process of concurrent planning[14] (pursuing separate but parallel routes for a child, aiming to reintegrate the child into the birth family, but simultaneously making adoption plans should reintegration fail) is current best practice.

Children who are 'looked after by the local authority' may be accommodated (with foster carers or in a residential placement) with the agreement of parents, and the local authority does not share parental responsibility in this situation.[15] If the child is subject to a Care Order, then the local authority shares parental responsibility and may allow the child to live with the parents or may remove the child and place them in a foster home or other placement.

Parents who voluntarily relinquish a child for adoption retain parental responsibility until the adoption order is made. However, once a child is 'placed for adoption' the adoption agency shares parental responsibility.[16]

Types of placement required

The range of placements required for children and young people who cannot live at home extends from supportive daycare, through respite care, transitional family-based foster placement, long-term family fostering, residential care, specialized fostering projects for older children and young people (e.g. remand fostering and community parent placements), to work promoting and supporting independent living in care leavers. These placements may be provided by local authorities, voluntary agencies (such as Barnardos or NCH) or independent foster care agencies. Placements should be seen as a continuum of substitute parental care for children, provided according to their needs.

Desirability of maintaining contact with family

It is important to balance the child's need for permanence and stability with other emotional needs.[17] Older children may have a well-established attachment to an abusing or mentally ill parent, and it may not be in the child's best interests to make the decision for adoption. However, the child's need for permanence (of placement, consistency, warmth, safety, etc.) may be met by a combination of a family or residential placement with regular home visits or supervised contact, depending on the age and needs of the child. Many children in the care system worry about their parents and are greatly reassured to be able to see them from time to time, even though the child knows they do not want to live with their parents.

It is an expectation that a child who is looked after by the local authority will have contact with parents promoted by that authority, unless it is clearly harming or distressing to the child.[18] If permanent placement away from the birth parents is the only reasonable long-term plan for the child, there is an obligation on the local authority to explore the possibility of placement with an extended family member before considering an unrelated family.[19] The birth mother is involved in the process of selecting a new family whenever appropriate.

Prospective adopters are encouraged to accept the possibility of direct or indirect contact after adoption.[20] This is sometimes face-to-face contact, but more often involves accepting cards and letters for the child when they reach 18 years of age, or sooner, and by providing reports and sometimes photographs yearly to the birth mother via the adoption agency.

Health needs of looked-after children

The medical and health needs of looked-after children are greater than average, and are often poorly assessed and met. There is a greater risk of complex health and social needs, associated with previous experiences of neglect and abuse. Mental health problems, disorders or illnesses, and developmental delay are more common than in other children.[21] There are likely to be sibling groups with a range of different needs.

If looked-after children have problems with emotional adjustment to their distressing circumstances, they may display challenging behaviour.[22] This may result in placement breakdown and a move of carer, which may establish a cycle of poor attachment, superficial relationships, poor self-esteem and lack of emotional resilience. The outcomes include a greater risk of exclusion from school, truancy or school refusal. This means that looked-after children miss health-promotion messages (on contraception, safer sex, relationships, smoking, alcohol and drugs) and health protection (BCG, MR, meningitis C and tetanus immunizations) offered at school. They also have poorer access to continuity of primary healthcare, including general medical and dental practitioners.

National initiatives[23, 24] have attempted to reverse these health inequalities, but have had limited effects. At September 2003 there were 44,900 children looked after by English local authorities who had been looked after continuously for at least 12 months. The data showed that 72% of these looked-after children had their immunizations up to date, 75% had a dental check and 75% had an annual health assessment.[25] A survey of the mental health of looked-after young people in England[26] found that 45% of those aged 5–17 years had a mental disorder, which is five times the risk of children living in private households (about 11% with mental disorder).

Health and social outcomes for children who remain in public care until care-leaving age remain poorer than those of other young people;[27] they have few educational qualifications, and higher rates of criminal conviction, teenage pregnancy, sexual exploitation, substance abuse and homelessness. Legislation requires services to be provided to this group of young people.[28]

Role of the paediatrician in fostering and adoption

In all types of fostering and adoption placement, the medical role is similar and relates to each relevant part of the triangle. The overall aim is to assess the child's physical, psychological and developmental well-being, delineate the health needs of the child, carer and family in the context of the social situation, and identify how health services should be provided and coordinated with the aim of improving health outcomes.

The role of medical advising in adoption and for looked-after children requires skills and experience in fostering and adoption, developmental paediatrics and child protection. Expertise in child mental health is also desirable. The medical adviser is likely to be a senior member of a consultant-led community paediatric team (Boxes 13.1 to 13.3).[29]

The paediatrician must ensure that a comprehensive health assessment is performed for the child,[30] including physical, mental and emotional health, development and educational issues, health promotion, health prevention, and the wishes and feelings of the child. Continuity of medical information should be established by accessing past medical and GP records, a healthcare plan should be formulated, and appropriate interventions and follow-up offered. The healthcare plan should inform and dovetail with the overall care plan and the timing of the statutory review.

The paediatrician's role is to work with other health professionals (especially nursing and child and adolescent mental health services), social services and education to ensure that services are planned, configured and monitored such that these particularly deprived children receive the care that they need. It is worth remembering that the usual quality control (parental pressure) on a service is absent for this group of children. The skills of advocacy for children are greatly required in this work.[31]

A medical adviser to the adoption agency is required by legislation.[32, 33] The medical adviser has a full role on the adoption panel and has duties relating to health issues in each part of the adoption triangle – the child needing adoption, the birth family and the adopters.

Health assessment of looked-after children is a legal requirement. This must be done yearly for children aged 2 years and over, and every 6 months for children under this age.[29]

In many areas this service is provided by a multidisciplinary team of specialist looked-after children's nurses, who work in a team with the paediatrician to provide coordinated health and medical advice and planning. This process should ensure that children are well served in terms of quality of medical and dental provision, access to primary healthcare, immunizations and developmental screening, school health services, mental health services, sexual health services, secondary care services (including those for attention-deficit hyperactivity disorder (ADHD) and autism, speech and language therapy, occupational and physiotherapy as required), as well as the provision of a health record that travels with the child,[34] timeliness of medical reports and responsiveness to the social care planning process.

The report provided for fostering or adoption should contain a summary of any health or developmental problems that might arise in the future based on the family history. Any special needs or emerging diagnosis should be fully delineated as far as possible, and an assessment must be given of how this is likely to affect the child in the future (i.e. whether special educational placement or ongoing intervention is likely to be needed), together with a quantified risk of a child developing a condition such as schizophrenia or deafness. As well as affecting the planned placement of the child,

BOX 13.1

Service aims

The medical input for children requiring substitute parenting should:

- assist the assessment and planning process for the child
- ensure the coordination and continuity of healthcare for the child who has to move
- empower the child to take responsibility for his or her own health at the appropriate stage
- assist the assessment process for, and promote health support for, substitute carers
- promote appropriate health support and information for birth parents
- ensure that current medical knowledge is disseminated to inform policy- and decision-making for interagency work relating to children needing substitute care, their carers and families.

BOX 13.2

Medical adviser's role regarding the child needing adoption, foster or residential care

- Ensure appropriate health assessment, including medical examination, functional and developmental assessment, health promotion and protection as needed.
- Ensure development and implementation of healthcare plan.
- Ensure appropriate educational and psychological assessment.
- Liaise with other health professionals involved with child.
- Assess family history and its implications for healthcare of child.
- Provide medical report for adoption panel, care plan or care proceedings.
- Advise and attend adoption or fostering panel as required.
- Offer consultation and support to carers regarding child health issues that may impact on placement, including disclosure of new information emerging after placement.
- Provide updated reports for court proceedings.

BOX 13.3

Management of the service

The medical adviser leading the service must ensure mechanisms for monitoring and evaluating work, as well as the maintenance of professional standards and good interagency working. This can be achieved by:

- regular review and appraisal of own job plan and competencies (including specific skills in fostering and adoption, child protection and specialist expertise such as that in ADHD, autism, etc.)
- regular interagency review of roles and responsibilities and documentation of interprofessional roles
- participation in multiagency strategic planning of services for children requiring substitute care
- liaison with other statutory agencies (especially social services, child and adolescent mental health services, and education)
- regular monitoring and review of statistical information, involving outcomes where possible (e.g. immunization rates, adoption breakdown rates, coverage and quality of reports to social services)
- participation in medical and interagency audit, including agency and panel function (in the capacity as medical adviser to the adoption agency)
- membership of an appropriate professional body with the aim of furthering knowledge and improving standards in fostering and adoption (e.g. British Association of Adoption and Fostering)
- participation in research studies and dissemination of the findings in order to improve outcomes
- improving the profile of the work by making presentations at clinical meetings, and teaching and training other professionals at pre- and postgraduate levels.

the contents of this report will affect the actual care given (e.g. avoidance of anaesthetic in children from families where there is a history of hyperpyrexia).

Some children requiring respite care away from home for more than 30 days per year are, by definition, looked-after children. As a matter of good practice, respite care projects, often run by voluntary organizations such as NCH or Barnardos, often follow the same health assessment process for all placements.

Post-adoption problems

There are often predictable problems after adoption, even if psychological adjustment is initially good, and even if the child was placed as a baby. There is often a period of psychological distress when the child is between 7 and 9 years old. This can be attributed to the child's processing of the knowledge of adoption at that specific psychodevelopmental stage, the development of concrete operational thought[35] and the increasing ability to deal with the abstract. Put simply, the child perceives that, as well as being 'special' and 'wanted' by their adopters, this is because they were 'unwanted' by their birth parents. This can produce serious effects

on self-esteem and can be seen as a specific 'complication' of the 'whole-child transplant operation' of adoption. Adoptive parents can be supported in helping the child discuss the issues[36] and deal with emotions, using books and stories related to adoption or fostering (*Paddington Bear, Harry Potter, Tracey Beaker*). Post-adoption support and counselling from a professional experienced in adoption may be necessary.

THE BIRTH FAMILY

Any family history of illness or health condition in birth parents, their extended families, and particularly the child's siblings and half-siblings, should be considered. A specific history should be taken to elicit whether the birth mother used neurotic medications, alcohol or psychoactive drugs during pregnancy, as such exposure may have implications for the growth and development of the child during childhood,[37] increasing the risk of ADHD and language disorders. In some situations where the mother has had possible exposure to the human immunodeficiency virus (HIV), it may be helpful to engage her via the social worker and ask her to consider accepting counselling and HIV testing (which is in both her interest and the child's) in order to avoid having to test the child.

Inheritable disorders

Good links with departments of medical genetics are important as more information on inheritability of many conditions becomes available,[38] especially conditions such as ADHD, autism spectrum disorders, language problems, learning difficulties and mental illness. The gathering of any specific information or testing for inheritable disorders should be considered carefully before it is undertaken. Any testing must be demonstrably in a child's best interests and must be consented to by a person or body with parental responsibility. Diagnostic testing for treatable inheritable disorders during childhood is entirely appropriate. However, predictive genetic testing, for conditions that may arise later in childhood or later life (e.g. Huntington's disease) is an invasion of autonomy, does not benefit the child and should not be done.[39]

Medical information that comes to light after an adoption placement should be passed to the paediatrician advising the adoption agency so that it can be shared appropriately (e.g. a diagnosis of muscular dystrophy in a child placed for adoption or a discovery of hepatitis B carrier status in a relinquishing mother). In all situations, consent should be established for the forwarding of information. Legal advice may be necessary in some cases. Multidisciplinary peer group discussion of ethical issues can assist decision-making in complex situations.

THE SUBSTITUTE CARERS

Health issues and the approval process

Prospective adopters, foster carers and day carers will present with a range of medical conditions, which the medical adviser will be asked to comment on for the relevant approval process. The general principle here is to assess how the condition is likely to impact on their ability to give care to the child.[40]

Thus, a situation such as a woman treated for breast cancer in the past year will have very little effect on her ability to offer occasional respite care, but will have more effect on her capacity to foster. It might be appropriate to advise restriction to guaranteed transitional foster placements until the likelihood of recurrence is clear. It could be expected that such a medical history would have a profound effect on approval as an adopter because of the risk to any child who was placed having to repeat the experience of loss of a parent. If there is a reason to put a child in a high-risk placement (e.g. a sibling is already there or the child has an existing attachment to the carer), then the agency should be advised to develop a written contingency plan, which may for instance involve the firm commitment of the partner to give up work to look after the child, or the involvement of another family member or friend to take over the parenting role in the event of serious disability or death.

Many successful adopters and foster carers have medical conditions, illnesses or disability. It is not the absence of problems that is desirable, but the ability to provide a stable and child-focused environment for the child for the required period of time. Some conditions will give grounds for special plans to be made to ensure that appropriate supports are in place in the event of something adverse happening.

Gathering information on prospective carers

The medical adviser must always assess the GP medical report, and should attempt to get as much information as possible from any specialists treating the individual. Cardiovascular risk should always be assessed. If there is an illness or condition present, specific specialized information will be required, always pursuing objective questions such as the 5- and 10-year survival figures for an individual with that exact type and stage of disease, and effect of the condition and treatment on activities of daily living. The presence of illness or disability does not in itself constitute a contraindication to approval for adoption or fostering. However, a condition that has a profound effect on life expectancy or the prospective adopter's ability to parent the child should be carefully considered by the adoption or fostering panel before a decision is made. Approval is a panel (not exclusively medical) function.

Conditions that may affect prospective carers include: renal failure and transplantation, spina bifida, multiple sclerosis, Klinefelter's syndrome, epilepsy, depression, manic–depressive psychosis, schizophrenia, alcoholism, heart failure, hypertension, visual impairment and blindness, and various malignancies. Obviously, a paediatrician cannot be an expert in all these areas, and skill in consulting other physicians and surgeons is vital. It is worth remembering that physicians treating adults will be inclined to

promote the interests of their adult patient; it is the paediatrician who must promote the interests of the child. This can be done by ensuring that the questions asked are precise, and relate to factual information. This will allow the medical adviser to make an accurate and factual estimate of the likely risk to the placement, and thus to the child.

Intercountry adoption

The infertile childless couple often wishes to adopt a healthy baby to recreate the 'natural' experience they would have had. Now that very few babies are being given up for adoption in the UK, some couples are turning to other countries, such as China, where social pressures (the one-child policy, the social preference for male children) have generated a situation where there are many abandoned baby girls in orphanages. The Chinese government allows international adoption of these children. An extensive discussion is outside the scope of this chapter, but the medical adviser should be aware of the health-screening needs (for infectious diseases) of babies coming from abroad.[41]

Prospective adopters need to demonstrate the same competencies as for a domestic adoption, as the demands on adopters taking on a transculturally placed baby, which may have undiagnosed special needs, are no less than for a domestic adoption. The health assessment of the adopter should be performed as part of the adoption assessment, and the same health principles should apply.

The whole process should be demonstrably in the child's best interests, although regrettably this is not so in certain parts of the world, where there has been evidence of illegal selling of babies.[42] Anyone considering this step should be advised to contact governmental authorities (Home Office, Scottish Parliament, Welsh Assembly Government, Northern Ireland Assembly) for regulations.

CONCLUSION

The paediatrician has an important clinical role in promoting the healthcare and health of children who are looked after by the local authority or requiring adoption. Health needs must be properly assessed, and appropriate health services offered and coordinated for the child, their carers and their birth families. The medical adviser for adoption or looked-after children has a vital role in facilitating interagency understanding so that all the health needs of a child, their carers and families are addressed.

14

Chapter Fourteen

Sex education – whose baby?

John Rees • Alex Mellanby • John H. Tripp

SUMMARY

Sexual health, especially of young people, in the UK could be regarded as a national crisis. High rates of unwanted and unintended pregnancies, and soaring rates of sexually transmitted infections are well documented, with acknowledged health costs. The largely unacknowledged financial, educational, social and emotional costs of underachievement at school, emotional illiteracy, reduced likelihood of long-term parenting relationships and social exclusion are even more significant.

Despite the consequences and future costs of this 'time-bomb' there has been little cohesive response from health or education to address the issues. Localities have been set targets and are expected to deliver behaviourally effective sex and relationships education. However, the lack of proven resources and finance leaves commissioners, teachers, parents and health workers vulnerable to the vagaries of 'local initiatives'. These initiatives are often not theoretically sound, are frequently intuitive and are seldom adequately evaluated to assess likely impacts on health.

This chapter describes the rollout to 150 schools of a sex and relationships education programme (APAUSE), which independent evaluation has demonstrated increased knowledge, maturity and healthier behaviours among students, and supports the professional development of teachers and community nurses.

FATAL ATTRACTION?

Sex is one of the most powerful human drives. Anthropologists have argued that consciousness of sexuality is an important distinction of humanity from other mammals, and psychologists have based whole systems of psychology on sexual awareness and functions. Literature related to sex, sensuality and sexuality provides sensationalist, erotic and interesting reading; both beautiful and tragic poetry is available in all written languages. Popular music, advertising and other media, especially electronic, makes sex, sexuality and attractiveness the overt or subliminal focus of much communication. Love, desire and compulsive fascination with the human form are enduring and common to all cultures. Despite such undoubted benefits, the damaging consequences of sex are evident. Sexual desire and jealousy are central to much popular drama and are common reasons for violence. Sexual coercion causes misery and subjugation, frequently for women and children when sex is for sale. Unwanted and regretted sex-related contacts cause major medical, social, emotional and financial problems.

NOT IN FRONT OF THE CHILDREN

In the UK especially, anecdotes and jokes tell how parents avoid mentioning 'sex'. The heading to this paragraph reflects a common reality: few parents find sex and sexuality, either their own or their children's, easy to talk about in meaningful or informative terms. Many parents still rely on euphemisms and prefer vague terminology for 'private' body parts, pubertal maturation and even 'spending a penny'. The 'ostrich position' illustrates how many adults deal with teenagers' emerging sexuality, and describes a common situation: 'the parents bury their heads in the sand while the teenager hopes the sand will not blow away' (attributed to Bell). When discussing human sexuality, teachers remain concerned about lesson content and how to deal with students' questions; questions about emotions, relationships or, even more difficult, about different sexual practices. Primary care professionals often find it difficult to respond to the needs of adolescents, particularly those in their early teens, and to square the circle of promising confidentiality while not disempowering parents from supporting their child.

Adolescents find many of these groups of adults difficult, even those providing dedicated services for teenagers. Young people often find it easier to talk and learn about sex from people their own age and outside their family. Few adults believe that the teaching of sex, negotiation of sexual relationships, determination of personal values and understanding of behavioural norms should be left entirely to the whim of playground acquaintances. Society, including parents and young people, and health, education and media professionals, must be prepared to take radical steps to improve public sexual health, to commit funding to research and to implement the best available educational technologies. If this is not achieved, future generations are likely to remain at the mercy of playground gossip, misinformation and 'media myths'. Our young people deserve better than this if they are to avoid sexual ill health and if we are to achieve the pro-social, health-improving changes desired by parents, and meet government targets.

KNOWLEDGE AND ITS APPLICATION

Despite living in a highly sexualized society where sexual knowledge and experience is not only 'cool' but expected, young people's knowledge of sexual health and awareness of accurate social norms remains poor. Common misinformation includes a failure to appreciate that many contraceptive methods do not have any role in preventing the transmission of sexually transmitted infections (STIs). It seems strange that we do not have a word for 'contra-fection'. Many young people overestimate the efficacy of barrier methods in preventing STIs and many have an inaccurate understanding about the timing of ovulation – 25% of 15–16 year olds believe that midcycle (the most fertile days of the menstrual cycle) constitutes the 'safe period' for avoidance of pregnancy. Few believe that blindness will result from masturbation, but older fables have been replaced by newer 'mythunderstandings', bringing their own potentially damaging misapprehensions of the real world. Thus, currently, the vast majority of teenagers believe (incorrectly) that most of their peers are sexually active before the age of 16 years and that human immunodeficiency virus/acquired immune deficiency syndrome (HIV/AIDS) is the most common STI. This latter belief, together with the fact that, even today, few have direct knowledge of anyone with the disease, results in the misapprehension that STIs are extremely rare. The belief that most young people under the age of 16 years are sexually active not only normalizes this expectation for an individual but facilitates the teasing and pressurizing of virgin heterosexual boys and girls. Despite increasing societal tolerance of same-sex relationships, lesbian and gay people still suffer prejudice and rejection, and their needs are seldom met within sex and relationships education (SRE).

WHAT IS THE AGENDA?

Until relatively recently a vociferous and influential group of educationalists and policy-makers regarded the role of sex education in school as one of giving knowledge and skills. This view ignores the influence of certain sectors of the media, which appear to be promoting unhealthy choices, unfettered by such 'moral' considerations, while others, sometimes within the same newspaper, lament the promotion of sex and contraception, without moral guidance. A media focusing on circulation figures rather than the public interest may provide unhelpful and 'unhealthful' mixed messages, and happily misrepresent responsible research under titillating headlines or distort and polarize debate in the desperate search for 'good copy'.

The mixed messages that young people receive from adults and society's inability to engage in mature discussion about the role of sex, and the purpose of SRE, almost inevitably leads to anxiety in schools and confusion for young people.

Many, if not most, adults want a successful, caring, exclusive, long-term sexual relationship to be an important component of their lives. This is seldom reflected in the media, where immediate gratification, and short-term but intense sexual relationships are portrayed as the norm and to be sought at almost any cost. Such unrealistic expectations of hedonism confuse us all, and for most young people relationships, short and long, are complicated enough without involving sex. A legitimate aim of SRE could be to provide young people with the knowledge, skills and social environment where it is not only possible, but recognized as desirable, to avoid the unwanted social, emotional and health consequences that can result from unplanned, unconsidered or pressured sex. Another aim might encourage the positive aspects of a wide range of relationships. These will include promoting mutually supportive relationships with parents, peers, teachers, employers and siblings as well as intimate, physical relationships, irrespective of gender or sexual orientation, which acknowledge the positive aspects of sexual relationships and those that involve physical intimacy but do not necessarily involve full intercourse.

Despite increasing evidence of the importance of parental support, the agenda for sex education at home is frequently very limited. Parents, usually mothers, may discuss puberty and menstruation with daughters, but frequently skip briefly over sexual intercourse to pregnancy and childbirth. Boys, especially when denied consistent, positive male role models, often have extremely limited sex education from either parent, which may be confined to 'You will take precautions won't you?' when their parents guess them to be sexually active. It has been internationally accepted that young people have a right to health-promoting and pro-social SRE. Schools, where the vast majority can access education, are the logical place to ensure provision of such an entitlement.

In schools, SRE is usually perceived by students to be confined to the biological aspects of sex, with substantial time devoted to anatomy, menstruation, contraception and STIs. However, as part of their sex-education policy, many schools will include discussion of personal relationships, but a lack of clear policy substantially affects what individual students receive in the classroom, promoting a current description of SRE as 'more patchwork than pattern'. Despite efforts to develop the National Healthy Schools Programme and continued professional development for teachers and community nurses, there is little evidence that significant expenditure has had any positive outcome on either professional practice or young people's health.

Parental and educational objectives often conflict with messages from the media, which portray 'sanitized' sexual intercourse as a normal consequence of relationships. Short acquaintances are shown to result in intense physical excitement, with minimum personal interaction, and are followed rapidly by intercourse. An average adolescent television viewer may see many hundreds of simulated heterosexual sexual encounters in any one year, with sexual intercourse portrayed as a casual activity rather than as part of a relationship. Contraception and STI prevention is not discussed or portrayed. Sex is not preceded by gradually increasing physical intimacy developing over a period of time in a relationship or even foreplay. Media images traditionally fit the stereotypical male, rather than female, sexual response, although female orgasm is increasingly portrayed.

There remain pervasive double standards in relation to sexuality that accept, condone and almost expect boys to have sex 'when they can get it', with multiple partners and using high-status descriptions, such as 'stud', to describe them. Despite 'girl power' and 'ladette' attitudes, girls who have multiple sexual partners or change partners within their same social circle are still often treated with disdain. These attitudes are not confined to teenagers; studies have shown that not only do teenage boys receive far less parental supervision (e.g. their whereabouts, time to be home, activity), but that parents have expectations that boys will be sexually active and that girls will not.

Thus, whatever the agenda might be for SRE, it is increasingly unlikely that today's teenager is growing up to believe that society considers sex to be something participated in by two equal individuals who have strong, long-term commitments to each other and that is for their mutual enjoyment and satisfaction.

WHOSE RESPONSIBILITY?

It is clear that the responsibility for sexual and relational health is one borne by society as a whole, although while governments bemoan the situation, their expectation that parents and educators should be active in trying to prevent adverse outcomes for young people is clear. The state has previously considered that sex and marriage are private matters in which it has a limited role. The burden of termination of teenage pregnancies, unintended parenthood and the increase of STIs, including HIV/AIDS, requires a re-evaluation.

Government departments are addressing the medical and social consequences of dysfunctional sexual relationships exemplified in the stubbornly persistent rates of unwanted and unintended pregnancies, and the increasing incidence of STIs. In the UK, we have recently seen the formulation of a National Sexual Health Strategy, ironically preceded by a 'Teenage Pregnancy' strategy. Despite considerable investment in initiatives to reduce teenage pregnancy, halfway into a 10-year strategy little progress has been made towards the identified goals, and funding to improve sexual health remains focused on treatment rather than prevention or health-promotion work.

The fact that the children and young people most likely to suffer high levels of health risk are generally those least likely to benefit from the modelled behaviour of their parents, means that the role of schools in health prevention is increasingly recognized. Given the nature of very young teenage relationships and the inconsistent use of contraception, it is unlikely that SRE will be able to make their sexual relationships 'safe'.

WHERE DO TEENAGERS LEARN ABOUT SEX?

Sex education is a broad but compartmentalized subject. Teenagers still want parents to supply much of the information, certainly practical help with menstruation for example, and they continue to look to parents for guidance on morality. While young people remain adamant that their parent(s) would be their ideal sex and relationships educators, professionals must engage with parents to attempt more than telling girls about periods and actively promote their espoused relational values and behaviours. Both society and families directly or inadvertently promote a wide range of moralities. Parents and young people often underestimate family influences, while recognizing the influence of peers. Although young people learn about sex and relationships informally and in settings such as youth clubs, one of the most important places during adolescence is school. Parents and young people expect that schools will contribute significantly to SRE, and its potential for public health improvement should not be ignored.

TEENAGERS' VIEWS OF SCHOOL SEX EDUCATION

Only a minority of teenagers rate their school sex education as 'OK' and few feel that it meets their needs. Nearly 80% of teenagers who have been asked about school-based SRE wanted 'visitors' to be involved in the teaching. They cite a wish for 'easier' and 'more comfortable' discussions, problems of asking known staff difficult questions, the embarrassment of some teachers and the perceived veracity of local (sexual) health professionals. Teenagers are also concerned about confidentiality and the fact that teachers are authority figures within schools.

Virtually all children in the UK attend full-time education at the age of 13–14 years. Although the teaching of citizenship is mandatory, the content of SRE beyond the confines of the Science National Curriculum is largely optional, and remains a controversial subject that, from time to time, has its profile raised by outrage or disaster. It is serious enough to require a separate school policy, but apparently of insufficient importance to be standardized or interrogated with any rigour. The public health aspects of SRE, including education in relation to HIV/AIDS and teaching about contraception to reduce teenage pregnancy, are compulsory, but parental withdrawal is allowed when these discussions go beyond the National Curriculum.

CURRENT PROVISION

Many primary schools still choose to deal with SRE from an exclusively medical perspective or fail to provide age-appropriate education, leaving children ill equipped to face puberty or anticipate rapidly changing social structures. Health education is not a main subject in the undergraduate curriculum for teacher training.

Science teachers often choose not to stray from the biological into the emotional, because this might raise the issue of parental withdrawal and because it is not covered by an examination syllabus with attendant grades or league-table scores. Despite the seriousness of the problems associated with early teenage sexual behaviour, and the efforts of many schools and their teachers, the result has often been a further marginalization of non-biological sex education. Teachers of religious education, physical education or other curriculum areas (sometimes those with little curriculum time) find themselves responsible for social, moral, spiritual and cultural education, with little training or support. Despite the recommendations of Ofsted, the school inspection service, for specialist staff teams, many schools still require whole school staffs to teach sex education in tutorial time. A teacher, with little training or support and concerns about legality, parental reaction, young people's preciousness and a host of other curriculum pressures, may find this a lesson worth avoiding.

The appropriate timing and content of SRE has caused considerable controversy and occasionally has resulted in public debate in the media. Good SRE needs an incremental curriculum from preschool to post age 16 years. Young children usually receive guidance about 'sharing', 'friendships' and other pro-social values, but need information about anatomical differences and functions before puberty. In this context lessons may be less likely to be associated with embarrassment for children or difficulty for teachers. Such information will undoubtedly, however, require 'revisiting' as children become more aware of their bodies in late childhood and early teens. There is wide variation in age of physical development, exaggerated by the fact that girls develop secondary sexual characteristics earlier than boys. The result is that teaching of SRE in school cannot be optimized to an appropriate age of either physical or psychological development. A further complication in the classroom is that, without skilful management, such differences provide opportunity for personal comments, put-downs and teasing, which may then undermine the whole lesson.

While some children will be sexually active in National Curriculum Year 9 (age 13 years), the number is relatively small (probably less than 5%), and this is probably an appropriate year group in which to build on previous input and to base the majority of SRE. The disadvantage of failing to teach it earlier is that there will already be role models within the year who will suggest a perceived normality of sex experience in early teens and will pressure others. In contrast in Year 8 many of the children simply will not be sufficiently aware of the relevance of learning about intimate relationships to find the subject of use.

Schools may make use of external agencies such as health to assist with SRE, and GPs, school medical officers, school nurses or health visitors may be asked to support in the planning and delivery of lessons on specific subjects related to this curriculum. Such contributors to the school curriculum are unlikely to have had any training in classroom management, do not necessarily have any theoretical basis for the structure of their delivery, may rely on knowledge-based approaches, and may have insufficient knowledge of the level of understanding or the social, cultural or educational needs of the children they are teaching.

A limited amount of sex education occurs in youth clubs and other settings, but involves only a small minority of the population and is frequently directed at older teenagers, concentrating on promoting the use of condoms to avoid STIs and pregnancy.

Despite the 'guidance' from the Department for Education and Skills (DfES),[1] the Qualifications and Curriculum Authority (QCA) and Ofsted[2] in terms of learning outcomes, the picture is of a fragmented system with no overall established curriculum and few replicable, reliable programmes to ensure delivery. Individual teachers, schools or even local authorities expected to create and implement their own individual approaches are unlikely to be able to provide SRE that results in healthier attitudes or behaviours. Even if individuals did succeed in achieving such rare outcomes, replication in neighbouring, much less all, schools is improbable. This disjointed patchwork is mirrored by steadily increasing rates of sexual activity among young teenagers, dramatic increases in STIs and minimal, if any, decrease in teenage pregnancies in spite of government efforts and investment to improve accessibility of contraception together with the now widespread use of emergency contraception.

THE ROLE OF HEALTH SERVICES

Since the benefits of SRE may include reduced health expenditure, such education is an entirely justifiable call on health budgets. This requires a radical reappraisal of funding and the subjection of all interventions to which funds are devolved to a proper assessment of effectiveness in achieving behavioural goals. The adoption of the

Health Development Agency's work by The National Institute for Health and Clinical Effectiveness (NICE) renders this achievable.

Health personnel may need to accept significant responsibility in delivery of SRE, both to assist teachers improve their knowledge base and to discuss clinical information, especially accessing services, with appropriate relevance to teenagers. As with teachers, however, for this to be a successful intervention the health staff involved need appropriate training. They require not only adequate medical information and to be taught appropriate skills for the classroom, but the literature is clear about the theoretical basis required for effective interventions.

The so-called 'medical model' of teaching in which facts are given and risk identified has not been shown to have any effect on adolescent behaviour. Young teenagers, at the 'concrete stage' of cognitive development, simply do not translate such information into beliefs that affect behaviour. While they may accept the veracity of the facts taught, young people will not act on them.

The situation is further complicated by the fact that teenagers may not trust information in this area when it is given by adults, believing that adults have a vested interest in 'frightening them off'. This is becoming a genuine concern following the introduction of selective and inaccurate information in some 'abstinence' sex-education programmes, which fail to meet young people's human rights entitlement and have not been shown to have their desired effects.

There are, nevertheless, two advantages of using health staff to support schools in SRE. The training and expertise of health staff will allow accurate and standardized information in subjects covered. Health staff also provide representation of, and links to, (sexual) health services. They provide veracity and credibility of information and can 'bring alive' the process of a health consultation, even using role-played situations, and reassure young people of the confidentiality of medical practice.

Health involvement might be criticized as 'medicalization' of SRE, but this may be required if the aim of SRE is healthier behaviours rather than simply improved knowledge. Concerns have been raised that this involvement is simply a pragmatic capitulation to teenage sexuality, an attempt to promote contraceptive pre-scription in the classroom; even financial motivation has been suggested. Although sexually active teenagers clearly need assistance with contraception and 'contra-fection' their SRE should not imply that sexual intercourse is an expected activity for young teenagers. Any medical involvement, especially in the classroom, should provide very positive support for those who do not wish to have sex. Verbalization of this support is probably currently inadequate. Medical input to the classroom needs to be part of an overall SRE programme that provides comprehensive skills and the creation of an environment where teenagers are expected to negotiate healthful relationships. Some of these skills and values and the creation of a healthful environment may be to maintain relationships, increase tolerance, and to reduce sexism and homophobia, and some will be to enable young people to resist unwelcome pressure.

WHAT WORKS?

Pupil ignorance and misinterpretations are powerful drives for adults to supply information to children, predicting that the better informed will make better and safer choices. 'Informed decisions' require perception of vulnerability that may be at odds with adolescents' detached personal interpretation of themselves or their feelings of invulnerability. Too many health-education interventions rely on adult thinking, believing that teenagers will base rational behaviour on knowledge of risk, while failing to acknowledge that the risk most frightening to teenagers is being disrespected by their peers.

Only programmes based on social learning and associated theories (social cognitive theory and the theory of planned behaviour) have been shown to effect any measurable change in behaviour in the vast numbers of interventions that have been reported in the literature, whether related to tobacco, substance abuse or sexual activity. The update of a key 1994 review in 2001 reached almost identical conclusions about the key components of effective interventions. Reflecting on 20 years of experience in the field, Kirby[3] introduced one other key issue, that of connectedness between teacher and learner, a concept that is entirely consistent with social cognitive theory. Both the RIPPLE[4] (experimental) and our own APAUSE[5] (rolled out in service) peer-assisted programmes have demonstrated the possibility of achieving delay in first intercourse.

It is one thing to know what should work, and quite another to deliver it to a population. While such delivery, with evidence of effecting the necessary changes in beliefs, normative expectations and behaviours, has been achieved, it has been reported in few programmes. All were based on one of the above theories and all were peer assisted. Yet another major step is required before such an intervention can be considered effective, as opposed to efficacious, since the programme quality has to be maintained while delivering it to a whole population of young people.

The view that the key issues are openness about sexual issues, together with good sex education and easy access to contraception has been widely promulgated in the UK, with frequent reference to The Netherlands, where these factors apply, and teenage pregnancy rates have been much lower than here. There is, however, only circumstantial evidence for these widely accepted conclusions, and it seems at least equally likely that the much stronger culture of the family, intrafamilial passing on of moral codes, strictures against teenage pregnancy and greater religiosity are important associations. The apparently religiously based fervour for 'abstinence until marriage' associated with absence of education about contraception, which has been strongly supported by two Republican administrations in the USA, has also received a great deal of critical comment from experts in the UK. There have also been reductions in the benefit support for single mothers. While such vociferous opposition to this approach may be justified in the name of liberal values and young people's rights, we should be aware that this giant and uncontrolled social experiment does appear to have been temporally associated with reduced teenage pregnancies and without the explosion of STIs seen in the UK.

THE APAUSE PROGRAMME

Since the late 1980s we have developed and trialled an experimental, school-based SRE programme as a partnership between health and education services and with a significant peer-education component. The Added Power And Understanding in Sex Education (APAUSE) programme was based on our literature review, conducted in 1990, to identify strategies associated with

health benefit. We concluded that an optimal programme would be delivered jointly by health workers, teachers and peer educators (slightly older teenagers who have received appropriate training). The programme aimed to counteract myths, encourage sensitive yet safe discussion in mixed gender groups and classrooms, and to develop a shared understanding between young people that would facilitate later negotiation between couples.

A controlled study demonstrated the efficacy of this programme, and a recent external evaluation, carried out on behalf of the Teenage Pregnancy Unit by the National Foundation for Educational Research (NFER),[6] shows that it has been possible to retain the effectiveness when it was rolled out to 150 schools. The responses of all stakeholders and the quantitative analysis showed that they thought the programme appropriate, applicable, acceptable and effective, even though some of the experts did not. An intermediate experiment confirmed that peer educators were much more effective in correction of misunderstood norms than adults delivering an as near as possible identical programme.

Our own evaluations confirmed by the independent analysis of the NFER[6] shows that young people participating in APAUSE have better knowledge about sexual health and relationships (including contraception and STIs), are more mature in their beliefs about sexual relationships for young people, and are less likely to believe that sexual activity before 16 years of age is normal or to have experienced sexual intercourse. There was a correlation of perceptions of having been taught assertiveness skills (a key programme component) with increased use of contraception amongst those who are sexually active.

Case studies are used as a vehicle to promote discussion, and it is the active discussion of sensitive matters within these that is one essential component of social learning. In simple terms, if a teenager in a class, surrounded by classmates, states that teasing and exploitation are unreasonable methods of getting sex, they will find it harder to do those things outside the classroom – especially since their proposed 'victim' could well have been present in the same or similar lessons.

Teachers and health workers are provided with training and materials to implement a framework that is sufficiently flexible to respond to the diverse social, physical and cultural needs of young people.

Learning and practising skills to resist pressure and creating an environment where it becomes socially acceptable to implement such skills are essential if a teenager wishes to be able to stop or slow the physical progression of a relationship or insist on barrier contraception if that relationship involves penetration. Cross-age peers are effective in helping younger teenagers to learn to be assertive and develop refusal skills, because they are given permission by the class to bring role plays and engage class members in active roles. They act as 'role models' to provide genuine support for younger teenagers who may wish to say 'no' or say 'yes' safely. For example, a girl might feel that 'having sex is just the price of going out with a boy' but hears from an older teenager that 'having sex is a personal decision and no one should make you do something you don't want to do'. Additionally, she will learn the verbal and emotional skills within a supportive social framework, and is more likely to be able to use them in practice. A young man will learn how to defend himself from peer jibes about his failure to 'persuade' his girlfriend to sleep with him.

The peer leaders have their own credibility and confidence raised by a structured training programme. Slightly older, they have less image concerns in the classroom than the students they are teaching. They do not have to resort to mythology or insult to maintain their street credibility – they know what they are talking about, and observing teachers refer to their 'professionalism'. Many schools and colleges have also been prepared to commit time and resources to supporting this model of peer education because of the many and varied positive gains for the peers themselves. They almost invariably report gains in their own knowledge and understanding, improvements in presentation skills and assertiveness and self confidence, and improvement in their own relationship skills, in addition to a very helpful contribution to their university and/or employment interviews.

APAUSE remains the only service programme in the UK with evidence of health gain and educational benefit. The costs of the programme are not insignificant, but may represent good value for money with significant gains in staff development, young people's personal development and almost certainly a long-term cost benefit to health services. Government policies, first not to support any one approach or programme, and second to expect schools to buy in any support they need for SRE from what are usually very minimal budgets for personal social and health education, have meant that the number of participating schools grows only slowly and that most young people in the UK are denied access to the programme.

A FULL CIRCLE

At the beginning of this chapter we discussed the power of sexual drives and how teenagers turn from embarrassed adults to people their own age for information, social norms and cultural expect-

ations. Teachers and health professionals using the approach we have described are empowered by the same processes of peer influence. The peer component is preceded and often followed up by adult-led teaching, which provides a backbone of information, links to health services and establishes an appropriate classroom environment for discussion of these sensitive issues.

Informed and trained teenagers may be one of the best and most effective means of assisting younger teens to develop skills for successful sex and improved relationships. Such skills, values and ethos may also be harnessed to promote other healthful behaviours, and our internal training evaluations indicate that teachers and health professionals use the skills learned and networks established in other curriculum areas.

There is an urgent need to find a solution to enable delivery of a theoretically sound and peer-supported programme if we are to expect a health benefit from school-based SRE, and forthcoming changes to local sexual health promotion mean that the programme is unlikely to continue beyond those areas in which it is already established. Such a failure to capitalize on a proven, if emergent, technology appears to us to be folly.

So whose baby? Probably SRE should be everyone's baby – it is better to deal with the concept than the issue!

CONFLICT OF INTEREST

Note both J. Rees and J. H. Tripp are, and A. Mellanby was, involved in the origination, development and promotion of the APAUSE programme.

Chapter Fifteen

Delinquency: the role of paediatrics in management and prevention

Elspeth Webb

SUMMARY

'Delinquent' is a legal rather than a medical concept, applied to young people who have broken the law, and is one manifestation of a spectrum of antisocial and violent behaviours seen in a group of young people, some of whom will have had conduct disorder in earlier childhood. Delinquency conceals two distinct categories: 'life-course-persistent' and 'adolescence-limited' antisocial behaviour. Life-course-persistent delinquency, with which this chapter is mainly concerned, is part of a developmental continuum that is manifested in different ways throughout childhood and young adulthood. It is associated with impulsivity, low intelligence and attainment, family criminality, poor parental child-rearing behaviour, poverty, and socially disorganized communities. Paediatricians have important contributions to the prevention of serious antisocial disorders, in the care and management of children with established difficulties, and in advocating for a seriously disadvantaged group of children and young people. These are discussed in detail, with particular reference to poverty, child protection, attention-deficit hyperactivity disorder and learning disability.

INTRODUCTION

'Delinquent' is a legal rather than a medical concept, applied to young people who have broken the law. Delinquency, i.e. criminal behaviour, is just one manifestation of the broader concept of antisocial behaviour in adolescence, which includes antisocial attitudes, dishonesty, aggression, drug and alcohol abuse, gambling, sexual promiscuity and violence. For the purpose of this chapter I use the term 'delinquency' to include these broader aspects, and the term 'conduct disorder' for antisocial behaviours in childhood. These two phenomena overlap considerably. Conduct-disordered children have a very high (around 40%) likelihood of subsequent delinquency.[1]

EPIDEMIOLOGY

Prevalence

The prevalence of conduct disorder is fairly stable across most developed industrialized countries at around 10%, with more boys affected than girls. Adolescent delinquency is much more common.

Moffit[2] argues that delinquency conceals two distinct categories, each with a unique natural history and aetiology. One group, comprising around 5% of the Dunedin cohort (one of the longest running longitudinal cohort studies of development), engages in antisocial behaviour at every life stage, whereas a larger group (around 20%) is antisocial only during adolescence. Moffit has called these two phenomena 'life-course-persistent' and 'adolescence-limited' antisocial behaviour. Sex comparisons showed a male to female ratio of 10:1 for childhood-onset delinquency, but of only 1.5:1 for adolescence-onset delinquency.[3]

Aetiology and risk factors

Life-course-persistent antisocial behaviours.

For this group, adolescent delinquency is part of a developmental continuum (Box 15.1), which is manifest in different ways throughout childhood and into young adulthood.[4]

Conduct disorder and delinquency have multiple associated risk factors that can be classified into genetic/biological and environmental factors. Not all these will be causal, but simply act as markers for risk. Teasing out which factors are causal, which are merely symptomatic and which are confounding is a complex task. In the Cambridge Study in Delinquent Development,[5] the most important childhood predictors of adolescent delinquency were:

- antisocial child behaviour
- impulsivity
- low intelligence and attainment
- family criminality
- poor parental child-rearing behaviour
- poverty and socially disorganized communities.

In the Dunedin study childhood-onset delinquents had childhoods of inadequate parenting, neurocognitive problems, and temperament and behaviour problems in infancy.[4]

A more recent study looking at a group of 41 young people referred to a Youth Offending Team in the UK found that, of the 29 who were of compulsory school age, 15 (52%) had special educational needs and 19 (66%) had difficulties with basic literacy/numeracy. Living arrangements were described as 'complex' by the authors: 9 (24%) were not living with their birth parents (being either fostered or in residential accommodation); 2 (5%) were homeless; 6 (16%) were living in overcrowded accommodation lacking basic amenities; 11 (29%) were resident in deprived households; and 8 (21%) were living with known offenders.[6]

Delinquency is claimed to be more prevalent in ethnic minority communities; but families belonging to these communities

Developmental continuum of life-course-persistent delinquent adolescents

- **Infancy**: 'difficult, demanding'.
- **Nursery years**: oppositional behaviours; aggression; deviant or delayed early development.
- **Mid-childhood**: aggression; lying; stealing, bullying; 'troublesome, disruptive' (i.e. conduct disorder); learning difficulties.
- **Adolescence**: antisocial attitudes; truancy; dishonesty; aggression; drug and alcohol abuse; gambling; sexual promiscuity; violence and law breaking; poor educational outcomes.
- **Young adulthood**: drug and alcohol abuse; gambling; sexual promiscuity; violence and recidivist criminal behaviours; unemployment.

experience racial discrimination, and are more likely to be unemployed or in low-paid jobs, to live in poor housing, to have significant disparities in health, and to have children who attend poorly resourced schools. It is highly unlikely that ethnicity itself is an important primary risk factor, but simply a marker for social disadvantage and discrimination.

Adolescent-onset delinquency

Adolescent-onset delinquents, male and female, do not share the pathological backgrounds found for those with life-course-persistent antisocial behaviours.[3] Moffit suggests that this phenomenon is a consequence of what he terms 'a contemporary maturity gap', in which, in modern postindustrial societies, sexually and physically mature individuals are infantilized by extended education and delayed work opportunities, resulting in antisocial behaviours 'that are normative and adjustive'.[2]

This is an important issue. Around 25% of British men under 25 years old will have accrued criminal records to accompany them through their adult life, of which over half will have been adolescent-onset delinquents.

Relationship between attention-deficit hyperactivity disorder (ADHD) and the development of delinquency.

Hyperactivity is an irrefutable risk factor for delinquency.[4, 5] The term ADHD first appeared in DSM-III-R, and is still current in DSM-IV. It includes children with hyperactivity/impulsiveness, children with inattentiveness, or children with both, this latter group being equivalent to hyperkinetic disorder (HD), which is current in ICD-10. However, only those children with hyperactivity and impulsiveness have an increased risk of future social dysfunction. The diagnosis is a clinical one and is based on behavioural criteria. In epidemiological studies carried out by trained and knowledgeable professionals, about 1% of children will fulfil criteria for primary HD,[6] with a few per cent more fulfilling criteria for ADHD (hyperactive–impulsive subtype). Hyperactivity disorders have very high rates of comorbidity, of which the commonest comorbid diagnosis is conduct disorder.[7]

THE ROLE OF THE PAEDIATRICIAN

Paediatricians have important contributions to the prevention of serious antisocial disorders, in the care and management of children with established difficulties, and in advocating for a seriously disadvantaged group of children and young people.

Role in prevention

The paediatrician's role in prevention of serious antisocial disorders can be split into five areas:

- recognition of at-risk children
- effective child protection
- parenting programmes
- initiatives to reduce poverty and the impact of social disadvantage
- effective services for hyperactivity and related developmental difficulties.

Each of these is discussed below.

Recognition of at-risk children

Paediatricians and other child health professionals have myriad opportunities to meet at-risk infants and young children – in the neonatal unit, the acute ward, casualty, and outpatients, as well as in the investigation of possible abuse or developmental problems. Paediatricians should be aware of risk factors, in the child, the family and the wider community, and be able to link families in with appropriate local support services. They need also to be aware of children whose social circumstances increase the likelihood of their at-risk status being unrecognized, and take steps to ensure that marginalized and socially excluded children are not missed in child surveillance.

Effective child protection

Given the strong links between early experience of violence, abuse and harsh parenting regimes with later development of conduct disorder and delinquency, it is crucial that children are protected effectively from harm. Although, currently, social services take a lead role in child protection, health professionals, particularly paediatricians and health visitors, are crucial elements of the multiagency child-protection team. As the one service that links in with all preschool children, either within neonatal services or child surveillance, health professionals may be the only members of the multiagency team who are in a position to recognize such harmful, or potentially harmful, situations and set in motion the child-protection process. It is imperative that robust measures are taken that not only address immediate physical safety, but also incorporate a long-term view of minimizing the emotional harm that accompanies domestic violence and other emotionally abusive family contexts.

Parenting programmes

Harsh and inconsistent parenting has already been mentioned as strongly associated with delinquency. Unsurprisingly, there is a great deal in the literature on parenting programmes, although much of it relates to programmes directed at families in which there are children with established difficulties.[8, 9]

Parents have long been held responsible for the antisocial behaviours of their offspring and the social ills that accompany them.[10] Common sense would suggest that improving parenting would go some considerable way to reducing adolescent delinquency, and there has been a recent refocusing on these measures, both in the literature[11] and in government policy.[12] But parenting happens in context. If that context, i.e. extreme poverty, homelessness, violence and social disintegration, ensures that adults cannot function effectively as parents, then interventions that focus exclusively on parenting will fail. As Taylor et al.[10] eloquently point out:

> the current interest in parenting arises as a result of the apparent increase in behavioural problems, child abuse and neglect, juvenile crime, and delinquency. The emergence of (these) social problems is accompanied by explanations that, as they did at the turn of the century, focus on individual rather than societal causes.

Parenting in the UK, as in the USA, also occurs in the context of a society in which parenting is a low-status occupation. This is linked to the low status of women, given that most parenting continues to be provided by mothers. Many western governments, particularly in Scandinavian countries, have a long history of policies that underpin the importance of good parenting to society as a whole. These have included protecting parents in the work place, with employment policies that acknowledge the dual roles of working parents and enable parents to both contribute to the wider economy and parent effectively. The UK has a poor record in this area.

Effective parenting programmes must be implemented in ways that address these contexts. They need to be accompanied by initiatives that increase community cohesiveness and increase the capacity of communities to respond to the needs of children. They must be asset based, i.e. take into account not only the faults but also the strengths these families and communities have, and make broad use of community members in the delivery of services. This will lead to more effective support and empowerment of families to work in full partnership with agencies providing services. The Sure Start programme[13, 14] is one example of an intervention that aims to improve parenting by supporting communities in this broad-based manner. Although Sure Start is somewhat limited by being geographically based, thus excluding many poor families, it is important for community paediatricians to establish active partnerships with their local Sure Start projects.

Initiatives to reduce poverty and the impact of social disadvantage

The UK has a poor record in keeping children out of poverty in comparison to other northern European countries. Although there have been improvements since 1997 in this area, it still has one of the highest rates of child poverty of any industrialized nation.[15] A review of the role of child health professionals in initiatives to reduce the impact of social disadvantage and poverty upon health and development is beyond the scope of this chapter, but is available elsewhere.[16, 17]

Services for children with neurodevelopmental difficulties

ADHD

Ideally, primary hyperactivity disorders should be recognized before children present with established behavioural difficulties. Management should be according to a recognized protocol, of which a mainstay is stimulant medication.[18] As some children with ADHD have comorbid neurodevelopmental disorders, paediatric-

ians working with these children should be experienced in their diagnosis and management. They must also work with schools to develop appropriate responses to these children's needs. It is preferable for children to be recognized as having difficulties rather than to be labelled as 'bad'.

Although there is very good evidence for the effects of stimulant medication on the symptoms of ADHD, medication alone does not appear to affect long-term social and educational outcomes. However, these findings may simply reflect the increased severity of ADHD in medicated children. Medication combined with a positive parenting style is associated with good outcomes.[19]

Intellectual disability

Children with cognitive impairments require care from a complex multidisciplinary team, of which paediatricians working in a community setting will be members. Their role, in partnership with colleagues within Child and Adolescent Mental Health Services (CAMHS), includes the continuing management of behavioural difficulties and emerging conduct problems, which are common. In addition these children have an eight-fold higher risk of hyperactivity than do children of normal intelligence.[20] There is increasing recognition that such children require specialized and differentiated psychiatric care, although such services are in general lacking. In the absence of these services, paediatricians in community settings may be unfairly expected to fulfil this role, including the administration of psychoactive medication to children with serious and at-risk behaviours. Practitioners need to be mindful of the not insignificant clinical governance implications of this.

Role in the care and management of affected children and adolescents

Delinquency and conduct disorder associated with hyperactivity

Growing up with abuse and violence can lead to both anxiety and attachment disorder, both of which may lead to children fulfilling list criteria for ADHD/HD without necessarily having primary hyperactivity disorder.[6] These children also have high rates of conduct disorder. Some children with primary HDs will also be abused, or subject to poor parenting, itself a risk factor for delinquency and for poor outcomes in ADHD (Fig. 15.1). Clinically, this complex interrelationship between abuse/poor parenting, ADHD and conduct disorder/delinquency can be an extremely challenging diagnostic task, requiring the input of a skilled and experienced multidisciplinary team with expertise both in child mental health, paediatrics and child protection.

Learning disabled children in the criminal justice system

Low intelligence and low attainment has already been mentioned as a risk factor for delinquency. Although there is, theoretically, a comprehensive developmental surveillance system in the UK,[21] it does not reach all children; there is plenty of evidence to show that children living in aggravated poverty, and thus at risk of delinquency (e.g. children passing through refuges for domestic violence[22]) are those most likely to have slipped through the net and missed some or all of the surveillance programme. Add to this a move within educational psychology services from an emphasis on assessment to one on advice, it is unsurprising that some of the young people with learning disability who get caught up in the

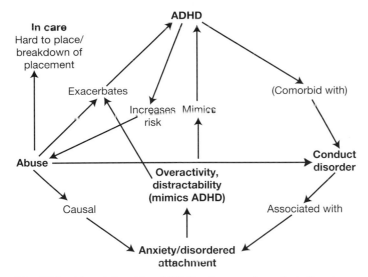

Fig. 15.1 Interrelationship of ADHD, abuse and conduct disorder.

criminal justice system have either never had their low cognitive abilities recognized, or this information is lost or unavailable.

A recent survey in South Wales used the Hayes' Ability Screening Index (HASI)[23] and the Strengths and Difficulties Questionnaire (SDQ)[24] to screen a random sample of 46 young people aged 11–18 years who had committed crimes and were receiving support for the local Youth Offending Team: 67% of these had HASI scores requiring in-depth assessment of possible learning disability, of which over half also had abnormal self-reported SDQ scores (Pippa Mundy, personal communication). These young people had either never had their needs recognized or had, at some point, been 'lost' by statutory services.

Such children and young people are extremely vulnerable within the court system and in detention. It is vital that personnel working in child health, including within 'looked-after' services, establish good links with CAMHS and youth offender teams to ensure that such children are recognized, appropriate steps taken to ensure that their general and mental healthcare needs are addressed, and that the courts are informed as to their cognitive level and the implication this might have for their ability to understand the legal process and be held responsible for their criminal activity.

General child health services

Children and adolescents with significant antisocial behaviours require support from professionals with a variety of skills, necessarily drawn from a range of disciplines and agencies. These young people will be of school age, with most having a statement of special educational need and probably educated outside mainstream settings. They may be in the care of the local authority; a few will be in secure accommodation or prison. As well as emotional and behavioural difficulties, some may also suffer from chronic illness or be disabled. Some will require inpatient treatment for surgery, acute illness, accidental or non-accidental injury, alcohol intoxication and drug overdose. A small proportion will develop very serious mental health problems requiring admission to specialist units.

All paediatricians, whether working in a community setting, such as school health or with looked-after children, or in hospital-based services, such as an endocrine clinic or the intensive care unit, will from time to time be required to provide care and support to what are, in the main, seriously disadvantaged and often distressed individuals, many of whom have suffered considerable adversity in their lives. It is important that all practitioners work in ways that respect the rights and integrity of these young people, and strive to attain good standards of care, despite the challenges that may present in terms of poor compliance. Services offered must be appropriate to their maturity and accessible to this socially marginalized group. Many with chronic illness (e.g. asthma, chronic middle ear disease, diabetes) may have a long history of suboptimal management of their condition, partly a function of their own anti-social behaviours, but also subsequent to their social disadvantage.

Paediatricians must be able to work effectively with professionals from other disciplines and agencies including, for example, genitourinary medicine clinics, obstetric and gynaecology services, police, probation officers, psychiatrists, psychologists, and professionals working in social services and education, in order to respond effectively to the needs of affected children and young people.

Young people in prison The few adolescents that are in prison are currently a cause of great concern. Around 3,000 under 18 year olds were recorded to be in prison at the end of 2002.[25] The number of 15 and 16 year olds on remand or in prison tripled in the 10 years leading up to 2002; in the same period the number of children placed in secure accommodation increased by 58%.[26] Although some progress has been made since then, for example, girls under 17 years old are no longer placed in prison,[27] there are few resources made available to provide dedicated and appropriate healthcare to this population. Apart from general health needs, their sexual vulnerability and often established drug habits put them at risk of hepatitis (B and C), HIV and other sexually transmitted diseases.

Advocacy

Advocacy is a core professional duty for paediatricians,[28] and in particular in representing the needs of children for whom discrimination and social disadvantage have contributed to their poor health and healthcare.[29]

Individual advocacy Delinquent behaviours are unattractive, and make it difficult for clinicians to empathize with their rude and antisocial adolescent patient. Dishonesty and aggression are not conducive to establishing good doctor–patient relationships, and can impede the provision of necessary therapeutic interventions or appropriate social and educational support. Despite this, paediatricians must view their delinquent patient as a young person in need first and foremost, and persuade other professionals to follow suit.

Group advocacy It is something of a lottery whether these young people are labelled 'sad, bad or mad'; depending on which they could end up with social services, child mental health services or in the criminal justice system. Most will be struggling to some degree or another, whether they are life-course-persistent or adolescence-limited, and need support, not censure, to address their offending behaviours and any underlying causes. Imprisonment is inappropriate for children and young people, with non-governmental organizations such as the Howard League for Penal Reform[30] consistently arguing for its abolition. Antisocial behaviour orders, also with an underlying agenda of punishment and humiliation, are equally censured:

We fear that current legislation has the effect of widening the net of the criminal justice system, by criminalizing naughty children ... Anti-social behaviour legislation relies on a low burden of proof. It does not rely on an objective test of behaviour but on the reaction to that behaviour by others. Yet anti-social behaviour legislation uses the criminal justice system if the original order is breached. There is a blurring of the boundaries between civil and criminal law which has serious implications for due process and the rights of the child.[30]

Children and young people who have committed very serious crimes, particularly violent crimes, are very likely to be victims and require intensive therapeutic support to come to terms not only with the consequences of their offences, but also their own experiences of abuse. We have a duty to speak out for these young people, to persuade government and politicians to acknowledge that the blame lies not just with children, their parents or their teachers, but has roots in attitudes and policies that create social conditions in which delinquency is inevitable.

Chapter Sixteen

Drug misuse: conception into childhood

Pamela A. Cairns

SUMMARY

The substance-abusing mother and her baby are at increased risk of adverse outcomes, both in pregnancy and long term. These may be due to the pharmacological effects of the drugs (e.g. causing fetal withdrawal in utero), comorbidities (e.g. sexually transmitted diseases) or associated social factors (homelessness, poverty, domestic violence, etc.). The aims of antenatal care in this population are to engage the family, stabilize the mother's drug use, screen for comorbidities, assess the social background and educate the mother. This is best achieved through multidisciplinary team working.

In the postnatal period babies should be carefully observed for signs of neonatal abstinence by using a standard scoring tool. Non-pharmacological means should be used to treat mild withdrawal. Morphine or methadone are both appropriate treatments for opiate withdrawal but may be less effective in other drugs. Chlorpromazine can be effective, either as a single agent or in combination with an opiate. Seizures should be treated with morphine if they are due to opiate withdrawal or phenobarbital if they are due to non-opiates.

The long-term outlook for children of drug-abusing parents is largely related to the environment of upbringing. The increased risk of neglect and physical abuse persists throughout childhood.

INTRODUCTION

Drug use is becoming more common in the UK, and the pregnant population is not exempt from it. Both the substance-abusing mother and her baby are at higher risk of adverse outcomes than non-drug-abusing people. The antenatal exposure to illicit drugs may have a relatively small influence on outcome, with persistent adverse social factors also being important.

BIOLOGICAL EFFECTS OF COMMON DRUGS

Opiates have been used for centuries for both their analgesic and stimulant properties. The main alkaloid derived from *Papaver somniferous* (the opium poppy) is morphine. Heroin, an acetylated derivative of morphine, is the most commonly abused opiate today. Heroin, morphine and methadone are all partially selective opiate receptor agonists. Heroin is the most lyophilized, and hence crosses the blood–brain barrier fastest, whereas methadone has the longest half-life. All cross the placenta to the developing fetus.

Cocaine is the alkaloid extract from the shrub *Erythroxyloncoca*. It acts by inhibiting the reuptake of amines at the presynaptic monoamine transporters. The extracellular concentrations of tryptophan, dopamine and noradrenaline therefore increase. This leads to euphoria, along with hypertension and local vasoconstriction. Amphetamines act in a similar manner but also stimulate the release of serotonin, dopamine and noradrenaline from the synaptic terminal stores. The effects of amphetamines and cocaine are therefore similar. Both freely cross the placenta.

The active extract from *Cannabis saliva* (marijuana) is D-9-tetrahydrocannabinol. It acts by enhancing dopaminergic transmission in the midbrain, and hence activating the endogenous opiate systems.

Teratogenic effects

There does not appear to be a teratogenic effect of opiate or cannabis use. The evidence relating to a direct teratogenic effect of cocaine has been more controversial. A wide variety of abnormalities of the face, central nervous system, skeleton, heart, urogenital system and gut have been attributed to maternal cocaine use. However, a recent large case–control study did not find any difference in the type or number of congenital abnormalities observed on physical examination between exposed and non-exposed infants.[1]

Both cocaine and amphetamines are vasoactive. It has been suggested that this leads to an increased susceptibility to necrotizing enterocolitis, bowel perforation, retinopathy and cerebral infarcts leading to cyst formation.[2]

Obstetric complications

Pregnant drug users should be considered to be a high-risk obstetric group. While many have good antenatal care, a proportion will attend erratically, if at all. In addition to poor antenatal care, they are at risk of poor nutrition, sexually transmitted diseases and obstetric complications such as premature labour, antepartum haemorrhage and pre-eclampsia.[3] Although the obstetric complications are likely to be multifactorial in origin, there are drug-specific effects. While animal studies have been helpful in suggesting mechanisms of action of the individual drugs, clinical studies have been much more difficult to interpret. Many women use more than one drug, and many pregnancies are also exposed to the effects of nicotine and alcohol.

Heroin is hydrolysed to morphine, which is metabolized to codeine and 3- and 6-morphineglucuronides (M3G and M6G). M6G is analgesic, while M3G is excitatory. Morphine or M6G will block the effects of M3G. Both mother and fetus will metabolize morphine in this way. However, M3G is a larger molecule than M6G, and will therefore be transferred less readily back across the placenta to the mother. M3G will then accumulate in the fetus.[4] If a mother takes a larger than normal dose of heroin, the fetus may withdraw (due to excess fetally produced M3G), although the mother does not. This will lead to apparent fetal distress, with fetal tachycardia but an active baby on ultrasound assessment. A dose of opiate, such as morphine or methadone, to the mother will normalize the fetal heart rate if withdrawal is the underlying problem. Fetal withdrawal may contribute to the increased rate of meconium-stained liquor noted in these pregnancies.

It has been suggested that heroin-using pregnant women may have increased uterine irritability.[5] This may contribute to the increased likelihood of preterm delivery and to shorter lengths of observed labour.

Cocaine use in pregnancy leads to an increased risk of prematurity, placental abruption and intrauterine growth restriction. This may be due to the direct effect of placental blood flow.

Early postnatal effects

Infants who have been exposed to illicit drugs antenatally may show evidence of neonatal withdrawal or intoxication. The clinical signs seen in a baby who has been exposed to opiates in utero indicate withdrawal, whereas those infants exposed to cocaine show signs of intoxication. Many babies have been exposed to a mixture of drugs, such as heroin, methadone and cocaine, along with alcohol and nicotine. The clinical picture is therefore due to a combination of effects. Clinical evidence of opiate withdrawal is more likely if the mother has been using a high dose of methadone or heroin and has taken it within 24 hours of delivery. However, there is marked individual variability, and it can be difficult to predict whether an individual baby will require treatment based on knowledge of the mother's drug use.

Clinical evidence of opiate withdrawal is said to occur in 60–90% of infants of opiate-using mothers. This will depend on the method of ascertainment of at-risk infants plus the criteria for assessing withdrawal. In Bristol, 50% of infants of self-reported opiate users require pharmacological treatment for withdrawal. The signs of opiate withdrawal are central nervous system excitability, gastrointestinal dysfunction and autonomic dysfunction. The initial signs are usually irritability and jitteriness (a stimulus-induced tremor that resolves with passive flexion of the limb). Clinical overt seizures occur in 1–2%, although abnormal electroencephalograms have been reported in more than 30%.[6] Other neurological signs include increased wakefulness, increased tone, a high-pitched cry, and frequent yawning and sneezing. The baby may have snuffles, increased sweating and temperature instability. Early signs of gastrointestinal dysfunction include diarrhoea and frequent feeding with an uncoordinated suck. As the infant becomes sicker he or she may not be able to feed and is at risk of dehydration.

The timing of onset of withdrawal varies from the first to the fourth day of life. Methadone withdrawal tends to occur later than that from heroin because of its longer half-life. It has been our experience that babies requiring pharmacological treatment will do so before the fifth day of life. While clinical signs may persist beyond this time, they are not severe. Infants suffering from neonatal abstinence may continue to have minor symptoms for up to 4 months, making them difficult, irritable babies.

The clinical signs observed in infants of cocaine using mothers relate to continued drug effects. The baby may have abnormal sleep patterns, with increased tone and tremors. Occasionally, seizures occur.

Late effects

The long-term effects of prenatal exposure to opiates or cocaine remain poorly understood. Studies are confounded by polydrug use, prenatal exposure to alcohol or nicotine, environmental factors such as social class, dysfunctional parenting, stability of caregivers and environmental violence.

Animal studies have suggested that antenatal opiates have a structural effect on brain development. Studies in rats have shown a reduction in dendritic arborization and axonal branching in rats exposed prenatally to opiates.[7] While it has been suggested that the brain reward system is permanently altered, work in this area has been inconclusive. Clinical studies have generally shown that infants of drug-using mothers have lower IQs, more behavioural problems and more school failure than controls. This may be due to issues relating to upbringing, as previously discussed, or to a direct drug effect. One study, which attempted to answer this question, compared children born to heroin-using parents and controls, with and without environmental deprivation. The children born to heroin-dependent parents had a lower IQ and higher incidence of hyperactivity and behavioural problems than controls. However, children born to heroin-using parents but adopted at a young age functioned similarly to controls.[8] This suggests that the majority of the developmental problems are environmental rather than in utero drug effects.

The long-term effects of cocaine have caused considerably more concern, with initial suggestions that the long-term effect of prenatal cocaine exposure would be catastrophic. This does not appear to be the case. A recent systematic review concluded that, in children under 6 years of age there is no convincing evidence that prenatal cocaine exposure is associated with developmental toxic effects, which differ from the sequelae of multiple other risk factors.[9] Cocaine appeared to have a specific negative effect on emotional expressiveness; exposed children showed less joy, sadness, arousal or interest.

MANAGEMENT

Antenatal management

The infant of a substance-abusing mother may be disadvantaged in many ways (Fig. 16.1). Substance abusers as a group demonstrate considerable heterogeneity. The drug-using mother varies from a well-controlled, employed professional with good social supports, to someone with chaotic drug use that is funded by prostitution and compounded by potentially abusive family and social contacts. The identification of a pregnant user is highly dependent on the perceived approach taken by professionals in their management. If mothers perceive that they are likely to have their infants removed,

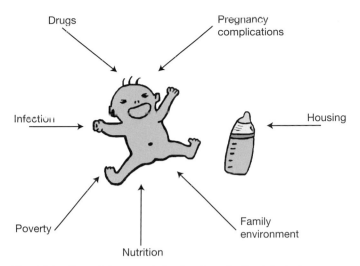

Fig. 16.1 Potential areas of disadvantage for the infant of a substance-abusing mother.

then many will either avoid antenatal care altogether or attend but conceal their drug use.

The goals of antenatal care are to engage the family, stabilize the mother's drug use, assess the areas described in Fig. 16.1 and educate the mother. These are best achieved with a non-judgemental multidisciplinary team. The team should consist of a drugs worker, specialist midwives with community involvement, a social worker, an obstetrician and a paediatrician.

The first goal is to engage the woman in order that good antenatal care may be provided. This may encourage subsequent future cooperation with health and social services staff involved in the care of the infant.

The second goal is to establish the mother's actual drug use and stabilize her on methadone if possible. Methadone is administered orally and has a half-life of 15–40 hours. Achieving control with methadone alone has the advantage of more consistent blood levels of opiate and a reduction in risk behaviour (intravenous injecting and illegal activities to pay for street drugs). Methadone treatment during pregnancy is felt to increase birth weight and head circumference in comparison to infants of those taking illicit drugs. It is not possible to differentiate between a direct pharmacological effect and that of improved maternal lifestyle.

The metabolic changes in pregnancy result in an altered volume of distribution of methadone and hence to lower levels. There are different approaches to methadone prescribing in pregnancy. One approach is to maintain the patient on relatively high levels of methadone, increasing throughout pregnancy in order to reduce the use of illicit drugs in addition. Others will keep the dose constant, thereby allowing the methadone level to fall gradually over the pregnancy. The third approach is to reduce the methadone and attempt to wean off if possible. There is no evidence to suggest which of these approaches is the best. Urine toxicology should be monitored throughout pregnancy in order to assess compliance.

Recently, buprenorphine, an opiate partial agonist, has been used as a treatment for opiate dependence. It readily crosses the placenta and passes into breast milk. It can lead to neonatal abstinence. At the time of writing it is not recommended for use in pregnancy. However, experience with it is increasing, and a number of small studies have shown promising results.[10]

The third goal is assessment, both medical and social. These women are high-risk antenatal patients and require careful monitoring of their pregnancies. They should be offered screening for sexually transmitted diseases, along with human immunodeficiency virus (HIV) and hepatitis B and C. Social services support should be available for help with housing or financial difficulties. While potential child-protection issues should be considered, it is not our practice to refer all identified drug users to social services. If the mother's social circumstances are known and acceptable, she attends regular antenatal care, is stable and has good support, then it may not be necessary to refer her for assessment. If there is any doubt in relation to parenting ability, domestic violence, etc., then referral should be made antenatally.

The antenatal period is a valuable time to educate the mother about the effect of drugs on her and her baby, in addition to education on breast-feeding and parenting, etc. Meeting a paediatrician antenatally to discuss the likely management of the baby after birth can be helpful.

Postnatal management

Although the clinical picture of neonatal abstinence is well recognized by experienced nurses and midwives, it is helpful to use a scoring chart routinely. This will aid consistency in deciding the threshold for starting and adjusting drug treatment. It can be helpful for the mother to see a reasonably objective assessment of her baby. Different scoring systems have been developed, such as those by Finnegan,[11] Ostrea,[12] Lipsitz[13] and Rivers.[14] These systems are based on opiate withdrawal and may not be entirely appropriate for the infant exposed to cocaine alone. A threshold above which drug treatment should be considered should be set. Mild withdrawal can be treated by non-pharmacological means, such as swaddling, cuddling and frequent feeds. It is our practice to treat a baby only if the score is above the threshold value on at least two occasions at least 2 hours apart. The aim of drug treatment is short-term relief of clinical signs. It is unknown whether neonatal treatment has any long-term benefit. Once the baby has been stable for 24 hours with abstinence scores below threshold, the drug dose should gradually be reduced. It is not necessary to wait until the baby is completely asymptomatic.

A number of drugs have been used. Oral morphine is effective in treating opiate withdrawal. The initial dose is 40 µg/kg given 4-hourly. The dose can then be increased or decreased depending on the clinical state. While infants suffering narcotic withdrawal appear to be less susceptible to the respiratory depressant effect of morphine, it is wise to nurse them with an apnoea alarm. Methadone has also been used. It should be started at 0.2 mg/kg 6-hourly until symptoms are controlled, and then 12-hourly. Clonidine is a potentially useful drug as it is an α-adrenoreceptor agonist that decreases sympathetic overactivity, which is felt to be the basis of the withdrawal syndrome. However, there are few data for the neonatal population.

Morphine, methadone and clonidine may be useful in treating opiate withdrawal, but are likely to be less effective for the alleviation of symptoms from other drugs. Chlorpromazine (0.5 mg 6-hourly) may be effective either singly or as an adjunct to morphine or methadone. It may increase the likelihood of seizures, however. Phenobarbitone (15 mg/kg) followed by (5–10 mg/kg once daily) relieves the central nervous system effects of opiate withdrawal but not the other effects. It may be the drug of choice for non-opiate-related clinical signs.

Seizures related to opiate withdrawal should be treated with intravenous morphine, whereas non-opiate related seizures should be treated with phenobarbitone.

Naloxone should never be given to infants of suspected drug abusers, as this will precipitate acute withdrawal.

General

If possible the baby should be kept with the mother, even if drug treatment is required. Bonding can be difficult, as the mother may be suffering from some symptoms of withdrawal herself, may feel guilty and the baby may give little positive feedback if he or she is also withdrawing. Keeping the baby with the mother will also allow assessment of parenting skills.

The baby should be screened for hepatitis B and C, and HIV if appropriate. We offer hepatitis B and BCG vaccinations to all infants of drug users, regardless of the mother's status, as they are at potentially increased risk of exposure to hepatitis B and tuberculosis in the long term.

The issue of breast-feeding should be discussed carefully with each mother, taking into account her HIV and hepatitis C status, use of illicit drugs and level of methadone maintenance. In general, we encourage breast-feeding if the mother is stable on 80 mg/day or less methadone, does not use cocaine, amphetamines or heroin

in addition, and is not HIV positive. There is no evidence that breast-feeding increases the risk of vertical transmission of hepatitis C.

A discharge planning meeting should be held before the mother and baby leave hospital. This should involve the parents, a paediatrician and the health visitor, and a drug worker and social services if indicated. This ensures that all agencies are aware of each other's role and that responsibility for follow-up and immunizations can be established.

CONCLUSION

There is a growing number of pregnant women using illicit drugs in the UK. They and their infants benefit from a coordinated, multidisciplinary approach to antenatal and postnatal care. The mother should be encouraged to stabilize on methadone during the pregnancy. Different units use different approaches, with no good evidence as to which is the most beneficial. It is unacceptable for infants to suffer extreme distress due to neonatal abstinence, and drug therapy should be used appropriately. Adoption studies suggest that the main factor in determining the outcome of these children is their environment of upbringing. Further research is needed into methods of improving the future of these children.

Chapter Seventeen

The role of the paediatrician in reducing the effects of social disadvantage on children

Nick J. Spencer

17

SUMMARY

Globally, poverty is the main determinant of death and poor health in infancy and childhood. In developed countries, although absolute poverty has been eradicated, relative poverty and low socio-economic status are associated with higher risks of death throughout infancy and childhood, higher levels of morbidity, poorer mental health outcomes and poorer educational attainment.[1] As adolescents, those from disadvantaged homes are at greater risk of teenage pregnancy,[2] smoking uptake,[3] truancy and school failure,[4] and criminal behaviour.[5] Socio-economic circumstances have a profound effect throughout childhood and into adulthood.

Paediatricians working with socially disadvantaged children and their families can become frustrated with the barriers to health created by low socio-economic status leading to a fatalistic view of the problem or a tendency to 'blame the victim'. This chapter sets out to explore ways in which paediatricians can help reduce the effects of social disadvantage on children, without becoming disillusioned or fatalistic about the future of poor children.

OVERVIEW OF THE EFFECTS OF SOCIAL DISADVANTAGE ON CHILDREN

In rich nations, children are one of the largest group in social disadvantage, and child poverty has increased in most countries.[6] Between 1979 and 2002, the proportion of UK children living in households with incomes < 60% of the average household income after housing costs rose from 1.9 million (14%) to 3.8 million (28%).[7] Since 1997, the UK government's measures to reduce child poverty, as part of its pledge to eradicate child poverty by 2010, have had some success, but currently available figures indicate that there are still very large numbers of children vulnerable to the effects of social disadvantage.

The social gradient in many child health outcomes is well recognized and well documented. Death is more common in low-income groups in infancy, childhood and adolescence.[1] The social patterning of mortality established in early infancy persists throughout the life course.[8] Low birthweight shows a strong social gradient, as considered later in this chapter. The risk of hospital admission for all causes, multiple admissions and admissions for specific conditions such as bronchiolitis is higher in children from disadvantaged families.

The social patterning of some childhood health-related outcomes is less well recognized and acknowledged. Parenting, the subject of much recent discussion, is strongly influenced by socio-economic circumstances and is sensitive to changes in the economic fortunes of the family.[9] Child abuse and neglect are known to occur in all social groups, but there is strong evidence linking it to social and material disadvantage.[10] Behaviour problems also show a social gradient, with a higher risk of these in disadvantaged children.[11]

Birthweight is a major public health issue, being the main determinant of infant health and a powerful health determinant in adult life.[12] Based on this work, standardized mortality ratios for coronary artery disease associated with birthweight > 3.7 kg have been estimated as 70, compared with 119 for birthweight < 2.5 kg. The extent and significance of the social gradient in birthweight has been underestimated.[13] Figure 17.1 shows the finely graded negative linear relationship between mean birthweight and increasing levels of material deprivation. Thirty per cent of births < 2500 g in the West Midlands could be 'statistically attributed' to social inequalities. In summary, social inequalities have a profound effect on health from birth through-

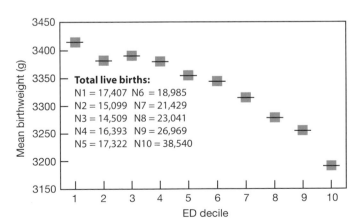

Fig. 17.1 Deciles created by ranking all enumeration districts (ED deciles) in the West Midlands health region by the Townsend Deprivation Index, based on the 1991 census. (ED decile 1, least deprived; ED decile 10, most deprived). (Source: OPCS data 1991, Births data 1991–1993.)

out childhood and into adult life. How can paediatricians contribute to reducing these adverse effects?

PAEDIATRIC STRATEGIES FOR REDUCING CHILD HEALTH INEQUALITIES

Child health inequalities are profoundly influenced by social and political decisions, which are beyond the control of individual paediatricians. Even relatively powerful medical organizations, such as the Royal Colleges and the British Medical Association, may have limited influence on social and health policy that determines the health of the population. The main determinants of striking improvements in child and population health in developed countries, and some less developed countries, this century are changes in living standards and nutrition rather than medical intervention. Wilkinson[14] argues that income distribution within a country is a major determinant of the health of its population. However, paediatricians and other health workers can promote the health of disadvantaged children in a variety of ways, including influencing local and national government.

Although good empirical evidence exists for the social and political policies that improve the health of poor children over a period of time, there is a dearth of evidence supporting health interventions designed to reduce the health effects of social disadvantage. Available evidence is summarized in a review prepared by the NHS Centre for Reviews and Dissemination,[15] but many of the studies provide very weak evidence of effectiveness. More recent work highlights what works in reducing child health inequalities.[16] Many of the strategies suggested below remain unevaluated. This is a limitation that needs to be overcome by further research. However, it should not stand in the way of paediatricians advocating for poor children and employing the proposed strategies.

Strategies for reducing child health inequalities can function at a number of different complementary levels: international, national, local and individual. Paediatricians might choose to focus on one or all of these levels, but will need to be fully informed of the magnitude and extent of health inequalities and committed to a non-victim-blaming approach, which accepts other disciplines and parents as equal partners. Political action and advocacy on behalf of poor families and children by doctors is not new. There is a long and honourable tradition of medical intervention on behalf of individuals and communities.

International strategies

Poverty has a powerful effect on child health in less developed countries. The World Health Organiztion and Unicef have developed a series of interventions aimed at minimizing the effects of poverty on the lives of children: primary preventive strategies include provision of clean water, adequate shelter and immunization against common childhood diseases; and secondary prevention includes measures to reduce the effects of diarrhoeal diseases such as the oral rehydration therapy (ORT) initiative.

The most successful strategies are those employed by governments to reduce income inequalities and improve female education: these have been highly successful in a number of countries, including Kerala State in India, Sri Lanka and Cuba. A recent Unicef report documents a trend in developed countries, with those countries with laissez faire market-based policies (such as the UK, the USA and New Zealand) showing a slowing or reversal of the gains in child health outcomes made during in the 1970s compared with continuing gains in countries, such as France, the Benelux countries and Scandinavia, which have welfare-based policies.[6, 17]

The 1989 UN Convention on the Rights of the Child (UNCRC), ratified by the UK government in 1993, makes specific reference to equity. Article 27 recognizes the right of every child to a standard of living 'adequate for the child's physical, mental, spiritual, moral and social development'. The Convention charges State Parties with providing material assistance and social security for children, and specifically emphasizes the importance of nutrition, clothing and housing (Articles 26 and 27). At the international and national levels, State Parties can be pressurized into addressing these issues, and the Convention can be a valuable advocacy tool. The Royal College of Paediatrics and Child Health (RCPCH) has established an Equity Project jointly with the American Association of Pediatrics. This has educational, practice and research components, and a complete course for health workers on the use of the UNCRC has been one of its first products.

Professor David Southall, Chair of Child Health at the University of Keele, has developed an international child health advocacy strategy that has included intervention on behalf of children in war-torn countries such as Bosnia, Iraq and Afghanistan.[18]

National strategies

In the UK, there is a particularly pressing need for health professionals to take political action on behalf of poor children and their families. Paediatricians need to confront the political nature of the solutions. The present UK government, in contrast to their immediate predecessor, recognizes the role of poverty and social disadvantage in the determination of health outcomes. However, professional groups, including paediatricians, will need to participate actively in the political process to ensure that appropriate child- and family-orientated policies are enacted. An example is the recent change in UK government policy on child care, which has been strongly influenced by the findings of systematic reviews undertaken by paediatricians (among others), demonstrating that good child care enhances child development and educational attainment.

'Healthy alliances' are encouraged by the government. In alliance with national groups such as the National Children's Bureau, Child Poverty Action Group, the Maternity Alliance and National Children's Homes, paediatricians, both individually and through the RCPCH, can bring research data to public attention and contribute to the development of alternative strategies for health gain. The RCPCH has established an Advocacy Committee with the remit of advising it on ways in which it can use its influence to advocate for health gain for children. The RCPCH has also recently appointed a Press and Parliamentary Officer, with a view to improving paediatricians' influence on behalf of children in the corridors of power. A child health advocacy network (CHANT) has been developed that is building alliances as part of its commitment to health gain for UK children.

Some countries have appointed Child Commissioners (in Norway and Sweden, known as Ombudsmen) whose task it is to represent the interests of children and monitor progress of the UN Convention on the Rights of the Child in their country. The British Association for Community Child Health (BACCH) and the RCPCH supported the establishment of Children's Commissioner posts in England, Wales, Scotland and Northern Ireland. The post for England has recently been filled by a leading paediatrician, Professor Al Aynsley-Green. In New Zealand, the Commissioner has been able to bring the needs of poor Maori and Pacific Island children to public attention, and influence policy related to the treatment of ethnic-minority children.

If paediatricians are to promote the health of children, they have to become more than just providers of treatment and care during illness. They must also be advocates for children in order to protect them from forces beyond the control of the individual child and family, which may damage their health and threaten their well-being. Advocacy for children is often limited to representing the child against its parents in child-protection cases. The limitations of this approach are discussed in more detail later, but advocacy can be a much broader concept. This broader concept of advocacy can be illustrated using two specific examples with an important relationship to health inequalities: the prevention of childhood accidents and the provision of affordable and suitable housing for families with children.

Childhood accidents are now the commonest cause of child death beyond the age of 1 year. Road traffic accidents (RTAs) become an increasingly dominant cause of death as children get older. Both RTAs and fatal accidents in the home show a strong social class gradient. Decontextualized health-promotion strategies have concentrated on the education of mothers. Recent evidence shows that health education alone is ineffective in reducing accidents. Strategies that modify the child's environment are needed in order effectively to prevent accidents. The incidence of RTAs is increased by proximity to busy roads, and strategies which separate residential areas and busy roads have proved effective. In the home, reliance on mobile gas and oil heaters, as well as structural problems and overcrowding, are associated with fatal accidents.

In the area of childhood accidents, advocacy must address the social context in which accidents occur. Advocacy might concentrate on the following issues:

- the evidence linking accidents to poor social conditions
- the evidence linking residence in poor areas and proximity to heavy traffic
- the evidence demonstrating the relative effectiveness of environmental change over education strategies
- the evidence linking home accidents to overcrowding, poor housing conditions and inappropriate forms of heating
- lobbying national and local government to modify children's environments using traffic-calming strategies and more long-term strategies that reduce reliance on the private car
- forming healthy alliances with local and national professional groups to influence transport and housing policy locally and nationally
- promote community participation and community diagnosis locally, which can identify from the perspective of community residents the main sources of danger to their children.

An initiative to prevent childhood accidents in Newcastle utilizes some of these approaches to advocacy. Of particular interest is the use made of a survey by local parents that demonstrated a lack of safe crossing points on the children's route to school. These data were used by a multidisciplinary group to lobby for environmental change.

Affordable and suitable housing is almost uniformly recognized as essential for the well-being of families and children. UK government policy over the last 20 years has drastically reduced the stock of affordable housing, and local authorities have been starved of capital for repairs, with the result that there has been an increase in homes that are unfit for human habitation. One result has been a sharp rise in homeless families, who are accommodated at great expense in privately owned hotels and guest houses. This accommodation is insanitary and overcrowded, with whole families living in one room and using inadequate communal washing and toilet facilities. Health workers have contributed to the challenge to government housing policy and have advocated for children living in homeless accommodation.

Paediatricians have a particularly valuable role as advocates for housing improvements. They are in a position to provide the following, which can be used by intersectoral groups and those, such as Shelter, campaigning for the homeless:

- data on the health effects of inadequate housing and homelessness
- data on the health effects of damp and mould
- data on the health effects of overcrowding
- data on the detrimental psychological effects of housing insecurity
- local data on the health hazards of inadequately maintained dwellings
- data collected through community participation related to the health effects of inadequate housing as perceived by the tenants themselves
- expertise to tenants' organizations in setting up surveys, carrying out interviews and data analysis
- support for individual families seeking rehousing on the grounds of poor housing.

Local strategies

The examples of advocacy given above have a strong local component, and the division between national and local may seem rather artificial. However, although national strategies are likely to be informed by locally generated data and strategies, those involved in developing strategies for overcoming health inequalities may not wish to dissipate energies in a national intervention but concentrate on the particular issues faced by poor families living within a specified area. Local communities may prefer to deal with their own problems rather than become part of a larger more impersonal national group. Equally, paediatricians may see their role as advocates on behalf of their local patients, not as national campaigners.

Health workers have considerable influence within localities, with access to data and the media and the power to 'unlock the doors of local power'. In alliance with local people they can influence the health of large groups by arguing for environmental change that will benefit those living in disadvantaged circumstances. A modest example was the intervention of local health workers, health visitors and community paediatricians on behalf of families living in unsuitable accommodation in the centre of Sheffield. Judicious use of the local media, whose interest was prompted by the involvement of health workers, induced the local council to move families to more suitable accommodation.

Community participation and community diagnosis have been mentioned above. These are techniques, initially developed in third world countries, designed to ensure that interventions and solutions, perceived by the community itself as irrelevant or threatening, are not imposed on communities by well-meaning but ill-informed outsiders. Participation has to be as a genuine partnership. The skills and experience of local people have to be respected and regarded as of equal value to those of the professionals. Community diagnosis moves away from the medical model of disease identification in individual patients towards diagnosis by the whole community of the main threats to its health. There are many different models of community participation and diagnosis, and it is inappropriate to prescribe rigid, generally applicable models. Approaches must be flexible and sensitive to the characteristics of the particular community.

These techniques have been applied on a deprived estate in Newcastle to identify the factors perceived by local families as influencing their health.[19] The families themselves identified worries about lawlessness and crime on the estate as the greatest problem, with personal health worries sharing equal importance with housing and the local environment. A health committee has been formed with local residents, and a health forum has been established that has specifically addressed the concerns raised by the local families. Further steps are being taken to develop a family health service more relevant to local needs.

Community-wide strategies for protecting children from harm

Child protection has been dominated by the investigation of child abuse and neglect and the prosecution of perpetrators. In part, this domination is the result of the focus on 'family pathology', with little regard for the societal processes that create the climate and pressures in which abuse of children is likely to occur, so that child abuse is narrowly defined within the confines of the family. Social policies that increase family poverty and impede child rearing are likely to lead to an increase in child abuse and neglect, along with other poverty-associated problems such as teenage pregnancy, school failure and truancy and drug abuse.

Community-wide strategies that foster social support and aim to reduce the overall risk of the whole population by reducing inequalities are likely to be the most effective way of protecting children from harm. However, there is an important role for local health workers and local decision-makers in promoting the development of local community-wide initiatives.

What are the key features of such initiatives? The following is a composite of the features of successful community-wide strategies:

- comprehensive and intensive
- needs-led flexible service rather than service-led service
- family and community orientated
- easily accessible
- staff with the time and skills to develop relationships of respect and collaboration
- social and emotional support, and concrete help with specific requirements
- participation and partnership with associated training and job opportunities
- full use of local resources.

Applying the above principles in practice requires a long-term strategy supported by all child-caring agencies locally and a shift away from crisis management as the main service response to child abuse. Child-protection crises clearly have to be dealt with appropriately, but failure to institute effective preventive strategies offering support to parents struggling with child-rearing in conditions of poverty is ensuring an inexhaustible flow of crises that are overwhelming the child-protection agencies.

Individual-level strategies

Many health workers work mainly with individual children and families, either in clinics or surgeries, or in the family home. Even at this level, strategies for reducing inequalities can be employed. Poor families often experience poor services as a result of the operation of the 'inverse care law'. The powerlessness associated with poverty and deprivation tends to lead to an unequal power relationship between client and health worker, and class, cultural and language barriers can further impede communication. As a consequence, access to good child healthcare may be relatively difficult for poor families, whose children are more likely to need specialist as well as non-specialist child health services.

Strategies at this level for reducing inequalities involve ensuring access of poor families to high-quality child health services. The basic principles are:

- accessible, flexible and relevant services 'free at the time of use'
- locally provided services of high quality, minimizing the financial burden imposed by the need to travel to specialist services
- paediatricians who respect parental skills and treat parents as genuine partners in the care of their children
- paediatricians who recognize the special problems of caring for children in poverty, and modify their case management and treatment regimens accordingly
- paediatricians who carry out non-discriminatory practice, respecting cultural differences and recognizing the 'double jeopardy' faced by ethnic-minority families.

CONCLUSIONS

The question must inevitably arise: With the understanding that we now have of health inequalities and the range of strategies available for reducing them, why are they continuing to widen? The first and most important response is the lack of political will, coupled with an ideological resistance to accepting the existence of relative poverty in society and its effects on health. Health is seen as an individual responsibility, and the health and safety of children the main (sometimes the sole) responsibility of parents, regardless of their material circumstances. As noted above, social policies, punitive to those families dependent on state benefits, are likely to be the underlying reason for widening child health inequalities.

Further barriers to the reduction of health inequalities, although less significant than the lack of political will and government social policies that exacerbate poverty, are organization and attitudes within the health services. The drive for increasing cost-efficiency combined with the 'NHS reforms' is shifting resources from patient care to financial management, and is tending towards a 'two-tier' service that will inevitably disadvantage the poor. Despite declarations of commitment to equity in service delivery, punitive and discriminatory attitudes to the poor and the disadvantaged remain a problem within the health services.

For paediatricians committed to health equality these barriers may seem insurmountable. However, use of some or all of the strategies outlined above will contribute to the pressure for political change and, at the same time, improve the capacity of parents and families to protect and promote the well-being of their children.

Chapter Eighteen

Promoting helpful parenting: the paediatrician's role

Jane Barlow • Sarah Stewart-Brown

SUMMARY

The *National Service Framework for Children, Young People and Maternity Services*,[1] *Every Child Matters: Change for Children*[2] and the public health White Paper *Choosing Health: Making Healthier Choices Easier*[3] all recognize the influence of parenting on the emotional and physical health and well-being of children and young people. Good-quality, timely support for parents is identified as important for improving children's health, and their social and educational development. Paediatricians have a key role to play in implementing such policy initiatives in their clinical work with parents and children, and in planning and developing parenting services in a multisectoral context. This chapter aims to support such implementation by describing the health impact of parenting, together with some of the parenting services of relevance to paediatricians that have been developed and evaluated in the UK.

PRACTICE POINTS

- Parenting is central to children's mental and physical health.
- Paediatricians have an important role to play in promoting helpful parenting:
  - by identifying need and helping parents to access the newly burgeoning range of services designed to support parenting
  - in ensuring the availability of universal and targeted services to support helpful parenting
  - in the development of interagency working between the statutory and voluntary sectors
  - in advocating for social and policy changes to support parents.

INTRODUCTION

A number of recent policy documents, including the *National Service Framework for Children, Young People and Maternity Services*,[1] *Every Child Matters: Change for Children*[2] and the public health White Paper *Choosing Health: Making Healthier Choices Easier*,[3] have all highlighted the importance of parenting for children's healthy development and pointed to the role of paediatricians in all specialities, in supporting parenting.

The aim of the present chapter is to explore the role that paediatricians can play in promoting helpful parenting. The first part describes what is known about parenting and its impact on child health and development. The second part aims to explore the paediatrican's role in a clinical context, describe parenting services developed and evaluated in the UK, and to address the paediatrican's role in developing such services.

PARENTING AND ITS IMPACT ON CHILD DEVELOPMENT

Paediatricians are in a position – in the clinic, in accident and emergency, and on the ward – to observe parents and their relationship with their children. Although these occasions are usually stressful for parents, observing what happens in such situations provides an important window into family life. The paediatrician may observe the level of sensitivity parents show their infants and children, and the extent to which they allow them an age-appropriate role in decision making about their health. They may also observe how parents speak to their children. Do they, for example, talk about them in the third person, do they criticize and belittle them, are they warm and affectionate or rejecting and angry?

Do these things matter? There are three strands of research that suggest that they do. One strand, which originated in the work of John Bowlby in the 1950s, has shown the importance of aspects of the mother–child relationship in infancy: maternal sensitivity and attunement. This research has concentrated primarily on mothers, but indications are that the findings are also applicable to fathers. Sensitivity and attunement allow parents to understand their infants and meet their needs, providing comfort and reassurance. It is also respectful of the infant's needs to explore and develop independence. Infants nurtured in this way become securely attached and internalize a sense that the world is a safe place to be. They learn to self-soothe, and develop resilience to distressing events. In contrast, parenting that is either intrusive and controlling, or unresponsive, leads to various manifestations of insecure attachment. Recent research has also shown that the mother's capacity to be 'mind-minded' (i.e. being able to read her baby's emotions or state of mind) is more important for later development than maternal education or employment.[4] Maternal mental health problems, such as drug abuse and postnatal depression, interfere with the development of such sensitive and attuned parenting.[5]

A further strand of research, being led by biologists and neurodevelopmentalists (including work with animals), has shown that mother–infant relationships in early life influence the architecture of the developing brain. The prefrontal cortex and limbic system (amygdala, hippocampus and cingualte gyrus), areas that regulate emotions, are different in the progeny of 'good' mothers of monkeys and rats. The differences in the brains of inadequately mothered animals are associated with an abnormal hypopituitary–hypthalamic response to stress, and in adult life are associated with behaviours that mimic those seen in children with emotional and behavioural problems.[6, 7] There is now a range of evidence, based on neuroendocrine imaging and post-mortem studies in infants, which confirms that such processes are pertinent to human as well as animal development.[8]

The third strand of research has focused on parenting 'styles' or 'practices' and parent–child relationships, after the first year of life. Lack of warmth, affection and 'positive regard' (thinking well of the child), inconsistent and harsh discipline, and poor monitoring and supervision in mid-childhood, have been shown to play a central role in the development of antisocial behaviour, delinquency, criminality and violence in adolescence.[9] In early and mid-childhood, authoritarian, permissive and neglectful parenting have been shown to predict the development of emotional and behavioural problems and school failure. Authoritarian parenting is restrictive and demanding of conformity above individuality, lacking in warmth and empathy. It can also involve highly punitive discipline practices. Permissive parenting is responsive, accepting and affectionate, but provides insufficient boundaries. Neglectful parents provide neither affection nor boundaries. In contrast, authoritative parenting is responsive, affectionate and provides boundaries in a way that is fair and consistent, and that takes account of the needs of both parents and children.[10]

Although genetic factors and child temperament play some role, parenting styles and practices are thus an unequivocal cause of emotional and behavioural problems and conduct disorder. These are now the most common cause of functional disability in childhood,[11] and their incidence is particularly high in children with chronic disease and other forms of disability, who are likely to be under the care of paediatricians. Children attending outpatient paediatric clinics are twice as likely to have emotional and behavioural problems as children in the general population.[12] Such problems increase the burden of caring for children with health problems, and impact negatively on the lives of siblings.

A number of studies now report an impact of parenting on children's physical as well as emotional health. These have focused on aspects of parenting such as praise, derogation[13] and rejection,[14] as well as early mother–infant interaction.[15] Effects have been demonstrated on 'health in general' as well as asthma.[16] Studies in adolescence suggest a role for parenting in the adoption of unhealthy lifestyles such as cigarette and alcohol use,[17] unhealthy eating[18] and teenage pregnancy.[19] 'Parenting styles' have also been shown to influence cognitive and psychological health in adolescence, with positive parent–child relationships (e.g. praise, encouragement, physical affection, good communication and time spent together) predicting school achievement, social acceptance, close friendships, prosocial behaviour and self-worth (see e.g. Desforges[20]).

Further longitudinal studies show that the health effects of parenting track through into adult life, providing evidence that parenting is predictive of mental health problems (depression, alcohol and drug misuse), psychosocial problems (poor work and marital outcomes, delinquency and criminal behaviour) and physical health (health in general, common physical symptoms and diseases, heart disease and cancer).[21]

Problem parenting is more common among families living in social deprivation, and factors such as poverty, unemployment and marital conflict make the job of parenting more difficult. However, the evidence that parenting and social deprivation are independent risk factors for poor health and social outcomes is strong. While the risk of poor parenting is higher in families living with deprivation, because problem parenting is common and there are many fewer children living in deprivation than not, the majority of children whose health is affected by parenting are not poor. Indeed, some of the studies that have tried to disentangle the effects of parenting and socio-economic stress have concluded that parenting mediates the relationship between poverty and poor outcomes.[22–24] This research suggests that parents who are able to parent well in unpropitious circumstances can protect their children from the effects of deprivation.

PAEDIATRICIAN'S ROLE IN CLINICAL SETTINGS

Recognizing and acting on unhelpful parenting

What then should paediatricians do when they observe unhelpful parenting or its consequences in the families of their patients? Parents are likely to be highly sensitive to criticisms of their parenting, and there is a real risk of interrupting the doctor–parent–patient relationship, and jeopardizing treatment and management of the child's health problem. Parenting practices are not necessarily constant over time, and what goes on in the clinic may be different from what happens at home. Parenting is known to deteriorate in stressful situations, and may therefore be worse during acute illness or exacerbations. It may differ with different children and may also be bidirectional (i.e. it can be influenced by the child's temperament). These factors make it difficult to judge when to intervene and when to do nothing. However, evidence suggests that parents who do receive help and support with their parenting are pleased to have received it,[25, 26] even those who have been referred to programmes under parenting orders.[27]

There are four steps involved in recognizing and acting on unhelpful parenting:

1. Suspecting that unhelpful parenting is playing a role in the child's problems (optimal parenting is probably uncommon, but seriously unhelpful parenting affects 20–30% of families, and frankly abusive or neglectful parenting affects 5–10%; see e.g. Cawson et al.[28]).
2. Gathering evidence from observation and questioning. Recent research has shown that the Strengths and Difficulties Questionnaire (a brief questionnaire that asks parents about their child's strengths and difficulties) can be helpful in this respect.[12]
3. Broaching the subject with parents.
4. Recommending solutions.

The third stage is likely to be the most difficult, but it will be made easier if the paediatrician has developed a supportive, non-judgemental relationship with the parents. For example, the parents need to know that the doctor is impressed with their ability to cope with aspects of their child's disease or disability, or to cope in very unpropitious social circumstances. They also need to feel that the paediatrician is empathetic and supportive. Under these circumstances, parents are more likely to be able to hear what might otherwise be construed as criticism. There is a management adage that suggests that people need to hear five genuinely positive things about their performance before they can accept negative observations in a positive frame of mind. If the subject is broached as information giving, in the same way that comments on treatment are offered, it is more likely to be well received. For example: 'Other parents and researchers have found that this problem gets better if you can do so and so'.

Knowing what services are available locally to help parents develop their parenting and how to direct parents to these services is important. In the next section, we outline the sort of services that may be available. However, the fact that these services are provided in a range of settings (including community and voluntary organizations, family centres, Sure Start programmes and the emerging children's centres), and that provision varies across the country can make it difficult to keep up-to-date information, and requires forward planning. Having to hand a series of resources (books, videos etc.) to show parents, and possibly to loan to them, can be helpful. An important distinction to bear in mind when gathering such information is that between 'support for parents' and 'support for parenting'. Many family services focus on support for parents. Such services help parents to feel less stressed, build their confidence and self-esteem, and help them develop supportive networks. These services play a vital role in support for parenting, but alone they rarely influence parenting styles or practices or improve parent–child relationships. Paradoxically, interventions that aim to support parenting need to be provided in a setting with approaches that support parents as well as supporting parenting.

Developing an awareness of available programmes

Programmes for parents can be divided into those primarily for the parents of infants, and those for parents of toddlers and older children. They can also be divided into those which have been developed primarily for high-risk groups and those that are suitable for all parents. There are fewer programmes and interventions available for the parents of adolescents.

Infant programmes
Home-visiting programmes

Programmes to promote parent–infant relationships are often provided in the home. They may begin during the antenatal period and continue for up to 2 years postnatally. They have been provided with a range of different goals, but many aim to prevent abuse and neglect. Possibly the best known example of a home-visiting programme that aimed to improve parenting is the Elmira home visiting study,[29] in which a group of high-risk women were visited during pregnancy and early infancy by a trained nurse who focused on promoting three aspects of maternal functioning: health-related behaviours during pregnancy and early childhood; the care provided to the children; and maternal personal life-course development. The results of a 15-year follow-up showed that women who were visited by nurses during pregnancy and infancy were significantly less likely to be identified as perpetrators of child abuse and neglect (i.e. 0.29 versus 0.54 verified reports, $p < 0.001$). This effect was greater for women who were unmarried and who were living in deprived households during pregnancy.[29]

The effectiveness of home-visiting programmes in preventing abuse has not been uniform,[30] and this is in part due to the wide variety of programmes being evaluated (i.e. in terms of their frequency and duration), in addition to problems with evaluation, including surveillance bias (e.g. in which more cases of abuse are identified in the intervention arm due to the extra surveillance).

There has been limited evaluation of the effectiveness of home-visiting programmes in the UK, but a recent evaluation of an intensive home-visiting programme that was delivered by specially trained health visitors during the ante- and postnatal period showed improvement in mother–infant interaction, and suggested increased identification of abuse in the home-visited group.[31]

It is important to note that some home-visiting programmes do not aim to improve parent–infant relationships. Many have had more practical aims, such as increasing immunization rates or uptake of well-child check-ups. Some, particularly those provided by volunteers, aim to support parents rather than to support parenting.

Despite the consensus about the deleterious effects of maternal depression on child development, there is still ongoing debate about the value of screening for postnatal depression. There is, however, good evidence that mothers who become depressed can be helped. Cognitive–behavioural therapy and non-directive (Rogerian) counselling have both been shown to improve postnatal depression. These have primarily been delivered in the home. Non-directive counselling involves trained health visitors offering women the opportunity to talk about their feelings to an empathic and non-judgemental professional, and to make decisions based on their own judgements. This intervention has been shown to be effective in improving both maternal depression and the mother–infant relationship.[32]

Group-based approaches

Other approaches that aim to address very early parenting are also being used in the UK. Some, for example NEWPIN, aim to prevent further abuse in families with children on the child-protection register. NEWPIN is a multidimensional, group-based parenting programme comprising an intensive 4-month intervention package that includes three elements: (i) group-based psychotherapy, which aims to draw links between the mother's past and current relationships and present feelings; (ii) supported activities with their children; and (iii) group-work focused on parenting topics. The aim of NEWPIN is to support the development of problem-solving and to work with the mother's strengths. The intervention is based on a partnership model, in which parental expertise about their child is encouraged. This intervention was evaluated with 21 mothers with severe parenting difficulties, including 12 children on the child-protection register. The results show that, following this intervention, 10 out of these 12 children had their names removed from the register, with the two remaining children subsequently returning to the mother's care.[33]

Programmes that have a universal as well as a targeted role include infant massage. This is being taught, by specially trained health visitors, to groups of both high-risk and low-risk parents, with a view to promoting sensitive and empathic caregiving. The potential benefits of this technique include improved bonding, communication, parental competence, fun and awareness through loving touch for the parent, and an improved sense of well-being, relaxation, love, acceptance and security for the infant. Infant massage has been shown to be effective in improving mother–infant interaction in a group of depressed mothers.[34] Infant massage can also be taught individually, and is one of the skills taught in some home-visiting programmes.

The Parents in Partnership Parent Infant Programme (PIPPIN) is a universal parenting programme aimed at promoting parents' emotional preparation for parenthood. PIPPIN is usually delivered by midwives and health visitors as part of antenatal and postnatal classes within the NHS. The PIPPIN programme starts during pregnancy, and continues postnatally with one hospital or home visit following the birth. A total of 35 hours of support is provided for each family through a series of weekly 2-hour group-based sessions that are facilitated by two parent–infant facilitators. The focus of the programme is on parent–infant communication and relationships, as opposed to the 'mechanics' of labour, delivery and infant care. Evidence shows that the PIPPIN programme can improve the psychological health of parents, increase their confidence in their ability to parent, and increase their satisfaction with the couple and parent–infant relationships.[35] PIPPIN is also effective in producing more nurturing child-centred attitudes to infant care.[35]

Other approaches

The Sunderland Infant Programme[36] was developed in the Sure Start at Thorney Close. It is an intervention aimed at the promotion of sensitive parenting through the early identification of attachment problems. Health visitors undertake a videotape recording of a 3-minute period of mother–child interaction during the early postnatal period. The aim is to identify mothers who are 'controlling' or, alternatively, 'unresponsive' in their caregiving. Mothers who are identified as having problems of this nature are provided with 'developmental guidance' and/or 'interaction guidance' by a specially trained health visitor, through feedback of the previously videotaped interaction. Parents who are identified as having more significant problems are offered parent–infant psychotherapy. Therapists work with both the mother and her infant to address issues such as trauma and loss, and maternal attachment. This often involves discussing the mother's own experiences of being parented, with a view to helping her develop a more 'mindful' approach to parenting. The results of a controlled study showed that mothers in the intervention arm were significantly more sensitive and that infants were more cooperative.[36]

The Peers Early Education Programme (PEEP) is one of a number of UK-based Early Years Education programmes that aim to help parents to encourage their children's early learning and cognitive development. This particular intervention consists of a home visit to all families with new babies living in deprived areas, following which parents are invited to attend weekly group sessions where they are offered mutual support and group-based interactive activities with infants. These activities include sharing a book every day, songs and rhymes, listening games, playing with shapes, and belonging to the library. PEEP also provides resources for parents to use at home, and endeavours to link up with families who are not able to attend groups. This intervention is effective in improving verbal comprehension, vocabulary, concepts about print, phonological awareness, writing, early number concepts and self-esteem.[37]

Toddlers and school-age children programmes
Group-based parenting programmes

Group-based parenting programmes are one of the main interventions available to develop parenting skills and address children's emotional and behavioural problems. Some parenting programmes have been developed for high-risk parents and some have been developed as part of a universal approach. A number of systematic reviews show that these programmes are effective in improving parenting practices, and children's emotional well-being and behaviour problems in both older (i.e. 3–10 years) and younger (i.e. 1–3 years) children.[38] Parenting programmes are also effective in improving maternal psychosocial health.[39] There are two main types of parenting programme.

Behavioural programmes are based on social-learning theory and aim to help parents to use positive methods of dealing with children's behaviour (i.e. ignoring bad behaviour and praising good behaviour). These programmes are targeted at parents whose children have behaviour problems, but are also helpful to parents whose children do not have overt behaviour problems.[26] Relationship programmes include all the non-behavioural programmes (i.e. adlerian, psychodynamic, communications, etc.), and help parents to recognize the reasons for children's behaviour, to become more effective listeners, and to reflect on the way in which they were parented and how this has influenced their own parenting practices. These programmes are usually suitable for all parents, but can also be helpful in high-risk groups.

Some of the programmes use both behavioural and relationship approaches. Programmes currently available in the UK include the Parent and Child Series,[40] Family Links Nurturing Progamme,[41] Family Caring Trust[42] and the Triple-P Parenting Programme.[43] There is an increasing body of evidence showing that both high-risk and low-risk parents enjoy and value these programmes and that they want more provision.

Other approaches

First-level preventive services for high-risk parents can take a number of forms, such as primary child mental healthcare clinics[44] and primary mental health teams.[45] The primary child mental healthcare clinics have been established as part of a community child and family mental health service based at six local GP practices, and comprise on-site clinics that are aimed at helping children with emotional and behavioural difficulties, and their families. The clinics are run by child mental health specialists and involve direct clinical work, case discussions, joint assessments and clinical advice to practice staff.

This educational project also comprises a fortnightly consultation service for day-nursery officers with a member of the mental health service team. This provides nursery staff with the opportunity to discuss their concerns about an individual child with someone who can give them specialist advice. An evaluation of this service is currently being conducted.

Leicestershire Child and Adolescent Mental Health Service have developed a new role of Primary Mental Health Worker (PMHW), whose main tasks are consultation, liaison, direct work and training of primary care staff. The Primary mental health team comprises 13 PMHWs and is an integral part of a comprehensive child and adolescent mental health service. The PMHWs support and enable primary care professionals in their work with mental health issues in children and families, thus promoting early recognition and management of child mental health problems and filtering of appropriate referrals for specialist CMHS intervention. Early findings suggest that this service decreases referrals to specialist services, deals with less complex problems, and supports primary care staff through consultation and training.[45]

Population-based approaches

The interventions described above have been evaluated and shown to be promising in a UK setting. Many other approaches that may also be worthwhile have not yet been formally evaluated. These include telephone helplines for parents, magazine articles, newsletters, books, videos and the increasing number of television programmes on parenting. The extent to which these approaches impact on parenting in individual families is largely unknown, but they are very likely to help by raising the profile of parenting and its importance, and by helping to create the belief that parents are not powerless and that they can have a positive influence on outcomes for themselves and their children.

Multiagency working, and promoting increased coordination and access to provision

The optimal model in terms of supporting parenting, including the prevention of neglect/abuse and emotional and behavioural problems, is now recognized to include both universal and targeted provision.[2, 3] While current government policy proposes universal support of the sort outlined in the above section on population-based approaches, given the wide range of outcomes that are potentially susceptible to improvement in parenting, and the evidence suggesting that optimal parenting is relatively rare, there are strong arguments for suggesting that group-based parenting programmes should be on offer to parents on an open-access or universal invitation basis beginning during pregnancy, and continuing throughout childhood. Such provision would provide a valuable backdrop to targeted provision for at-risk families,[43, 46] improve uptake of other parenting services by families who are unlikely to attend group programmes, and maximize the use of scarce resources. A recent survey[47] showed considerable geographical variation in the levels of services available to families, and identified significant gaps in provision at a national level, particularly with regard to support for families of children over 5 years old.[47] The survey also showed the need for greater coordination of service provision.[47]

A substantial proportion of family services are currently provided by the voluntary sector on uncertain funding, with some being funded (in part) by local authorities.[47] There is, therefore, a need for increased partnership working between statutory and voluntary (i.e. non-government) organizations.[46]

THE BROADER ROLE OF PAEDIATRICIANS

Paediatricians are well placed to take a lead in terms of being advocates for service development and ensuring the multiagency working that will allow wide access to the services that support the development of helpful parenting. Indeed, the absence of their voice in this debate is a deterrent to service development. At present, services are patchy, but they are growing rapidly (40% of services have been established in the last 5 years[47]). The emerging consensus in relation to parenting support is that effectiveness depends on the skills of the providers, and there is a great need for investment in and attention to the development and training of professionals and others who want to develop skills to help parents.[44, 46] This may include ensuring that such training and development is available for health visitors, midwives, school nurses and others who are well placed to provide them.

Paediatricians can also advocate for changes to social and health policy. This could include aspects of policy that would make the job of parenting less difficult. For example, a reduction of child poverty through social-security reform, improved child care and leave arrangements for parents, and transformations to midwifery and health visiting services.[48] The promotion of change to the legislative framework might include promoting children's rights, such as the prohibition of physical punishment. Changes of this nature will ultimately promote the development of a culture in which children are valued and their rights respected.

CONCLUSION

Parenting is now recognized to play a central role in the health and development of children. Paediatricians have a key role to play in helping parents recognize and value helpful parenting, and in directing them to services that could help them improve the way they parent. They also have a role to play in ensuring the development and coordination of these services, in promoting interagency working, and in advocating for the social- and health-policy initiatives that would support the development of helpful parenting.

Chapter Nineteen

Cot death: responsibilities of the paediatrician

Christopher J. Bacon

SUMMARY

When a baby dies unexpectedly at home, the paediatrician has a very important role to play, both in helping to investigate the cause of the death and in supporting the family. In 2004, the working group set up by the Royal College of Pathologists and the Royal College of Paediatrics and Child Health (The Kennedy Committee) recommended that every area should designate a paediatrician for this role, but implementation has been patchy. This work is invaluable for the families, and is professionally rewarding; it takes up little extra time, although availability poses problems. A multidisciplinary approach that includes cooperation with the coroner and the police is essential.

PRACTICE POINTS

- A paediatrician should be designated in each area to take on responsibility for dealing with cot deaths.
- The main objectives are to investigate the cause of the death and to ensure proper support for the family.
- Tasks include a home visit soon after the death, briefing of the pathologist, and holding a case discussion as soon as all details are available.
- A balance is needed between medical and forensic investigation, so it is essential to work in cooperation with the police and the coroner.

INTRODUCTION

In 2004, the Kennedy report[1] strongly reiterated the recommendation, first made in 1985 by the then British Paediatric Association and the Foundation for the Study of Infant Deaths (FSID), that a paediatrician, to be termed 'the SUDI paediatrician', should be designated in each health district to have responsibility for all aspects of sudden unexpected death in infancy (SUDI). In some places such a scheme has worked well, but in many others it has never really got started or has fallen into abeyance, and families report very variable experience of the support they receive from paediatricians.[2] Some paediatricians argue that they have more than enough to do dealing with children who are sick, and that dealing with babies who have died unexpectedly at home is not their concern. However, I would maintain that cot death is very much part of a paediatrician's business, on several counts:

- Paediatricians are best equipped to undertake the difficult and complex task of identifying the many possible causes of sudden infant death.
- Paediatricians have a responsibility to safeguard other children in the family, including those yet unborn, when unexpected death has arisen from inherited disease, such as a disorder of metabolism, or from covert maltreatment.
- Paediatricians are experienced in ensuring that bereaved families get all the support that they need, both immediately and when the next baby is born. A family whose baby dies unexpectedly at home may not otherwise receive the support from the paediatric team that routinely follows a death in hospital.
- The greatest reduction in postneonatal infant mortality in recent years has resulted from research led by paediatricians into risk factors for sudden infant death syndrome (SIDS). Further reductions should now be achievable.

Of course not everyone will have an interest in cot death or the time to pursue it. However, it seems reasonable to expect that in each health trust one person, who will often be a general or community paediatrician, should be designated to take on special responsibility for cot death. This person will need to have one foot in the hospital and in one in the community. This may be more difficult in those areas where hospital and community paediatrics are sundered into separate trusts, but should still be possible given good professional cooperation. There is something to be said for combining responsibilities for cot death and for child protection.

NUMBERS INVOLVED

The role has become more feasible now that the number of cot deaths in England and Wales has fallen to below 300 per year. For the purposes of this chapter, 'cot death' is taken to mean all sudden unexpected deaths in infancy, both the minority for which a cause is found, and the majority that remain unexplained and are classified as SIDS or as 'unascertained'. In 2003, the latest year for which figures are available, the Office for National Statistics recorded 175 sudden infant deaths and a further 117 infant deaths registered as 'unascertained'. This means that even large health trusts are unlikely to have more than four or five cot deaths a year, so the workload for SUDI paediatricians should not be excessive. On the other hand, by definition, the work will be unpredictable and will demand immediate attention, so that routine duties will have to be shelved or delegated at short notice. This will require colleagues to accept that this task merits the same overriding priority as other unforeseeable paediatric emergencies. Smaller trusts might combine to share the same team, and cover arrangements would be needed for sickness and holidays.

RESPONSE TO COT DEATH

The Kennedy report[1] detailed recommendations on how we should respond to cot death. These recommendations build on those arising from the study of SUDI carried out between 1993 and 1996 as part of the Confidential Enquiry into Stillbirths and Deaths in Infancy (CESDI),[3] which is the largest and most comprehensive study of its kind yet undertaken in the UK. There are two main requirements in the aftermath of a cot death: the need to investigate the cause of death, and the need to support the family. These requirements are of equal importance and must be pursued in parallel, neither being overemphasized to the detriment of the other. Combining the two may at times seem uncomfortable, but families will accept the need for full investigation – and indeed will usually welcome it – so long as they are given enough explanation and support.

ROLE OF THE SUDI PAEDIATRICIAN

To meet the requirements, the SUDI paediatrician will need to take the following steps:

1. Make sure that there is a notification system that will inform him or her of any unexpected infant death in his or her area in less than 48 hours. The system will need to tap all sources that might first learn of the unexpected death of a baby, such as GPs, health visitors, the ambulance service, accident departments, paediatricians, mortuary attendants, pathologists and coroner's officers.

2. Ensure that the accident departments to which cot death victims may be taken are properly versed in how to manage the situation, and in particular in how to cope with the family (FSID has produced a very helpful leaflet for this purpose). Some SUDI paediatricians will want to be called immediately, regardless of the time, so that they can become involved and meet the parents soon after they have come into the accident department. Sometimes a death is certified at home and the body is taken straight to a mortuary rather than to a hospital. It will then be more difficult for the paediatrician to become immediately involved and to provide early support. If this is a frequent problem, it may be necessary to try and persuade GPs of the advantages of always sending cot death victims to the hospital, as recommended in the Kennedy report.

3. Arrange to visit the home of the bereaved family as soon as possible after the death, preferably within 48 hours, for the purpose of gathering information and initiating support. Experience in the CESDI SUDI study showed that families welcome such an early visit, and that the traditional practice of waiting until later is mistaken. A home visit is far more acceptable than a consultation in the accident department or the paediatric clinic, which most families find alien, rushed and unrelaxed. The SUDI paediatrician should preferably make this home visit himself; alternatively, it might be made, under his direction, by a specially trained health visitor or community paediatric nurse. Although it might seem simpler for the family's usual health visitor to make this visit, this extremely difficult task requires special training and experience. It is helpful if the family's health visitor can make the introduction. The Kennedy report includes a checklist of all the information that should be gathered, but the family must be allowed time to tell the story in their own way and at their own pace, and to ask the questions that are teeming in their minds. All this will take at least an hour, sometimes much longer. Before leaving, the paediatrician (or specialist nurse) must ensure that the family is put in touch with people who can support them, for example through the FSID's network of befrienders.

4. Assemble all relevant records about the baby and the family. These will include maternity, paediatric and accident department notes, as well as any records from the GP and the health visitor, and sometimes from the social services. The child-protection register should also be consulted.

5. Compile, from the information obtained at the home visit and from the previous records, a full briefing for the pathologist who is doing the post-mortem. Pathologists will tell you that the single most helpful item in elucidating the cause of an unexpected infant death is a good history. This report must be produced very rapidly; it may sometimes be better to delay the post-mortem for 24–48 hours to ensure that it is complete. Liaison between the SUDI paediatrician and the pathologist is invaluable; there should be no problems here when the local paediatric pathologist is involved, but there may be more difficulty when a forensic specialist is called in.

6. Attend the post-mortem examination. Direct discussion with the pathologist sometimes throws up new ideas about the death. It also promotes future liaison, helping to ensure that the most suitable pathologist does the post-mortem and that the recommended protocol is followed.

7. Organize and chair a case discussion as soon as all the results of pathology investigations are available, which will usually be about 6 weeks after the death. Participants should always include the GP, the health visitor and the pathologist, and sometimes other professionals such as a midwife or social worker. Attendance by the primary care team is essential, so the meeting should be held at a time and place that best suits them. The agenda should include all the antecedents and circumstances of the death, possible causes and contributory factors, lessons for professionals and for carers, and support for the family, both in their present bereavement and for when they have another baby. Sometimes the complete picture of a death only becomes clear when all those who know the family have met to join up their pieces of the jigsaw.

8. Cooperate with the police and coroner throughout. Because this is an important and contentious issue, it is discussed at greater length below.

9. Oversee the implementation of the CONI (Care of the Next Infant) scheme within your area.

10. Participate in collaborative studies of cot death. Following the reduction in incidence, research can yield meaningful results only if data are aggregated.

COOPERATION WITH THE POLICE

Now that cot deaths are fewer, concerns about the proportion that result from maltreatment have come to the fore.[4] It is impossible to be certain how large this proportion is, but the best estimate is likely to come from large-scale studies that are population based and consider this question systematically. The CESDI SUDI studies, which meet these criteria, suggest that the figure may be between 5% and 10%.[3] Anxiety is heightened by the evidence that parents who kill one baby may go on to harm another if they are not identified.[5] Because of these concerns, in some parts of the country the police and forensic pathologists are taking over the investigation of all sudden infant deaths, natural and unnatural alike. Such a predominantly forensic approach brings the serious risk that causes of natural deaths, which still constitute the large majority, may not be adequately explored, and that families may be treated inappropriately.

The Kennedy report recommends a collaborative interagency approach, involving a paediatric pathologist in most cases. Paediatricians are in the best position to ensure that the medical and humanitarian aspects of cot death are given sufficient emphasis, that there is a proper balance between forensic and medical investigation, and that the families receive appropriate advice and support. However, the paediatrician will only be able to achieve these goals if he or she cooperates with the police and coroners. If the paediatrician tries to work independently, he will provoke antagonism and be ignored. They should not be deterred by the vagaries of the media, which at one moment call for more thorough investigation and at the next castigate those who carry it out. Some paediatricians may regard liaison with the police and coroner as uncomfortable, and perhaps inappropriate for a doctor, although the procedures for child protection provide a precedent that is now well accepted. Discussions with the General Medical Council (GMC) and with the Medical Defence Union suggest that there would be no ethical objection if the doctor is acting with the coroner's authority, and if his cooperation with the police is made clear to the parents from the outset. The parents could then choose not to talk to him, but experience suggests that this would not happen often.

The exact form that this cooperation takes will vary from place to place, since neither coroners nor police forces follow central direction but make individual arrangements within their patch. The SUDI paediatrician will need to introduce himself to the coroners in his area and to the senior police officers responsible for the investigation of infant deaths. Following recent publicity several police forces are now devising new procedures, and paediatricians may need to move fast to influence their shape before they become established. In some areas, for example, it is usual for the home visit and collection of information after any cot death to be done entirely by police officers, with no input from a health professional. Since most cot deaths result from natural causes, this cannot be appropriate. In other areas a paediatrician and a police officer make the visit together, a practice commended in the Kennedy report. In some police forces the investigation of cot deaths is carried out by officers from their child-protection or family-liaison units, who are experienced in dealing with sensitive family issues and in working jointly with other agencies. This seems a helpful development.

In the wake of the Laming report,[6] it has been proposed that each area should have multidisciplinary child death review teams. Such teams could provide the mechanism for ensuring that all cot deaths are investigated in the comprehensive and standard manner recommended in the Kennedy report. FSID, widely regarded as the champion of bereaved parents, has for some time been campaigning for better investigation of all cot deaths, which would then be categorized as SIDS only after the most thorough scrutiny. Surveys show that most parents would accept this as long as the reasons were explained. For families the overriding need is to find out why their baby died. More thorough investigation would also help remove the stigma that has sometimes been attached to the term SIDS. Ideally, the SUDI paediatrician would build a relationship with his opposite number in the police that ensured cooperation and consultation at every stage. If they visited the home separately they should confer about the information obtained and its interpretation. Similarly, they should cooperate in the collation and interpretation of the medical records, and in the provision of the report to the pathologist.

Paediatric participation from the outset should help to head off misguided police action after a death that the paediatrician could readily identify as natural, and to ensure that the family was always treated and supported in an appropriate manner. On the other hand the paediatrician must accept that the police have a responsibility to investigate any death that might be unnatural, and that the distinction between natural and unnatural often cannot be made for some time – sometimes never. This dilemma calls for extraordinary skill and sensitivity on the part of everyone involved. There might be advantages if a police officer routinely attended the subsequent case discussion; this would follow the precedent of child protection, and would help to build mutual experience and trust.

There is a danger that recent high-profile court cases and GMC hearings will deter people from getting involved in this kind of work. It is vital for effective child protection that paediatricians do not shy away. They will not incur credible criticism so long as they are always careful to take a balanced approach and do not express opinions that go outside their expertise or beyond our limited knowledge of covert homicide in infancy.

COOPERATION WITH THE CORONER

The position of the coroner, who has statutory oversight of the investigation of unexpected death at any age, is crucial. The Coroners' Society takes a keen and well-informed interest in infant deaths, but the Society, although it may make recommendations, is not in a position to determine the behaviour of individual coroners, who enjoy a large measure of independence. It is therefore sensible for the SUDI paediatrician to meet the coroners in his area and discuss how they would like cot deaths to be handled. Some coroners may need to be persuaded of the advantages of a joint investigation by health professionals and police. Others may need no persuasion, and may wish to be kept informed at all stages, receiving a copy of the paediatrician's initial assessment in addition to the report of the pathologist, and even perhaps chairing the case discussion.

Doctors might feel more comfortable in cooperating with the police if they knew they had the coroner's approval. It is the coroner who chooses the pathologist, and the paediatrician may need to remind him tactfully of the advantages, as spelt out in the Kennedy report,[1] of instructing a paediatric pathologist for cot deaths. Unfortunately, there are not yet enough of them to do all the cot death autopsies throughout the country, but undoubtedly they could do more if coroners were so persuaded and referrals to specialist centres were more frequent. If a general or forensic pathologist has to be chosen, it should be one who has had at least some paediatric training. The SUDI paediatrician is also well placed to ensure, in consultation with the coroner, that parents are routinely asked whether they are willing for tissues to be retained after the autopsy for the purposes of later investigation and for research.

RESOURCES AND PRIORITIES

There seems no immediate prospect that extra money will be forthcoming to fund the role of SUDI paediatricians. However, people in many parts of the country are doing the work already, regarding it as one of their more important responsibilities. Ultimately it is a question of priorities. The Royal College of Paediatrics and Child Health has endorsed the Kennedy report in principle, but has expressed reservations (which some would regard as niggardly) about the extra resources required. Meanwhile I hope this chapter may encourage individuals working in an area where there is no SUDI paediatrician to consider taking on the task. They would find it as interesting and rewarding as anything else they do. Above all, failure by paediatricians to become involved will do families a great disservice.

Chapter Twenty

Bereavement support following sudden and unexpected death in children

Andrea Nussbaumer • Robert I. Ross Russell

SUMMARY

Dealing with families who have suffered a sudden and unexpected death is a skill that may be needed by any paediatrician. Offering a bereavement follow-up meeting to such families is part of accepted practice, and is perceived to be of value in helping the family to come to terms with the loss. Unfortunately, there is very little guidance on the objectives for such a meeting, or the training required to help staff conduct such meetings.

In developing such a programme, staff need to understand the basic theories of grief, as well as have a practical approach to their objectives during any meeting. This should include consideration of the best timing for any meetings, information sharing, sibling support, ward visits and pathological reactions.

PRACTICE POINTS

- Morbidity following child bereavement is substantial.
- Siblings may be more affected, and for longer, than adults.
- Objective evidence of benefit from bereavement programmes is poor.
- A structured approach to bereavement meetings may help.

INTRODUCTION

The death of a child is unlike any other loss. Regardless of the age of the child, it is one of the most traumatic experiences a family can suffer.[1, 2] This is particularly true when the death is sudden and unexpected.[3] Its impact on relatives (and particularly the mother[3, 4]) is often more pronounced than that of a death after a prolonged illness, during which they have had time to prepare themselves. Many units provide support for families in this situation, but there are few data to guide the best way of providing support or defining the specific aims of a bereavement programme. In this chapter we reflect on such information as is available, and set out suggestions for the key elements of such a programme.

THE PROBLEM

There are several specific features of sudden and unexpected death that affect the ability of a family to adjust. The most obvious issue is the lack of preparation. This requires families rapidly to assimilate information about the cause of death and the care that their child may have been receiving at a time when they are emotionally unable to do so. Not surprisingly, people who are suddenly bereaved often require more support and counselling than those who have known for some time that their relative is dying, yet they usually receive less.[5] Secondly, unexpected deaths

will usually occur in hospital, either in a resuscitation room or in an unfamiliar high-dependency or intensive care unit (ICU).[6] This adds to the confusion and isolation of families, who may well be (at the time) poorly supported by friends and relatives.

How information about the illness or death is delivered will also have a lasting effect on family and friends, and may affect their ability to come to terms with the death.[5] In unexpected death, for example in the resuscitation room, there is often very limited time and space to take families through any careful discussion or interview. Active resuscitation may be going on in front of the parents or siblings, who often do not want to leave the scene.[7, 8] Indeed, there is some evidence that being present at resuscitations may help in long-term recovery,[9] but it certainly impinges on any possibility of quiet discussion. Similarly, in the ICU, decisions about critically ill children, and the management of the dying process make important differences to the families involved.[10]

BEREAVEMENT THEORY

It is important to distinguish between the terms 'grief', 'mourning' and 'bereavement.'[1] Grief is the normal process of reacting both internally and externally to the perception of loss. Different types of reaction may be seen, which may present in a number of different ways (Table 20.1). Mourning is the process by which people adapt to a loss. Different cultural customs, rituals or rules for dealing with loss may be followed, and are influenced by one's society. Bereavement is the period after a loss during which grief is experienced and mourning occurs. To be bereaved implies being robbed or deprived of something or someone of value. The length of time spent in a period of bereavement is dependent on the intensity of the attachment to the deceased, and how much time was involved in anticipation of the loss. Mortality in parents following the death of a child, from both natural and unnatural causes, has been shown to increase.[4]

Table 20.1 Different elements of grief reaction

Type of reaction	Reactions seen
Psychological/emotional	Anger, guilt, anxiety, sadness, despair
Physical	Sleep difficulties, appetite changes, somatic complaints
Social	Feelings about taking care of others, desire not to see friends or relatives, work avoidance

The classic work of Kübler-Ross[11] and Parkes[12, 13] describes the phases in the process of grief resolution. These phases do not necessarily occur in a given order and may take many years to complete. Initial shock and disbelief is usually followed by expressions of grief such as anger, guilt and somatic complaints. The phase of disorganization and despair is typified by feelings of emptiness and depression. Many parents experience a loss of meaning in their life. The final phase of reorganization suggests recovery from the loss. However, Parkes[12, 13] acknowledged that, in part, parents may never fully recover from the loss of a child, and that they learn to cope with rather than 'get over' their loss. The American psychologist William Worden adds to this model the concept of tasks of mourning, which relate to each of the phases.[14] This encourages both mourner and helper to recognize the potential for aiding the grief work. At the same time, the idea of a task suggests a necessary degree of resolution before the next phase can be negotiated and the whole process can be successfully completed.

Research has shown that the loss of a child through death is a unique and particularly intense type of grief, more severe than other types of bereavement, and it results in symptoms that last longer and present a wider variety of serious symptomatology. Researchers have suggested that all stages of development, from infancy through adolescence and beyond, are equally difficult stages during which to lose a child.[15] Despite the devastating nature of parental loss, research also suggests that appropriate professional intervention at the time of loss can significantly improve the chances of successful grief resolution.

COMPLICATED GRIEF

Complicated or pathological grief reactions are maladaptive extensions of normal bereavement. Grief that becomes pathological is often identifiable by the increased duration of symptoms, the increased disruption of psychosocial functioning due to the symptoms, or by the intensity of symptoms (e.g. intense suicidal thoughts). Risk factors for pathological grief include suddenness of loss, gender of the bereaved,[16] and the existence of an intense, overly close or highly ambivalent relationship to the deceased.

GENERAL ASPECTS OF GRIEF THERAPY

There is a growing body of evidence suggesting that bereaved persons whose grief and pain are not addressed may become 'secondary victims', as they are more at risk of a variety of problems, such as severe mental disorders, alcohol abuse and violence.[5] Many centres have therefore advocated and developed programmes for supporting families in this situation.[17–23] Similarly, dealing with families who have suffered a sudden and unexpected death is a skill that may be needed by any paediatrician,[18] yet many doctors and nurses feel inadequately trained to deal confidently with the bereaved. Few guidelines on either the structure or the process of support are available, and a clear understanding of the objectives of a bereavement support programme is difficult to achieve. To be effective, hospital staff must be knowledgeable about the parental and sibling grief process, the effects of the grief experience on the family, and the kind of interventions that are helpful in facilitating resolution of grief.[10, 15] Part of the solution is the development of adequate communication skills.

Most of the support that people receive after a loss comes from friends and family, but physicians and nurses can identify and orchestrate mechanisms for support and healing and make an important difference. Gudmundsdottir et al.[20] have studied the habits and practices developed by families following the unexpected death of a child, and offer helpful advice on the manner in which the death is assimilated into that family's experiences. For those who are experiencing particularly difficult problems in their bereavement, specific interventions may be considered. All interventions by staff will influence the overall grief reactions during this difficult and critical phase,[1] and of course cultural and religious backgrounds are important considerations in dealing with the bereaved family.[17] Guidelines on the key elements of a bereavement service have been published, which may help units develop such services (Box 20.1).[18]

BOX 20.1

Proposed key elements of a bereavement programme[1]

- Bereavement meetings should be delayed for 8–12 weeks following the death of a child.
- All new information should be discussed with the family, and an opportunity given to review any of their clinical questions or concerns.
- Issues related to childhood death, such as support for siblings or professional help needed by families, should be specifically discussed.
- Revisiting the ward where a child died can be of particular importance, especially if some family members were unable to visit during the child's illness.
- Staff undertaking bereavement meetings need to recognize signs of 'pathological' grief.

AT THE TIME OF DEATH

Bereavement support needs to start at the time of death or even before.[18] Some units maintain prepared packs to give to all bereaved families, containing a leaflet explaining the processes that follow death (including post-mortem examinations, referral to the coroner, registering the death, etc.) as well as a selection of leaflets from bereavement support groups.[18] Chaplains can assist in comforting parents, extended family, friends and hospital staff.[5] A separate private room to mourn should be available. Whenever possible, representatives of the family faith should be contacted and asked to assist the family. Appropriate religious rituals should be offered.[5]

AFTER THE DEATH

After the death of a child the relatives may have many questions to ask, and they may want to return to the hospital to discuss these with the doctor or nurse who cared for their child. This may be an important step in the grieving process.

Delaying the meeting

Cook et al.[18] found that bereavement meetings may work better if delayed for 8–12 weeks following the death. Information that may have been unavailable at the time of death (e.g. post-mortem results or other blood results) should be accessible prior to a meeting. The delay allows families time to reflect on the events surrounding the death, and to generate questions that they need clarifying. Delaying for too long, however, can cause its own problems. Families can feel uninformed and excluded, and this can generate anger towards the hospital.

Sharing of questions and of information

This is a critical element of the bereavement interview, which needs to include all new information that has become available as well as providing an opportunity to review any clinical questions or concerns. Frequently, reassurance is wanted that the family themselves are not to blame for the death (e.g. by not taking their child to hospital earlier). Anger is common, and in some situations it is essential that this anger (and the questions that underpin the anger) is resolved before grief can be progressed. Similarly, particular circumstances associated with the death may be important.[22] Children who have donated organs or those in whom care was electively withdrawn may raise very specific anxieties in the family after their death.

Visiting the ward

For children who die in hospital, coming back to the hospital (especially if it is not their local hospital) can be very traumatic for their family. It can be helpful to meet the family at a distance from the area where their child died, but revisiting that area can be of particular importance, especially if some family members were unable to visit during the child's illness. For these people, the visit to the wards can be an essential part of their memory of their child's last illness.

Issues related to childhood death

Support for siblings or professional help needed by families should be specifically discussed. Discussing the reaction of siblings and offering advice or the names of specific support groups may be of benefit, as are specific days each year for bereaved siblings to come together and to discuss issues that may be worrying them.

Identifying pathological reaction

This can be a very difficult element of any meeting. The range of 'normal' reactions to grief is vast. In the course of a 1–2 hour meeting it can be very difficult to clarify the 'abnormality' in any individual. Prolonged grief, excessive depression or unresolved anger may all be seen, and might prompt further discussion with other carers, such as the person's GP.

SUPPORTING THE BEREAVED SIBLING

Controlled studies based on population samples have confirmed that bereaved children have a significantly increased risk of developing psychiatric disorders, and may suffer considerable psychological and social difficulties throughout childhood and even later in adult life.[18] A child's grief may appear more intermittent and brief than that of an adult, but in fact it usually lasts longer because children cannot rationally explore all their thoughts and feelings as adults can. In addition, children often have difficulty articulating their feelings about grief. Support for these children may need to be addressed repeatedly at different developmental and chronological milestones. Since bereavement is a process that continues over time, children will revisit the loss repeatedly, especially during significant life events.

Several factors can influence a child's grief. This includes (amongst others) the child's age, previous experiences with death, stability of family life, parental styles of coping with stress, and the availability of consistent relationships with other adults. There are interventions that may help to facilitate and support the grieving process in children.

Explanation of death

This should be kept as simple and direct as possible. Each child needs to be told the truth, with as much detail as can be comprehended at his or her age and stage of development. Questions should be addressed honestly and directly. Children need to be reassured about their own security.

Correct language

Any discussion about death must include proper words(e.g. 'cancer', 'died', 'death'). Euphemisms (e.g. 'passed away', 'he is sleeping', 'we lost him') should not be used because they can confuse children and lead to misinterpretations.

Planning rituals

After a death occurs, children can and should be included in the planning and participation of mourning rituals. As with bereaved adults, these rituals help children to memorize loved ones. Although children should never be forced to attend or participate in mourning rituals, their participation should be encouraged.

DOES BEREAVEMENT SUPPORT WORK?

Oliver et al.[5] describe the beneficial effects of a hospital bereavement intervention programme after traumatic childhood death. They found that many parents continued to grieve for months and years after the death, and lived essentially without hope. These parents felt that 'feeling good' would be a betrayal of their child and would indicate that they had forgotten that child. The Bereavement Intervention Programme (BIP) was organized around four chaplain–parent interactions: family contact at the hospital; a home/funeral home visit within 1 month of the death; an educational meeting with parents and 15 supporters at a restaurant within 2 months of the death; and an in-home interview/survey with parents 12 months or later after the death. Parents need supporters to remember their child and to appreciate the significance of their grief. However, long after supporters have worked through the emotional upheaval caused by the child's death, parents will still have a lot of work to do.

However, there is very little good evidence of a major benefit from bereavement programmes. Schneiderman et al.[24] found four randomized, controlled trials in a literature search back to 1964. Two of the studies showed benefit, and two did not. The review concluded that there is little sound evidence either in favour of or against bereavement programmes. Rowa Dewar[25] undertook a systematic review of controlled studies to see whether interventions make a difference to bereaved parents. The provision of bereavement support for parents who have lost a child is based on the assumption that it will lead to better subsequent adjustment. No overall benefit for the interventions was shown. However, for highly distressed mothers, psychological symptoms and marital dysfunction were significantly reduced. Applied to practice, these findings suggest that only some bereaved parents benefit from

bereavement support programmes. The author feels that a targeted approach may therefore be the best use of resources.

Dent et al.[26] looked at bereaved parents' perceptions of care after the sudden, unexpected death of their child in 11 health districts in seven regions of England and Wales. The results from postal questionnaires sent to both parents showed that most parents felt that community care was inadequate, leaving many feeling isolated. In contrast, questionnaires from health visitors and GPs in the same health districts showed that they believed that they were the most appropriate professionals to give follow-up care, but as there were few policies to guide them and little training provided, they felt unable to offer support. Families saw home visits as especially valuable.

SUMMARY

The loss of a child (or young sibling) is devastating and can have life-long effects. However, the benefits of bereavement programmes systematically to improve those outcomes remains difficult to demonstrate. Those of us who are establishing such programmes need to recognize the problems we are trying to deal with and generate rational programmes that both address specific issues of concern and allow objective assessment of outcome. At the same time, the lack of objective measures of improvement in this difficult and highly subjective area should not detract clinicians from offering help and support to a fragile and vulnerable group.

Chapter Twenty One

How to break bad news

Amanda Billson • Clare Edmonds

SUMMARY

Breaking bad news is never easy. There is no right way to do it. However, it is a vitally important communication skill, which we should be helping junior doctors to learn. In the past, doctors have tended to learn by experience and there has been little or no formal training in this important area. While there is no substitute for experience, we highlight features of good practice in the way we communicate with our patients. We also identify common faults in the breaking of bad news.

INTRODUCTION

Breaking bad news is not easy, but is an inevitable part of a doctor's working life. It can be demanding and daunting, and may come at the end of an emotionally draining resuscitation. Individuals often feel uncomfortable being the bearer of bad news. Causing distress in another person can cause distress in ourselves, particularly if we know the child and family well, and feel we are somehow letting them down. All these aspects are made worse if you feel ill-prepared. There is the temptation to avoid or shy away from the task.

All interactions with patients and their families rely on good communication, and this lies at the heart of a sensitive approach to breaking bad news. The consultation will have a major impact on the patient's and parents' ability to cope with the information given to them. They will remember much of the consultation for many years to come.[1] Being as prepared as possible will help the patient, their family and other members of the team to feel more confident in the doctor, and hopefully lessen the distress for everyone involved.

In this chapter we highlight some key points for good practice in the three phases of breaking bad news:

- preparation
- breaking the news
- follow-up.

DIFFERENT TYPES OF BAD NEWS

There are many different situations in which a paediatrician may have to break bad news. There is the sudden catastrophic event where the family is not previously known to you; for example, an infant found dead in their cot. There is the diagnosis of a malignant disease or the recurrence of a malignancy that had been thought to be cured. Then there are situations where there is ongoing bad news, for example an extremely premature infant on the neonatal unit, or an adolescent with a chronic illness such as cystic fibrosis. There are also situations where bad news evolves over months or even years from initial uncertainty, as with a child born with hypoxic–ischaemic brain injury, where the exact degree of disability cannot initially be predicted.

Ongoing bad news is best broken by a familiar and trusted member of the team, who has already built up a rapport with the family. Maintaining a good level of communication is vital in these situations.

Although, when we talk about 'breaking bad news', we tend to think about situations involving terminal illness, sudden death or the difficulties of telling parents their child has Down syndrome, most doctors are responsible for giving families information in their day-to-day work which may be perceived as 'bad news' by parents and patients. The doctor, however, may not always recognize it as such. The 'trivial' heart murmur mentioned at a newborn baby check may not strike a junior doctor as a particularly significant piece of news, but to a new parent it may be devastating. Their reaction will depend on their past experiences, cultural beliefs and attitudes, and level of knowledge, as well as the way the news is broken.

PREPARATION

When time allows, make sure you have prepared as well as you can (Box 21.1).

BREAKING THE NEWS

Key points for good practice when breaking the news are listed in Box 21.2.

Difficulties with breaking bad news

Although, ideally, both parents would be present, it is sometimes impossible to avoid giving bad news to one parent alone. For instance, the mother may be on the ward with the child and you want her to ring the father to ask him to come in so you can talk to them both. She will probably want to know why. The parents

BOX 21.1

Key points for good practice: preparation

- Are you the right person to give the news? Do you need someone more senior to answer questions? If so, when would they be available?

- Is it the best environment – ideally a quiet, comfortable, private room? Is this always possible? Does your ward or neonatal unit have a quiet room available?

- Minimize interruptions – try and make sure someone else holds your bleep for you, consider diverting phone calls if there is a telephone in the room.

- Do not appear rushed or in a hurry.

- Know as much about the case as you can (social circumstances of family, other children, etc.). Read through the medical notes before you enter the room!

- Consider who should be there. Both parents if possible – other children, the child themselves, nurse or other member of the team?

- If the child is going to be present, consider their developmental level. Who will you be talking to – the child or the parents?

- Consider whether you need an interpreter. A professional (or stranger) is better than family – a relative may not interpret everything you say if they feel the parents will be upset by the information.

- Consider whether there may be cultural attitudes that will affect how the family reacts.

- Introduce any members of the team (e.g. trainees) who are with you.

- Brace yourself for an emotional task.

BOX 21.2

Key points for good practice: breaking the news

- Explore what is known by the patient/family already.

- Give information with honesty but sensitivity – not abrupt, brutal honesty.

- Try to use simple language, avoiding medical jargon and euphemisms. Use emotive words like 'cancer', 'malignant', etc., with care. Try to avoid being too certain or too vague.

- Take care with prognostication. Never give specific time periods.

- Do not take all hope away – find some reason to be optimistic.

- Allow time for questions. Reply honestly to all questions (including 'I don't know' if that is the case).

- Listen to what the parents say. Try to think of the unasked questions that they may be worrying about, e.g. 'Is my child going to die?'.

- Do not be worried by periods of silence.

- Learn to recognize and cope with denial – respect the individual's response, but do not be party to the denial.

- Recognize and cope with family denial – 'Don't tell him doctor, it will kill him'. This can lead to a conspiracy of silence – the sufferer often knows that their condition is terminal or serious but is unable to talk about it. Do not impose the truth, but if the patient asks, do not lie.

- Avoid false reassurances.

- Acknowledge that dealing with uncertainty is often harder than knowing the diagnosis.

- Try not to let your own opinions interfere, even if parents push you to make a decision for them, e.g. whether or not to terminate for fetal abnormality. Give the parents sufficient information to be able to make any decisions with you.

- Recognize and acknowledge the feelings the parents or patient may have, e.g. anger.

- Acknowledge the fact that parents may respond differently depending on the age/developmental stage of their child, e.g. if a congenital abnormality is identified in the newborn period, one or both parents may feel ambivalent towards the infant.

- Show empathy but do not lose control.

- Try not to overload parents with too much information on the first meeting.

- Do not stay too long. Closure can be difficult – make sure you have arranged follow-up (see Box 21.3) then leave the room, preferably leaving a nurse with the parents for a period of time. Most consultations last 15–30 minutes. Some consultations may need to be more prolonged, but over an hour is generally too long.

may be separated or one may be working abroad. There is no easy solution, but ask whether the lone parent has a friend or another relative with them, and always have a supportive nurse present. Consider whether tape-recording the consultation and giving the tape to the parent to play to other family members would be appropriate.[2] If you have to talk to a parent alone, back it up with an offer to see both parents together as soon as possible, if appropriate.

You may feel uncomfortable breaking bad news if you feel that the family will lose confidence in you, especially if you are going to be closely involved with their future care. You may have found yourself endlessly reassuring a very anxious parent and have, therefore, initially overlooked pathology. Parents are nearly always appropriately concerned for their children. We are sometimes too eager to label the very anxious parent, who is constantly presenting with new concerns, as a 'difficult' parent. Asking a colleague to talk to the parents with you in this situation can be helpful. Be honest if things have gone wrong

Communicating with the child

Although their level of understanding is age-dependent, children have a right to be involved in decision-making as much as possible. Young children may misinterpret information that they hear their parents being given, e.g. the child who thought they were going to 'die of beatties' when newly diagnosed with diabetes. They need information communicated to them clearly and at their level. A play therapist can be helpful to ensure that the information is given in an age-appropriate way. The Royal College of Paediatrics and Child Health 'Child in Mind' teaching programme has some useful resources for improving information sharing with children.[3]

There is evidence that older children and teenagers expect their healthcare professional to talk to them directly and not via their parents.[4, 5] Children often cope much better than anticipated. They may actually try to protect their parents from bad news.[6]

When a child is seriously ill and likely to die, parents may want to talk to their child themselves or may prefer you to speak to them. It is best to encourage the parents to talk openly with their child. If the parents ask you not to discuss things with their child, make it clear that if the child asks you questions you will give them honest answers. Family members may fear the child's ability to cope with bad news, and so ask you to avoid telling them a likely prognosis. Full discussions should be encouraged to prevent the risk of a conspiracy of silence.

Young children think in more concrete terms than adults, and may not have grasped the finality and irreversibility of death. However, there is also growing recognition that even young children who face death personally may have a better understanding than is often assumed.

Other family members

Other family members may be affected by the news you give. Grandparents, in particular, are often very distressed in these situations – they are worried not only for the child, but also for their own son or daughter (the child's parent). Their anxieties can be heightened because they only receive information second hand from the child's parents. They may be given only some of the information – either because the child's parents do not want to upset their relatives or because they have only taken in half of the information they have been given themselves. It can be helpful to offer to speak to other relatives in the presence of the parents, but remember you need parental consent to discuss the child's care with other relatives. Again, it may be helpful in these circumstances to consider audio-taping the consultation, so that other family members can hear a direct account.[7]

A written account of the consultation for the parents, either a copy of the letter to the family doctor or a letter written to the parents direct, is one of the objectives in the NHS Plan for all consultations. This written account may highlight an area of the consultation that the parents have misunderstood. Siblings may feel left out and need to be appropriately involved when their brother or sister is unwell. A child may even feel that they are in some way to blame for their sibling's illness.

FOLLOW-UP

After breaking the bad news it is essential to offer the family follow-up (Box 21.3). If further test results are awaited, it is important to let them know when and how these will be available.

There are numerous parent and patient support groups that can be contacted by the family if they wish. Having a departmental 'bereavement folder' with information about local groups is invaluable. Much information is now available via the internet, but it may be helpful either to search for appropriate information for the parents or give them specific websites so that the information they receive is relevant to their child.

BOX 21.3

Key points for good practice: follow-up

- Arrange a review appointment relatively soon (e.g. on the following day or within a few days). You may need to have a series of review appointments. Make the family aware of who to contact if they have questions in the meantime (e.g. ward staff, yourself).
- Make sure the parents know if there are further results awaited and how they will get these.
- Provide written information if available (e.g. patient information leaflets, support group literature).
- Suggest to parents that they write down any questions they think of before the next meeting.
- Document in the notes what information the parents have been given and who was present.
- At review appointments update the news (e.g. if further test results are available).
- There may be ongoing bad news to communicate. It is vitally important to build up a relationship with the parents and to see them also at times when there is no bad news. In this way you can avoid being seen as 'the messenger of death'.
- Offer to talk to other relatives (e.g. grandparents), in the presence of the parents, if they would find this helpful. However, beware of demanding relatives – your first responsibility is to the child and his or her parents. Remember confidentiality.
- Liaise with the primary health care team (GP, health visitor) and any other relevant professionals.
- Consider a debriefing for the staff involved (do not forget interpreters).
- Find out about local services for bereaved people so that you can provide relevant information about bereavement support or make sure there is someone else within your organization who can do this (e.g. the hospital chaplain).

Communication with other members of the team, including the GP and health visitor, is also vitally important, and in the event of the death of a child, this is essential.

COMMON FAULTS IN THE BREAKING OF BAD NEWS

Although there is no right or wrong way to break bad news, there are a number of common faults that you should try to avoid:

1. Not doing it and hoping someone else will pick up the pieces – avoiding the patient, never seeing them alone, always being in a hurry.
2. Putting off the evil hour – e.g. by ordering more (unnecessary) tests.
3. Being economical with the truth to avoid upsetting someone you may have got to know well.
4. Deliberately not picking up patient cues.

5. Getting the child's name wrong – read the notes thoroughly before talking to anyone.
6. Fidgeting.
7. Looking out of the window.
8. Going into undertaker mode – there is always something positive to say, even in the most gloomy circumstances.
9. Being smug because you have got the diagnosis correct.
10. Identifying with the patient or parents so that your own personal feelings get in the way.
11. Saying things like 'I know exactly how you feel', 'Try to look on the bright side', 'You can always have another baby', 'You'll get over it'.

CONCLUSION

We have tried to highlight some key points that will help doctors to break bad news sensitively and appropriately, with empathy and understanding. Experience will help trainees to recognize the different situations in which they may be faced with breaking bad news and to understand the different ways that parents may react to bad news. Experience in the breaking of bad news is hard to gain at a junior working level, and more formal teaching is being encouraged. Although it is rarely appropriate to video a 'bad news' consultation, video-taped consultations are being used more often to help develop general communication skills. Role play can also be helpful to simulate some situations.

As well as formal training, we can all learn to communicate better by listening to our colleagues communicating and thinking a little more about our own approach, incorporating valuable learning points from others' experience. Reflecting on your day-to-day practice and seeking feedback from colleagues, trainees, and nursing staff will all help to consolidate your skills. You may find some families give you feedback in time – they may never have forgotten the experience, and positive feedback from parents and patients can be particularly rewarding.

ACKNOWLEDGEMENTS

We are very grateful to the participants of a one-day workshop at the RCPCH Psychiatry and Psychology group meeting in February 2000, which workshop led to the development of *A Trainer's Package on Breaking Bad News*.

22 Chapter Twenty Two

Parental reaction to the diagnosis of disability

Tammy Hedderly • Gillian Baird • Anna Boyce • Helen McConachie

SUMMARY

How the diagnosis of a child's medical condition associated with significant disability is communicated to the family has long-lasting effects. Circumstances in which the diagnosis comes to light over a longer time period are highlighted as particularly difficult for professionals to manage well. Guidelines for disclosure of a diagnosis are detailed, with reference to *Together from the Start*.[1]

The use of models of adjustment can help professionals to appreciate the impact of the diagnosis on the family and how to follow up the initial disclosure. The main findings of research on coping with disability are highlighted with emphasis on the importance of the multidisciplinary team.

INTRODUCTION

There have been major changes in the professional understanding of parents' reactions to their child having a disability. In the 1970s, the literature concentrated on 'handicapped families' and parental reactions such as guilt and overprotection. Now there is a greater understanding of the diversity of parents' reactions, which depend partly on how and when they are told of a diagnosis and, importantly, on the resources and coping strategies they bring to the challenges facing their child and the family.

DISCLOSURE OF DIAGNOSIS

All parents remember the moment when they first learned that their child had a disability. There have been a number of studies of the satisfaction or dissatisfaction expressed by parents concerning disclosure of diagnosis.[2–6] Such reports tend to look separately at the empathy and language of the person responsible for the disclosure, the circumstances in which it took place, and the information and follow-up offered. A high level of empathy elicits a greater degree of satisfaction than is seen with other aspects of disclosure, although the information given is also important. Parents appreciate that professionals have tried their best.

We still know a limited amount about the process of giving parents a diagnosis. Researchers have used discourse analysis[7, 8] to illuminate how professionals use language in the interview and the theoretical frameworks that determine judgements on how optimistic to be about the future, whether to emphasize biological or educational interpretations of children's difficulties, and how to negotiate a joint view with parents. Abrams and Goodman[7] noted that professionals shied away from an explicit use of labels. 'See-sawing' was observed, in which, when parents were despairing, the professionals tended to hold out hope, and when families were optimistic, professionals became more blunt and pessimistic.

Following repeated literature reports on poor parental satisfaction with disclosure[9] there have been drives to improve this aspect of medical training. 'Breaking bad news' is now covered in the medical-school curriculum and often involves sessions of role playing with actors. There are specific workshops available to specialist registrars training in paediatrics, and the topic is also addressed in the paediatric logbook training record. Similar training is needed for other key professionals in the community or specialist clinical team, such as clinical psychologists, physiotherapists, health visitors, and speech and language therapists. Diagnosis should be a team effort, with professionals taking time to reflect on their practice together afterwards.

The second area we know little about is whether guidelines actually make any difference. There seems to have been only one study that has audited the introduction of guidelines to a service, in this case how to manage a disclosure of diagnosis of Down syndrome.[2] This showed that dissatisfaction is not inevitable, despite professionals giving what most parents find devastating news soon after the birth of a precious new baby. However, the authors noted that, after staff changes, the policy was not closely adhered to, and dissatisfaction was again expressed by some parents.

Different types of impairment and their aetiology result in different circumstances and mechanisms for the detection and assessment of children's difficulties. Guidelines relate to those particular circumstances and are less relevant in others. Children with Down syndrome are usually identified within hours of birth, and thus the parents are usually available in hospital for the interview to take place. The condition is clear even if the prognosis is variable. For children with conditions such as cerebral palsy, autism and muscular dystrophy, the process of detection is much less certain. Parents often feel aggrieved that they were the first to notice problems and that their observations were not acted upon by professionals; for example, 86% of parents of young children with cerebral palsy had been the first to suspect a problem.[5] When the process of coming to a diagnostic conclusion is 'evolutionary',[10] parents need their concerns to be listened to, even if the ensuing advice is to 'watch and wait'. Parents need to feel that watching is a joint process and that appropriate help for the child is available.

Guidelines for professionals working with children from birth to 3 years of age, including good practice in diagnosis, are included in *Together from the Start*,[1] published by the Department of Health in 2003. The guidance aims to encourage multiagency working in the delivery of services to very young children with disabilities and their families.

GUIDELINES FOR DISCLOSURE OF DIAGNOSIS

The way in which information is shared by professionals should empower and support parents. All professionals should acknowledge and respect individual and cultural needs and differences. It is important to continue to review and modify guidelines as a result of practitioners' and parents' experience. It will also be important to develop an evidence-base for guidelines on discussion of diagnosis with children themselves.

Preparing for effective communication

- Families and their circumstances vary enormously so professional teams need to combine their knowledge of the family in order that the news is shared sensitively and effectively. When in doubt, ask families what they want.
- Professionals need to be well prepared and trained in communication skills; confident to share bad news, yet empathic enough to respond to parents' needs.
- Time and space should be available for parents to reflect, and reconvene with a member of the team if they wish.
- The telling should happen in a private place, without interruption from telephones.

Who should be there?

- Parents usually prefer to hear the news together:
- It may be appropriate for another family member or friend to be there to support one or both parents.
- If a parent cannot be accompanied, a member of the team should be present to support the parent during and after sharing the news.
- When an unaccompanied parent has heard the news alone, the other parent and family members should be informed as soon as possible.
- The number of staff involved should be kept to a minimum.
- A senior team member, who will be involved in the continuing care of the child, should convey the diagnosis.
- If an interpreter is required, care should be taken in the selection. A family member should not undertake this role.

Style and content

- Treat all parents' concerns seriously.
- Be aware of non-verbal messages conveyed through body language before you have shared your concern with the parents.
- Listen to parents and share information sensitively and honestly.
- Use plain, understandable language.
- Give opportunities to ask questions and check the parents' understanding.
- Remember that parents may not recall much detail from the first discussion.
- All children are unique; it is vital that professionals see the child first and the 'diagnosis' second.

- Wherever possible, keep your discussions about the child positive. Although many parents want some idea of the future, the clinician needs to be honest and acknowledge the limitations of prediction, while giving an opinion.
- If a baby is being discussed, try to keep the baby with the parents when sharing the findings and diagnosis – but ask first, as not all parents want this, and it is frequently inappropriate with an older child.

Next steps: practical help and information

- A record of the initial discussion should be made available to parents and their GP. This could be in written or audio format, but must be in the parents' first language.
- Contact details should be provided at the initial meeting, and parents encouraged to ask further questions as they arise.
- An early follow-up appointment should be arranged at the end of the initial meeting.
- Written information should be provided at an early stage about:
  - the child's condition
  - statutory and voluntary services
  - practical and emotional support
  - benefits.
- Support should be offered to parents to enable them to share the news with other family members and friends.

Telling the child or young person is an issue frequently neglected in both literature and practice:

- This should be done after discussion with the parents.
- The child's developmental age needs to be taken into account.
- The most suitable member of the team should do this; the physiotherapist or speech and language therapist, might, for example, have the best relationship with the child.
- The child should be offered further discussion, with or without their parents.

IMPACT OF THE DIAGNOSIS

After confirmation of the diagnosis, parents go through many stages of reaction and adaptation. Even if the diagnosis has been suspected for a long time, its confirmation can be a shock. Parents will be coming to terms with future uncertainty for their child and themselves.[11] They will also be trying to give information to friends and family members.[12] Their emotions may swing from despair and confusion to a desperate need to 'do something'. Further information about the diagnosis may be sought in order to control these emotions.[13] These feelings may be tempered with relief that their observations are confirmed and that something definite has been found; this includes a 'label', which can be seen as an access to information. Families increasingly use the internet as a source of information and support. (e.g. the Contact a Family website[14]).

An understanding of the common reactions of parents, and models of adjustment, helps professionals to provide appropriate support. Suggested models are based on stages of coming to terms with bereavement (Fig. 22.1).[15] A problem with such models is the assumption that all parents progress through the stages in the same way, that the steps are inevitable, and that it is a 'once and for all' process. The stages of reaction, from shock and denial, through adaptation and orientation, may occur again in response to new challenges such as finding an appropriate educational placement.[16]

Reactions   **Maladaptive responses**

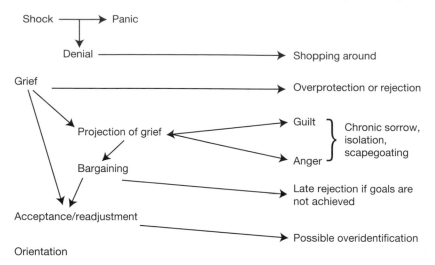

Fig. 22.1 Model for parental adjustment following disclosure of disability. (Adapted from Bicknell[15].)

Parents need accurate information about the child's condition and possible interventions (Box 22.1) because they are trying to make sense of a new way of thinking about themselves and their child. Therefore, it is essential that parents are given an opportunity soon after diagnosis to go over the information and ask questions of the same professionals, as well as receiving accurate and clearly written information. It is particularly the case in an 'evolutionary' diagnosis that parents report encountering a 'black hole' with regard to information and therapeutic support thereafter.[10] Furthermore, the clinician may need to work hard to understand the meaning of the diagnosis to the individual family, particularly if they already have a child with the same diagnosis, the child is adopted, or when the family is from a different cultural background to the clinician.

Follow-up appointments and additional referrals should be prompt, and involvement with established parent support groups for infants with disabilities can be suggested.

COPING WITH THE CHILD'S DISABILITY

The longer term impact of the child's disability varies across family members. Studies of the mental health of parents of children with an intellectual or physical disability have shown greater stress levels than are seen in other parents. The effect is usually greater in mothers than fathers, and autism seems to have the greatest impact on parental well-being.[17, 18] A child with behaviour problems and poor communication skills places a high demand on family members, the care load usually falling substantially on the mother.

There is also an impact on family finances. First, there are the increased costs of caring for a child with disability – additional heating, higher telephone bills and the expense of a suitable vehicle for transport, as well as clothing and bedding, equipment and house adaptations. Second, families have less income than they otherwise might have had, as parents are often less able to take up employment or promotion. Despite receiving some benefits, families may experience several years of financial constraint, this extending in some cases even into the period after the death of a child.[19, 20]

BOX 22.1

Key issues in the disclosure of a diagnosis

- Avoid any delay in disclosure.
- Use a direct approach with sympathy, clarity and hope.
- Allow time for disclosure and for questions.
- Use a quiet private environment, and offer the parents some time alone.
- Provide oral and written information about the child and the condition diagnosed.
- Provide written information about early services/agencies.
- Provide a contact name and number, and set up an early follow-up appointment.

Families find a variety of ways to cope with the demands arising from their child's disability, and research over the past two decades has provided ways of understanding individual differences.[21, 22] It used to be thought that there was an inevitable relationship between disability and stress for the whole family. We can now, however, think in a more complex way about the types of stressor that have the greatest impact, the external and internal resources that family members bring to the situation, and the cognitive coping strategies they adopt. We can examine how meeting the child's and family's needs by the provision of services contributes to family and individual well-being. It is also important to remember that, as with any child, bringing up a child with a disability is usually a very rewarding and positive experience for a family.[23]

The main findings of the research on coping are as follows:

- The type or severity of the child's condition does not in general predict the parents' well-being; instead, stressors such as behaviour problems, poor sleep and ill-health in children have the greatest impact.
- Life events that occur in any family (e.g. redundancy or the death of a grandparent) may tip the balance of coping in a family of a child with disabilities.

- The important material resources are a car, and a garden with a fence so that the child can play without constant supervision. The involvement of local housing departments, flexible employment arrangements for parents, and access to benefits are essential.
- Important social resources are practical and emotional support from family and friends, including the parents of other children with disabilities. Thus, if a family is isolated, services need to help to extend the social network through schemes such as link families and play schemes.
- Poorly coordinated services (health, education and social) can themselves be a source of stress. Communication between service providers is essential so that parents are not given contradictory advice. A 'key worker' approach to service provision is often recommended, and there are now detailed guidelines for implementation.[24]
- The impact on families has been shown to differ across racial and ethnic groups.[25]
- Services should consider how to meet the particular needs of families from minority ethnic groups,[26] for example the ways in which short term breaks are offered and arranged. The issue of equity of access is an important one for services to address.
- Research suggests that parents who feel empowered to problem-solve experience less stress. This implies a partnership between professionals and parents, allowing parents a choice in how services are provided. Negotiation of an appropriate partnership with community professionals is particularly important for parents of technologically dependent children, where the parents develop high levels of expertise.[27]
- Services should be provided with the aim of supporting the quality of life of the whole family, which could involve classes for fathers to learn signing, support groups for brothers and sisters, and so on.

The research findings summarized above lead to certain conclusions about the aims and organization of services for children with disabilities. They need to be based on a family-focused philosophy, with the ultimate aims not of only providing accurate assessment, diagnosis and treatment, but also helping families to maximize their quality of life.

This demands a team approach. A national study of parents' perceptions of their paediatricians' helpfulness[9] showed that these specialists were considered most helpful with issues directly related to the child's medical condition, i.e. diagnosis, and with information on general development. Only a small number of parents rated the paediatrician as being helpful in relation to common consequences of the impairments, such as managing behaviour problems, accessing benefits and liaising with voluntary organizations. Thus, the involvement of other disciplines and agencies is essential, including links between community child health, child and adolescent mental health services, and specialist social workers. The *National Service Framework for Children* has laid out the standards to be met by service providers, including services to children with disabilities.[28]

In all consultations with groups of parents, coordination and ease of access to services are mentioned, as are a lack of facilities such as respite care and access to leisure activities. Multiagency working, ring-fenced budgets for equipment and the provision of a key worker are suggestions that are made but continue to be difficult to implement within the current service structures. Interfaces between services need to be improved for seamless provision, which means equality of access not dependent on the type of disability, postcode or chance. Training and awareness raising and methods of coordination must be implemented in relation to other services such as dental care and acute hospital care, support in inclusive educational settings, and transitional care into adolescence and adult life. These are just some of the challenges involved in meeting the needs of children with disabilities and their families.

Chapter Twenty Three

Chronic illness:
the child and the family

Edward P. Sein

SUMMARY

The history of research in the care of children with chronic illnesses (CCI) is itself an excellent indicator of evolving themes in this area. In the 1960s there was recognition of emotional and psychological aspects of these illnesses, especially in the areas of death and dying, and in the 1970s there was an increasing awareness of the need to address the psychosocial needs of the children surviving chronic illness. The 1980s reflected the wider application of family and systems theories in the management of CCI. In addition, there was a growing recognition that the management of CCI should not focus solely on the negative impact of the disorder, but should draw upon the coping strengths and resources of the child and the family. This chapter reviews the trends and research evidence in the studies relating to the psychosocial effects of CCI on the child and the family, and management implications for professionals.

PRACTICE POINTS

- Research results may not be clear-cut, but paediatricians are bound to come across children with chronic illnesses (CCI) with psychosocial sequelae.
- Awareness of psychosocial issues is bound to enhance the overall management of CCI.
- Recognition and encouragement of families' coping strategies and strengths could prevent future dysfunctions.
- Close networking with mental health services could be of benefit.

EPIDEMIOLOGY

The estimate of the rate of children with chronic illnesses (CCI) in the community varies widely depending upon the definition used, method employed and the population studied. Overall rates of 10–20% have been found in a variety of studies.[1] There appear to be relatively stable incidence rates and prevalence at birth for most disorders, but in some disorders (cystic fibrosis, spina bifida, acute lymphocytic leukaemia, congenital heart defects) the survival rates have shown a considerable change over time. This increase in survival rates would have considerable impact in the estimate of population prevalence.

EFFECTS ON THE CHILD

The earlier assumption that chronic illness predisposes the child to psychological maladjustment appears to be less clear-cut. The discrepancies among the results could be due to various factors, including the measurements used, the reporters' perspective (parental more likely), the size of the population studied (the larger the size the more likely) and whether a single or multiple disorder is studied (multiple more likely). Therefore, larger epidemiological studies continue to support the evidence of an increased liability to behavioural, emotional and social competence problems, such as antisocial behaviour, anxiety/depression, headstrongness, hyperactivity, peer conflict/social withdrawal and immaturity/dependency.[2–4]

The effects on the child, such as pain and discomfort, fears and anxieties, isolation and stigmatization, appear to vary with age. In their longitudinal study of 5,362 children born in the UK in March 1946 followed up to 36 years of age, Pless et al.[5] showed that between 15 and 26 years of age those who had chronic illness in childhood reported more emotional problems, although their emotional well-being at 36 years of age showed no significant difference from those who had not experienced chronic illness in childhood. In addition, the majority of those who had chronic illness in childhood had very similar chances of marriage and becoming parents as those who had been healthy, and hardly differed in indicators of everyday social life. Another study indicates that additional factors of ongoing medical problems, and at least mild impairment in daily living, in addition to the chronic illness, imparts a higher risk of psychosocial problems.[6]

The effects of the diagnosis itself, as opposed to the physical components of the illness, were dramatically illustrated in a study quoted by Goldberg and Simmons,[7] where 56 children who were mistakenly diagnosed as having heart disease were studied. When the diagnosis was corrected and the children 'dislabelled', 35 of the 56 children were reported by their mothers to have positive behaviour changes.

Hawkins and Duncan,[8] in their study of 923 cases of children reported as abused or neglected, concluded that their findings support the contention that chronic health problems might place children at higher risk of abuse or neglect. It is important to bear in mind that chronic illness could also stimulate coping mechanisms in the child and family.

EFFECTS ON PARENTS

The parent–infant dyad is an interactive system wherein each participant's behaviour influences the other's. It follows that the behaviour of the child with a chronic illness such as in Down syndrome (reduced emotional expressiveness), young preterm (increased irritability) or congenital heart disease (feeding difficulties) could influence the behaviour of the caregiver.[9]

Most parents have to adapt to the child's chronic illness. Krener[10] mentioned five typical, but not obligatory, features of families with CCI. First, the constant recalibration to the ill child's needs makes it harder for the parents to read the child's developmental capacities. Second, symbiosis or regression of the parent–child relationship brings about a closeness and distancing from persons outside the caring dyad. Third, parents commonly doubt their own ability to meet the child's needs. Fourth, there may be a struggle between the parent and health professionals regarding the authority over the child. Fifth, the family may become socially isolated.

The effects on the parents of a child with chronic illness are not uniformly gloomy. A review suggests that, although parents of CCI experience more marital distress, research data do not indicate that they tend to become divorced.[11] Another study concludes that parents with CCI have increased rates of treatment for 'nerves' and an increased rate of maternal negative affect, but no increase in family dysfunction.[12] On the more positive aspect, mothers were found to score higher than fathers on strengthening of self and understanding of the medical situations.[13]

In their qualitative study of parents with CCI, Clements et al.[14] found that 70% of parents stated that the hardest time was at diagnosis. The authors provided some quotes from parents which provide some indications of the stresses placed upon them. When physical symptoms increased one mother recalled: 'When to call the doctor, when to start the antibiotics? Do you start if she sneezes once or do you wait till she sneezes twice?'. Another quote concerned individual parental responses after the diagnosis was made: 'And then that was when my husband told me he just couldn't get close (to their daughter).'

EFFECTS ON SIBLINGS

Studies regarding sibling adaptation preclude an easy summary due to the disparate aims and methods employed.[15] Earlier, more descriptive and smaller sample studies tended to emphasize the increased risks for healthy siblings of children with chronic illness, although more recent studies have not shown such clear-cut results. However, the general consensus appears to be that sibling maladjustment is selective and varies with age and sex, and that chronic illness is a stressor which, in interactions with other variables (family functioning, sibling relationships), may contribute to increased risk of psychological disturbance for some siblings.

Koocher and O'Malley[16] found that having a brother or sister with cancer had a profound impact on their siblings' lives, with feelings such as jealousy, resentment and fears about their own health being relatively common. However, other siblings reported positive aspects, such as enhanced feelings of closeness to other family members, and growth and development of own personal coping skills. Seligman[17] mentioned in his review that the presence of CCI might inhibit the family's communication, forcing the sibling to a kind of loneliness. They may also be burdened with a sense of responsibility for their ill sibling, and may harbour anger and resentment, depending on how much they resent the diversion of finance and parental attention to the ill child. Therefore, professional caring for the sick child should not overlook the psychological needs of siblings.

EFFECTS ON THE FAMILY

Among one of the most important basic tenets of the systems theory is the belief that change in one part is associated with change in all others. It follows then that chronic illness not only affects the child but also has ramifications for all the other members in the family system. It can be argued that professionals looking after CCI should not only be aware of possible implications for the whole family but indeed should adopt an orientation based on family systems and a socio-ecological model for understanding the coping and adaptation of a family with CCI. However, based on available research, there are few family assessment instruments that can be strongly endorsed as clinically or theoretically sound, and multiple methods, including self-report and interviews, should be used.[18]

It is important to differentiate between 'effect' and 'disorder or dysfunction'. Clearly, it would be difficult to accept that a major significant event such as a chronic illness in childhood would have no psychological effect on the child and family. However, this is not the same as saying that all families with CCI would have psychological disorders or dysfunctions. Rather, it is important to accept the presence of those effects that would then bring about attempts by the family system to re-establish equilibrium. The mechanisms employed by different families in coping with CCI are bound to be varied and, in addition, each family may interpret the same message differently, depending on historical, ethnic and cultural filters.[19] Furthermore, the mechanism employed may appear to be 'non-dysfunctional' within the context of a 'normal' family, but in actual fact may be an effective means by which the family copes and adjusts to the CCI. For example, the traditional view that 'denial' is pathological should be balanced against the normal healthy need for most people to minimize or focus on positive aspects in the face of adversity. Finally, it needs to be borne in mind that the family's reaction to a CCI does change over time.[20]

The clinician should also bear in mind that CCI may be serving a 'purpose' for the family in a way that is totally unrelated to the condition itself. It was noted in families with a child suffering from thalassaemia that parents and children often used the illness as the focal point for all their conflicts and as an explanation of their difficulties.[21]

IMPLICATIONS FOR MANAGEMENT

General remarks

With the increasing survival of CCI there are significant implications for professionals and planners alike. An increasing amount of professionals' time will be taken up with the long-term management of these children, and if the needs of the family are also to be addressed the time involved could increase even more dramatically. Training needs may have to be addressed, as inevitably professionals have to learn to deal with issues for the first time with various groups of children, for example coping with adolescence and early adulthood in cystic fibrosis and leukaemia. In addition to implications for the health service, there are bound to be other demands placed on education, social services, and voluntary and other agencies.

Physical versus emotional demands

It cannot be denied that medical procedures (infusions, operations, daily injections, etc.) can themselves be sources of stress and foci for conflicts. This is not to advocate a 'procedure-free' approach, but rather to highlight the need to take into account the emotional demands placed on the child and the family in trying to achieve a physical goal, regardless of how laudable or necessary the goal is.

It has often been argued that children with 'better' diabetic control show improved adjustment scores over those with 'poor' control. However, Eiser[22] has challenged this view, suggesting that efforts to maintain good control may be so demanding that children become more poorly adjusted (i.e. more depressed). It can therefore be argued that children should not be expected to achieve unrealistic levels of glycaemic control.

Liaison clinics

The mental health professional is rarely called in during the initial phase of chronic illness in a child. It is usually only when things are not perceived to be going well that the mental health professional is consulted. Although understandable, this process brings about the involvement of yet another professional, together with more appointments to be kept and tasks to be undertaken by a family with an already busy schedule. Ideally, the team of professionals looking after CCI should include a regular member from the mental health team. However, resource implications are such that this is not a practical option in most clinics in the UK at the moment. However, an increased readiness of physicians to recognize and then refer children and families to mental health professionals who, in turn, are willing to accept referrals not necessarily only in time of 'crisis', could be of immense help to the families.

The child

Clearly one of the main aims of management should be to help the child cope with the reality of having a chronic illness. Self-esteem is an important aspect of the coping mechanism, and it could be promoted through intellectual and creative skills, as well as through physical activities such as play and sports.[23] A supportive atmosphere that encourages expression of feelings is also a powerful coping strategy.

The parents

One or both parents almost always accompany a child during hospital appointments and admissions. It may be of immense benefit to the overall management of the child's health if the professional also bears in mind the emotional needs of the parents. The professional should try and gauge the emotional well-being of parents and likely stressors, if any, that may be impinging on the

parents and the wider family. The emotional well-being of parents impacts not only on the management of the chronically ill child, but also on other family members. A tired, depressed and irritable parent would be less tolerant of the child, leading to a downward spiralling of relationships in the family. The professional should have access to a network of other professionals and agencies that could provide additional support for the parent, such as mental health services and respite care facilities.

The family

Chronic illness in a child not only impacts on the family but, in turn, the family members are often brought into the network of carers for the child. Griffith and Griffith[24] describe the need to address the four aspects of family structure:

- boundaries – which can be affected by the need for some family members to care for the child, thereby giving rise to enmeshment
- hierarchy – whereby some children find ways to dominate their parents by strategically producing symptoms of illness
- alliances and coalitions – where the primary carer and the ill child may bond together in an intimate relationship while other family members may unite to oppose them
- symptomatic behavioural sequences – an example of which is an asthmatic child who may predictably wheeze whenever the parents start fighting.

The importance of having a family perspective is highlighted by Williamson,[25] who states 'the illusion of the dyad in medical practice can have a detrimental effect on treatment if the physician views the medical relationship as strictly a one-on-one encounter to the exclusion of other family members'.

Frey[26] postulates that in some adolescents the illness may assume a central role for longer than the expected initial phase in order that the family can avoid other issues that are more hurtful or threatening to the family structure. This could then lead to 'illness-maintaining behaviours' by the child in order to maintain the centrality of the illness in the family structure. Frey proposes a family/system approach to help the family adopt a different approach.

Society

In trying to understand the impact of chronic illness in a child on the family, Collier[27] advocates not only the use of a genogram (the composition of a three-generation family) but also an ecomap (the relationships between the family and outside systems, people, agencies and institutions that are important to the family).

Many parents found parent support groups to be of immense help. These groups not only provide a forum for exchanging information and education, but also the parents derived a degree of solace in the knowledge that other families share similar issues. Furthermore, the same information imparted by peers instead of professionals seems to have more impact. Hearing other parents relating similar problems helps dispel the 'I thought I was the only one' feeling, and seems to allow some parents to also express their own concerns, sometimes for the first time. Apart from being able to 'unburden' their feelings, this also allows other parents to come forth with practical suggestions.

Interestingly, there is a massive amount of information and a large number of newsgroups available on the internet, and anecdotal stories suggest that some families found this forum of sharing information to be very beneficial.

Professionals

It is difficult to believe, especially for those who recently entered the field of child care, that in the 1950s it was generally accepted by all that children with cancer should not be told of the diagnosis.[16] Current practice is based on truthfulness and sensitivity. Healthcare professionals should try and provide a framework within which the child and the family have a reference to the pros and cons of their coping mechanism, but should be aware of overdependence of the family, as this could be a barrier to the family developing coping mechanisms.[23] Professionals themselves need to be aware of certain issues when dealing with families with CCI. For example, the anticipation of loss holds attribution of failure, and the professional may either withdraw from the family or embark on a relentless pursuit for a cure. Professional training therefore needs to address both the technological and care-giving roles, and acceptance of the limits of our ability to control the uncontrollable.[19]

Regarding the awareness of primary physicians of the psychosocial adjustments of CCI and their families, Merkens et al.[28] found that the physicians' ratings of the impact on the child correlate well with the children's and parents' own assessment. However, the physicians' ratings of the impact on the family and on the parent did not correlate well with the parents' reports. The authors concluded that primary physicians are more aware of the psychosocial adjustments of the CCI than of their families.

In their study of parental expectations and the actual patient–doctor interaction, Lau et al.[29] found that a high proportion of parents (76%) expected the psychosocial aspects of care to be covered by the physician, but the parents rarely raised the issue themselves and in only 25% of visits were these issues actually discussed. They found that when these parental expectations were not met, parents had a greater degree of dissatisfaction. Finally, they noted that, whereas 80% of the discussions on physical symptoms were recorded in the notes, only 25% of the discussions on psychosocial aspects were recorded. The fact that parents rarely raised psychosocial issues during the visit may be because they did not feel that physicians would be interested in these issues or, even if they were, that there may not be a 'solution' offered; alternatively, it may be due to the deference of the parents. Therefore, parents should be encouraged to discuss these issues, and the professionals, in turn, should provide a suitable atmosphere for this to occur.

Among CCI, 11% had visited a mental health professional, and 38% of those at the extreme end of the score of the study had made such a visit.[1] The authors stated that the data indicated that most children at high risk were not seen by a mental health professional. Bearing in mind that the study was conducted in the USA, which is presumably better resourced than the UK, this point should be of concern for all health professionals and planners.

CONCLUSION

It can be argued that management of CCI should be family-orientated and should not just deal with the management of the physical aspects of the illness. The professional team (paediatricians, nurses, mental health professionals) should ensure that, at the least, all family members are made aware of the nature of the illness, the care it entails, and the likely associations of physical and psychosocial aspects. The family's coping and adaptation mechanisms should be acknowledged and seen in the light of the family's attempt to achieve an equilibrium, and should not be compared negatively with strategies employed by 'normal' families. Such coping mechanisms should be encouraged and fostered as long as they do not become pathological. Support from social structures and agencies should be made available when necessary.

Chapter Twenty Four

Autism spectrum disorder: how to help children and families

Rachel Brooks • Martine Marshallsay • Jaime Morey-Canellas •
William I. Fraser

SUMMARY

Children with autism spectrum disorder (ASD) have a social communication disorder with rigid or repetitive behaviours and poor imagination. They vary in intellectual ability, but they all have learning difficulties because of their ASD. We should be working toward the standards for diagnosis and support set in the National Autism Plan for Children (NAPC). All health professionals need a level of understanding of ASD in order to identify difficulties that may be due to ASD and to refer appropriately. There is also a need to tailor care to children with ASD, who may find interfaces with healthcare services for any reason extremely stressful. Understanding the child or young person with ASD depends on a basic knowledge of the spectrum and taking time to ask questions about the individual child. This chapter sets out to give some guidance to health professionals about ASD and what may be useful to ask and why.

PRACTICE POINTS

- The umbrella term autism spectrum disorder (ASD) covers children with widely varied difficulties and needs, despite having the triad of core impairments in common.
- Children with ASD need access to specialist services and advice.
- The National Autism Plan for Children (NAPC) sets standards for assessment and services.
- Parents can be hugely stretched providing care for these complex children and need multiagency support.
- Enquiring about and accommodating a child's ASD will promote optimum healthcare.

WHAT IS ASD?

The term 'autism spectrum disorder' covers:

- autistic disorder
- Asperger syndrome
- disintegrative disorder
- other autistic-like conditions (atypical autism or pervasive developmental disorder not otherwise specified (PDDNOS)).

These disorders all include the following triad of impairments:

- qualitative abnormalities in reciprocal social interaction
- qualitative abnormalities in patterns of communication (expressive and comprehension difficulties and non-verbal communication)
- restricted, repetitive and stereotyped patterns of behaviour, interests and activities.[2]

The child or young person with ASD is an individual whose presentation and level of difficulties depend on the severity of the impairments in each of the three above areas, and any associated difficulties, comorbid conditions and level of intellectual ability. Within the spectrum are children with a wide range of intellectual ability. Learning disability is more common in children with ASD, and the proportion of children with ASD increases as the level of learning disability increases.[3] However, all children with ASD have learning difficulties, however intellectually able they may be. The diagnosis encompasses able but socially gauche individuals who will find their niche in the world and manage independently, and those with severe learning difficulties and/or challenging behaviour who

INTRODUCTION

Each child with autism spectrum disorder (ASD) is first and foremost a child, with a need to be clothed, fed, kept safe and well, play, learn, and gain some form of independence. Any or all of these basic needs may present a specific challenge for the family of a child with ASD. To help families with these challenges all professionals who come into contact with them need to have an understanding of ASD and the ability to tailor care to the child as an individual.

This chapter sets out to: (1) discuss the wide variation in the autistic spectrum within a framework of the components of care and support we should be providing for all children with special needs; and (2) identify key issues and events that may require special consideration. It does not set out to describe in detail how to diagnose autism and the recommended time-scales for this process; this information is available elsewhere and is covered in the National Autism Plan for Children (NAPC).[1] Rather the aim is to describe autism in a way that allows all paediatricians to consider the diagnosis when appropriate, and to give consideration to the diagnosis when they meet children with ASD and their families.

will require intensive support at home or in a residential setting throughout their lives.

Common associated difficulties include:

- abnormal sensory responses
- hyper- or hypo-activity
- abnormal eating behaviours.

Co-morbidity includes:

- learning difficulties
- epilepsy
- vision and hearing impairments
- associated medical disorder (e.g. fragile X, tuberose sclerosis).

Psychiatric and/or behavioural comorbidity is frequent and can represent a challenge in itself. The more common problems seen in children are:

- depression
- anxiety
- attention-deficit hyperactivity disorder (ADHD)
- sleep difficulties
- Tourette syndrome
- conduct/oppositional defiant disorders
- psychosis.

FROM EARLY CONCERNS TO DIAGNOSIS

There is no screening test recommended for ASD. We must, however, listen to parents and take their concerns seriously, as they often suspect a problem early on.[4] Children still present at a wide range of ages. Young children whose language is not developing as normally should have this diagnosis actively considered. For children who also have moderate to severe learning difficulties the distinction between general delay and ASD may be more difficult, particularly in the very young child. The diagnosis of ASD may be very helpful in managing and understanding the difficulties of such children, and should be reconsidered at a later date if there is still concern. Children with Asperger syndrome may not present until junior-school age, when their difference from their peers becomes more acute.

DIAGNOSIS OF ASD

The diagnosis of ASD is discussed at length in the NAPC,[1] which sets out standards for the process, including the composition of the assessment team and the time-scales to achieve assessment. The current arrangements for assessment of children across the UK vary at present, but we should be working towards those standards. There are also a number of assessment tests that can feed into the diagnostic process. The items, in brief, are:

- a detailed developmental history, honing in on the development of social and communication skills and behaviours
- history and examination, to identify any associated conditions or comorbidity
- cognitive assessment, to be able to interpret behaviours in terms of their developmental appropriateness
- behaviour and mental health assessment

- observations in more than one setting (ideally including some settings with peers)
- speech and language assessment
- exploration of specific difficulties families are experiencing, in order to tailor advice and support.

Diagnosis may be made at a secondary level by a multiprofessional team, the members of which have appropriate training and experience. There should also be access to a tertiary service for difficult diagnoses and for children who require more expert help. The diagnosis may have been gradually emerging over a period of time, but for parents the confirmation of their belief (or fear) that their child has ASD is still a defining moment. Adhering to guidance about good disclosure of diagnosis will help parents accept and cope with this event and the future.[5] Parents need sound advice at this stage in particular, and will naturally canvas this from any health professionals they are involved with. However, conflicting and confusing advice is widely available in this field. Health professionals should be certain that they are giving accurate and up-to-date advice, or be honest that the area is not one in which they have expertise, and refer the question.

INFORMATION AND SUPPORT

Written information

There is a plethora of written information on ASD in book and leaflet form and online. It should be remembered that access to this information depends on parents' finances and literacy. Parents appreciate advice about how to select information relevant to their own child.

Case illustration 24.1

Joshua, 3 years old

Joshua has recently started nursery. The teacher has told his parents that he appears to be very much a loner, taking little interest in the other children; that he has poor eye contact with adults and peers; and that they have not heard him speak at all. Joshua's parents had also been concerned about him but had felt that he was merely shy; partly because his language development was not good (he has been referred to the speech and language therapist at the suggestion of the health visitor). Joshua is an only child and had little contact with other small children before starting nursery.

At an appointment to discuss the results of assessments, Joshua's parents were informed that he has a diagnosis of ASD. The implications of the diagnosis were discussed with the family, and they were given a leaflet including contact details for the National Autistic Society (NAS) and recommended books for parents with a newly diagnosed child. A team member arranged to see them at home, and they were given a contact telephone number should they wish to ask any additional questions prior to the planned visit. The family was also given a leaflet describing the EarlyBird Programme.[6] A letter was sent to the parents summarizing the discussion at the clinic appointment. With his parents' permission, Joshua was referred to the pupil support service for a statement of special education needs to be completed.

Case illustration 24.2

Emma, 8 years old

Emma has been assessed by pupil support services and has a diagnosis of dyslexia. Her teachers are concerned that she is falling behind her peers academically, and they have noticed that she appears at times to 'blank off' and be out of contact with what is going on in the classroom. Emma spends playtime on her own, walking around the lines of the netball pitch. Emma's teachers have noticed that she is rather old-fashioned in the way she speaks, and unlike her peers she is not interested in pop music and fashion but talks at great length and in detail about historical facts. Emma is noted to be both pedantic and clipped when speaking.

Emma has undergone the assessment process and, at a follow-up appointment, a diagnosis of Asperger syndrome has been confirmed. Information and support were provided in a similar way to that described for Joshua (Case Illustration 24.1), and the new information was sent to pupil support services. Emma's electroencephalogram (EEG) indicated that she was having absences; medication has commenced with good effect and a noticeable improvement in her concentration in school. Emma has recently told her parents that she knows she is different from other children in her class, and they are keen to provide age-appropriate information for her regarding her diagnosis. The team has suggested contact with the NAS, which also has information for siblings, as Emma has an older brother who has been asking questions. Emma's parents are keen for her to join the local Brownie Guide group, but are worried that she may not cope. The team advises that they contact the group leader and provide her with information about Asperger syndrome prior to Emma attending. The team also suggests that the group leader could set up a 'buddy' system for Emma, linking her with another child who is an established attendee and who could help her settle into the group.

Key worker

For children with ASD the key worker should have experience and training in ASD and access to tertiary-level advice, as well as being a member of the multidisciplinary team providing routine follow-up.

Membership of voluntary organizations

These include the NAS and Autism Cymru. These organizations may have local groups for support and education; they run (and advertise) training days aimed at parents and professionals on aspects of ASD.

EarlyBird

EarlyBird,[6] which is available in some areas, will answer the need of parents of children under 5 years old for advice and information. It is generally run by child psychologists and/or speech therapists that have been on a specific training course. Two places are offered to each family for weekly sessions on a 13-week course that includes home visits, group training and work around videos of their own child's behaviour. Outcomes are being fed back to ongoing evaluations of this course for the NAS and are encouraging. Parents value this opportunity.

INTERVENTIONS

Behavioural management and intervention

The behaviour of a child with ASD should be interpreted in the light of their core impairments, associated difficulties and developmental level. Understanding ASD and accessing information is helpful for parents. Early behavioural intervention seems to confer benefit. TEACCH (Treatment and Education of Autistic and related Communication-handicapped Children)[7] is almost universally used in schools, but more stringent approaches are costly in time and money to families, and they require expert advice prior to implementation.

Communication

All children with ASD need assessment by an experienced speech and language therapist. They require speech, language and social communication skills training built into life at home and at school where possible, with programmes devised and monitored (but not necessarily delivered) by the therapist.

The Picture Exchange Communication System (PECS)[8] is a valuable method of introducing the concept of communication to younger children who may go on to develop speech, and of providing a means of communication to children and young people who cannot develop spoken language. To be successful, this programme needs to be introduced stepwise under the management of a trained therapist who advises teachers and parents. Children with ASD do not apply skills learned in one setting to another, and PECS needs to be taught at home and at school to be successful in both settings.

Children with language may speak little or a great deal, but have no skills in conversation or interpreting situations using verbal, non-verbal or situational cues. Their understanding of language will be literal and concrete: saying 'give me your hand' may provoke a look of horror – clearly your hand is attached to your arm and therefore cannot be given without bloodshed! The speech and language therapist can offer programmes such as the use of Social Stories to help children and young people make sense of situations and interactions with others.[9]

Dietician

A restricted diet is common, although not universal, in children in the autistic spectrum. Chicken nuggets, strawberry yoghurt and Walkers (only Walkers!) prawn cocktail crisps may be all a child will eat at home, although he or she may eat other things in other settings (e.g. Granny's cheese sandwiches). A dietician can assess the overall nutritional value of the diet and reassure a desperate mother or advise supplements. Working to increase the dietary repertoire is difficult and slow.

There are many parents who wish to try eliminating gluten, wheat, dairy products and so on from their child's diet in order to try to improve his or her symptoms, especially if there are bowel problems. There is no evidence that these ingredients have any impact on the core impairments of children in the autistic spectrum.[1] Referral to a dietician can support parents and ensure that any diet is nutritionally balanced.

Psychopharmacology

There is no pharmacological cure for the core symptoms of ASD, and therefore psychotropic drugs should only be used to treat associated difficulties and comorbidities, either when all other interventions have been tried and failed or when the distress or behaviour experienced by the child renders it impossible to implement any other interventions. Methylphenidate, other stimulants and atomoxitine could be used to treat associated ADHD symptoms. Antidepressants could be used to treat symptoms of depression and anxiety. Melatonin, slow-release melatonin and other sedatives could be used to manage sleep difficulties. Antipsychotic medications have a role in the management of psychosis and Tourette syndrome. More specifically, low doses of risperidone have, in different trials, been shown to be safe and very effective in decreasing aggression, self-injurious behaviour and anxiety in children with learning disabilities. As stated earlier, these drugs should only be used when other interventions have failed, and ideally their prescription should be supervised by a psychiatrist with experience of using them in this population.

Life transitions

Times of transition will be especially difficult for a child with ASD and his or her family. Professional advice and support, both practical and psychological, should be provided. Each transition may bring its own specific difficulties and challenges, although common themes will be adjusting to changes in routine, venue, staff and other children, all of which will cause anxiety for the child and challenges for their family in supporting them through these changes.

A child's first day at school is an emotional milestone for parents. The transition from nursery provision to full-time educational placement, when a more structured routine and environment is introduced, will cause particular problems for children with short attention spans and/or who like to work to their own agenda. Provision should be in place on day one.

If a child attends mainstream school, the transition from primary to high school is another major life event. The move from a familiar environment with one teacher to a much larger school with changes of rooms, teachers and subjects throughout the day is likely to cause anxiety for a child with ASD. The noise level in corridors and the organizational skills required to 'change classes' may be daunting for the child. Practical help from non-teaching adult support may be necessary, or a buddy system may be appropriate.

Perhaps the most difficult transition for children with ASD and their parents is that from the educational system to adult life, and planning for this should start at 14 years of age. Interagency collaboration at this time is essential to ensure that all possible options after leaving school are considered. All professionals involved should attend annual review meetings following the child's 14th birthday. At this time the intellectual and social abilities of the young person with ASD will be major influences on the options available when entering adult life. It is essential that emotional support is available at this time, in addition to practical guidance. Leaving school is a poignant landmark at which the reality of ASD and its impact on life planning for the young person and his or her family is very sharply focused. Consultant psychiatrists with a special interest in learning disability may be available to provide ongoing management for mental health and behavioural issues. Access to social services support for adults has traditionally only been available to those with a sufficiently low IQ, despite many young people with ASD who are intellectually able being significantly disabled by their difficulties. The level of support and ongoing care available varies between areas.

Residential care

There are some children, with and without intellectual disability and ASD, who cannot be cared for in the family home as they get older. Making the decision that residential education and care is the correct solution for their child and the rest of their family is an enormous step for parents. Advice from specialist professionals will be part of this process.

FOLLOW-ON AND OTHER HEALTHCARE

This group of children may have particular difficulties that challenge the attempts of parents and health professionals to manage autism-specific, comorbid or incidental health conditions. These difficulties include:

- inability to communicate feeling unwell because of language delay or lack of help-seeking strategies
- high pain thresholds or no apparent reaction to pain
- high anxiety levels in unfamiliar surroundings (e.g. waiting rooms)
- sensory issues leading to extreme distress on being touched or on the application of dressings, etc.
- extremely limited repertoire of foods, and hence an inability to tolerate medication (or ward food!)
- extremely rigid routines, making alterations in medication problematic.

It is important to remember the triad of impairments when arranging appointments, investigations, and interventions for children in the autistic spectrum. It may be helpful to imagine how difficult it is for anyone visiting a different country and feeling vulnerable because the language is 'foreign'. For children in the autistic spectrum visiting an unfamiliar place and meeting unfamiliar people can be frightening, as they have difficulty understanding not only spoken communication but also gestures, facial expressions and the concept of why they are attending an appointment. Consideration of the following issues may assist children with ASD and their families in these situations.

Prior to appointment

Providing information to parents about what will happen at an appointment and who will be present will allow them to prepare their child as well as possible. Appointments should be planned so as to minimize the time the child must spend in the waiting area, particularly if the child is very active. Also, extra time should be allowed for appointments; e.g. a double appointment may be booked, especially if an examination or investigations are planned.

At an appointment

- At the beginning of an appointment ask the parents about their child's level of understanding and method of communicating their needs.
- Ask how the child prefers to be touched (e.g. lightly or firmly) before any physical examination.
- Ask if the child has any specific fears or sensitivities (e.g. loud noises, lights, others invading their personal space).
- If venepuncture or other intervention is necessary, ensure that this is carried out in a different room to the one used for discussion and examination, to avoid an association that may cause difficulties at future appointments.
- When speaking to the child use short sentences with key words, and be aware that the child may have a very literal understanding of language.
- Be prepared to remove any dangers in the consulting room, as the child may climb and explore without inhibitions or any sense of danger. Constantly minding the child will make addressing the issues in the consultation very difficult.

If at an appointment it becomes clear that an anaesthetic will be necessary for a planned investigation or procedure, share that information with the paediatrician dealing with the child's general care. This might be a rare opportunity to examine this child or perform another investigation under optimum conditions.

Following an appointment

Consider providing a written summary of what was said during the appointment, especially if new information was discussed, as parents may have difficulty in recalling the issues if their child required comfort and support during the appointment.

Admission to hospital

All the above is relevant if a child with ASD has to be admitted to hospital. Sometimes a large change in routine such as this provokes less anxiety than small, seemingly trivial changes. Parents can provide an insight into their child's difficulties and how the environment can be arranged to help them. The parents can also be asked to nominate a member of the team providing care for their child who would be able to give professional advice about any issue regarding the child's ASD and its impact on their health and healthcare.

Chapter Twenty Five

Supporting communication in the child with a learning disability

Helen Cockerill

SUMMARY

Learning disabilities can result from a range of genetic, social and specific medical conditions. In addition to a slow rate of learning, children may present with speech, language or communication difficulties of varying degrees. Associated physical, hearing or visual impairments will influence the nature and course of language development. Best practice in this area involves collaborative working between families, education and health professionals directed towards agreed functional communication goals. Augmentative and alternative communication techniques, such as signing, symbols and communication aids, can have a major role in the development of effective social communication, appropriate behaviour and curriculum access.

PRACTICE POINTS

- Children with learning disabilities form a heterogeneous group, with a range of aetiologies, abilities and needs.
- An early referral for speech and language therapy should be made for any child who is at risk of having speech, language or communication difficulties. A 'wait and see' approach is not acceptable.
- The management of communication problems in children with severe learning disabilities requires a team approach.
- The child and family must be central to any communication intervention.
- Augmentative and alternative communication systems do not hinder speech development but can increase communicative competence.

LEARNING DISABILITY

'Learning disability' is an umbrella term for a wide variety of genetic, social or specific medical conditions that result in a slow rate of learning. Children with learning disabilities share the common feature of scoring under 70 on IQ tests. Mental retardation, intellectual impairment and learning difficulties are other labels that have been applied to this group of children. Learning disabilities can be classified as mild, moderate or severe, again based on IQ scores, with the latter group including children with profound and multiple learning disabilities. Clearly, the severity of a child's cognitive impairment will influence the rate and course of language learning; however, an IQ score tells us little about a child's communication skills or needs. It can be difficult to carry out IQ testing with learning-disabled children, and indeed the validity of testing procedures for such children can be questioned. Instead, it may be more meaningful to profile a child's learning and communication skills, and the consequences for adaptive behaviour, independence and social functioning, using criterion-referenced assessments.

Children with learning disabilities frequently have additional impairments that impact on the development of communication skills, including hearing loss, visual impairment, motor impairment or social communication disorder. This chapter does not seek to describe the type of communication disorders that typically occur in specific conditions, but rather presents some of the themes and issues that commonly arise in the field, with particular regard to children with more severe learning disabilities and limited natural speech.

SPEECH, LANGUAGE AND COMMUNICATION

Speech, language and communication are highly integrated but separable systems. Using examples from outside the learning-disabled population it is possible to illustrate how these systems can be delineated. A typically developing deaf child, in a family in which sign language is the main means of communication, may have limited speech but would have a well-developed language system and be a highly proficient communicator within the deaf community. A child with Asperger syndrome may have no difficulties with speech pronunciation or grammatical sentence construction, but may have problems with the appropriate use of his language skills, resulting in a significant communication disorder.

It can be important to distinguish between these components in describing the abilities of children with learning disabilities, and in planning appropriate intervention and support strategies. A child may have specific difficulties with the articulation of speech sounds, resulting in limited intelligibility. Language skills may reflect cognitive skills or follow an atypical path and be more impaired than would be expected from a child's general intellectual level. Patterns of strengths and weaknesses may emerge within a language profile. For example, children with Down syndrome have been described as having strengths in vocabulary, but weaknesses in grammatical understanding and production beyond the two-word level. Receptive skills are in advance of expressive skills in many children with a learning disability. Communication, if defined as the sharing of information, needs, experiences, thoughts and feelings with others, may be as much a function of a child's family, school and community to support communication as of the child's own ability to utilize his speech and language skills for social interaction. Many children with learning disabilities will have speech, language and communication difficulties.

INTERVENTION

There is a bewildering array of intervention programmes and therapies for children with learning disabilities. These are based on a range of models of learning and many different philosophies of education and treatment. Some approaches are designed for specific conditions, with autism receiving particular attention. Many programmes make spectacular claims, usually with little published evidence to support them, both in terms of outcomes and in the range of children who might benefit. There is little research comparing the results of different programmes, and a dearth of studies that relate individual characteristics to outcomes. Most programmes include intensive, one-to-one interaction with parents or professionals, which may be the unifying and most important factor.

Many therapists and educationalists in Britain claim to follow an eclectic approach, drawing on aspects of a range of programmes and techniques in response to an individual child's strengths and difficulties. This may be rather incomprehensible and unsatisfactory for parents of children with learning disabilities. Many parents feel the need for explicit guidance on what to do to help their child. Highly structured programmes, particularly those that are well packaged and are the subject of unsubstantiated claims on the internet and in the media, may be more attractive to some parents, at least in the early stages, than the services offered by local professionals.

In addition to describing the abilities and impairments of children with learning disabilities, much research has focused on the behaviour of the parents (usually the mothers) and how this may influence the course of language learning. Studies have described the carers of children with learning and communication disabilities as being more directive than the carers of typically developing children, i.e. they give more commands, direct the child rather than following the child's focus of attention, employ more explicit language teaching such as asking a child to repeat words, etc. It was assumed that these behaviours were detrimental to language learning, and therefore many intervention programmes for preschool children with learning disabilities have been directed at changing the behaviour of carers. There has, however, been an increasing recognition of the complexities of early interaction and the contributions of both the child and carer. An infant with a condition associated with a learning disability may move, look around, make sounds and respond in a way that fails to trigger the parental responses seen in the early experience of a typically developing infant. It is hoped that future research will focus not just on the child or the carer, but attempt to look at the interaction between the two and how this can be facilitated. This is a difficult area to study due to the problems of early diagnosis in many conditions that may involve learning disabilities.

As children move through the education system the emphasis shifts from early communication and cognitive skills to a child's ability to access the curriculum. Traditionally, special schools have followed a developmental curriculum for children with severe learning difficulties, focusing on fundamental cognitive and communication skills in functional activities, with the aim of promoting independence. The move towards inclusive education and the introduction of a national curriculum has challenged teachers, in both mainstream and special schools, to differentiate a subject-based curriculum for children with learning disabilities. Academic subjects can be treated as contexts for developing cognitive or language skills; for example, setting targets for turn-taking or choice-making in the context of the classroom literacy hour, or developing an understanding of cause-and-effect in the context of a science lesson. In this way, children at different levels of ability can be taught alongside each other, each working on skills specified in his or her individual education plan. The overall aim is to provide all children with a broad and balanced curriculum, regardless of ability.

Possibly the most important development in intervention for children with learning and communication disabilities over the past 25 years has been augmentative and alternative communication (AAC). AAC is the use of non-speech modes of communication to supplement or provide a substitute for speech. Examples of non-speech modes include manual signing, pointing to picture symbols, and electronic communication aids with speech output.

In the past, it was felt necessary to evolve therapy and education protocols in which the decision would be made to work directly on speech and language, or to introduce AAC (usually only considered if speech was felt to be impossible due to oral–motor impairment). Current practice employs a more holistic approach, with the recognition that communication can be multimodal. With functional communication as the goal, rather than the development of 'normal' models of spoken communication, children with learning disabilities are often exposed to a total communication approach in which speech is augmented with manual signing, picture symbols and/or computer-based technology.

WORKING WITH FAMILIES

In the past, the family may have been seen as a useful resource, with professionals as the experts using parents and other family members to carry out therapy and education programmes. More recently, there has been a shift towards recognizing the family as a system with communication needs and skills in its own right. It is now considered good practice for professionals to provide services based on collaborative problem-solving methods.

A child's communication skills and needs can be described in relation to his or her communication partners and communication environment. For example, a child with a speech impairment may be intelligible to immediate family but unintelligible to the teachers at school. This would highlight the need for an AAC system at school, but explain why it may be rarely used at home. Another child may have behavioural difficulties when required to accommodate a flexible routine at home, while remaining calm in the more structured school environment. This would highlight the need for strategies to help the child adjust to events within the home setting. Different environments may place different demands on a child, offer different opportunities for communication and provide different supports for communication. As a child gets older, the circle of communication partners may widen to include carers other than parents, friends, health and social services professionals, and people in the wider community. The child's communication needs and the expectations of communication partners will change over time. Any communication intervention must take these factors into account and attempt to build a consensus regarding priorities and appropriate strategies at each stage in a child's life. Because of the high incidence of additional disabilities affecting communication in this population this is likely to require a team approach, with parents and other family members as core members of the team. Professionals involved may include speech and language therapists, psychologists, teachers, occupational therapists, paediatricians, physiotherapists, rehabilitation engineers, audiologists and ophthalmic consultants. As the child matures, he or she may also be included in this decision-making process. Many children with learning disabilities have strong views about their own communication needs and which strategies they find useful.

COMMUNICATION TECHNIQUES

While some children with mild-to-moderate learning disabilities may communicate entirely through the traditional oral routine, following a delayed but largely normal pattern, many children with severe disabilities will require the support of AAC techniques. Some commonly used techniques are described below.

AAC can be used to support a child's understanding of language, i.e. as an input system, and also to facilitate a child's ability to express him- or herself, i.e. as an output system. For some children AAC is likely to be a step towards speech, and for others it may have a permanent role. AAC can be used to build on a child's strengths and compensate for areas of difficulty. For example, children with Down syndrome, and those in the autism spectrum are known to have better visual-processing than auditory-processing skills. This can mean that visually presented language information can be more noticeable and more meaningful than spoken language.

Signing

Signing is the AAC method most commonly introduced to children with learning disabilities. Early intervention programmes from the 1980s onwards have recommended the early introduction of signing as a way of supporting the development of eye contact and attention skills, facilitating comprehension of spoken language, developing thinking skills, providing a means of expression, developing emotional stability, increasing confidence and facilitating social interaction. Numerous research studies have demonstrated that many children, at least in the Down syndrome population, go on to develop speech and stop using signs once spoken words are acquired. A range of other benefits is reported.

There are obvious limitations to signing, including the need for family and teacher training in the chosen sign system, the limited number of communication partners who will be able to use or understand signing, and the difficulties of accurate and intelligible sign production by children with motor impairments. Most children with learning disabilities will be seeing only keyword signing, i.e. a selection of vocabulary taken from a sign language or an artificially developed signing system designed to accompany speech, rather than a true sign language such as British Sign Language, which has its own grammar. They could, therefore, be considered as being exposed to impoverished linguistic input rather than a full range of linguistic features. The impact of this type of input on language development is as yet unknown.

Graphic symbols

Pictures or symbols can be used to represent speech, particularly for children whose motor impairments preclude the use of manual signing. Printed pictures or symbols arranged on communication charts or in books are, by definition, permanent, less transient than both speech and sign, and can provide a focus of shared attention. It is this aspect of pictures/symbols that is harnessed in programmes for autistic children in which instructions and important information is presented in both auditory and visual form (e.g. visual timetables).

When used as an input system it is thought that symbols can provide a bridge to language comprehension, helping the child to map spoken words onto the objects and events to which they refer. When used as an output or expressive system the child is able to give unambiguous messages, which can be interpreted by a range of communication partners.

The limitations of symbols, particularly picture symbols, include the difficulty of representing abstract concepts and linguistic features, and the speed of communication, particularly if the child is unable to point directly to the symbols due to a physical disability. Some children will access their communication systems through eye-pointing, requiring sensitive and skilled communication partners. Most children will not have access to role models who communicate through symbols. They will receive most of their linguistic input from speech but be expected to give their messages through symbols.

Again the impact of this input–output asymmetry for long-term language development is unclear. It would seem that there are qualitative differences in the linguistic output of symbol users compared to speaking children, such as telegrammatic sentences and atypical word order. It was assumed that these differences were due to the amount of physical effort involved in communicating through pointing to symbols. However, recent research with typically developing, physically able children suggests that such differences in style may also be related to the nature of a graphic medium, and the way in which it is processed, rather than simply the physical or learning disabilities of the augmented communicator.

It is thought that using graphic symbols may provide a bridge to reading skills, and the potential of symbols for involving children in literacy activities is a rapidly developing area of research.

Voice-output communication aids

Computer-based electronic devices are increasingly recommended for children with limited speech. Messages are stored in the device and spoken when the child selects symbols from a screen or overlay. Very simple devices that can store a single phrase may be used to provide a severely learning-disabled child with the experience of being able to give a spoken message. This can be a valid way of involving a child in a social situation such as saying 'Hello' within classroom circle time, 'shouting' for a turn, triggering the start of a favourite song, etc. The understanding that symbols can represent objects and events is necessary for the use of more sophisticated devices, where the child actively selects the message he or she wishes to give.

Voice output communication aids (VOCAs) are primarily used with children who have motor speech impairments. The extent to which a child will be able to use a VOCA will be determined by such factors as his or her cognitive and language abilities, as well as the physical ability required to access the device. Some children may be able to point directly to symbols on the screen or keyboard of a VOCA, while others will use switches to operate a scanning system.

There is some evidence that children using VOCAs are perceived to be more intelligent than children who are using low-tech systems such as communication charts. This may help to explain why many families may express a preference for VOCAs over communication charts and books. However, the high rate of VOCA abandonment suggests that families' initial expectations may not be fulfilled as the cognitive and physical demands of aided communication become apparent.

Presymbolic communication

Children with profound and multiple learning disabilities may not achieve the cognitive level required for the use of symbols (spoken symbols, graphic symbols or signs). Communication may be at a reflexive or reactive level, and the child may not develop the use of conventional communication signals. Such children will need a communication programme aimed at establishing consistency in the interpretation of the child's behaviour by communication partners, thereby facilitating the development of intentional communication. A range of sensory stimuli may be used to arouse attention, develop awareness of cause and effect, to reward desirable behaviours and to provide a context for social interaction. Carefully selected objects (known as objects of reference or tangible symbols) may be presented to a child in a systematic fashion in order to help that child anticipate familiar activities (e.g. a spoon for lunch, a small piece of towelling for swimming).

THE IMPACT OF AAC ON SPEECH

Many families, and some professionals, fear that the introduction of AAC will have a negative impact on speech development. Studies of Down syndrome children would suggest signing may have a facilitative effect on speech development. Similarly, studies of autistic children who have been taught to exchange pictures for desired objects also report speech development, and the consequent abandonment of the picture system, in some children. The situation is less clear in relation to children with motor speech impairments, although it would be difficult to postulate the neurological mechanism that would result in reduced speech if alternative modes of communication were used. Few studies have specifically examined the question of speech development in physically disabled children who are using AAC. In the few intervention studies where speech development outcomes have been documented, it would appear that children's natural speech production remains the same, or is slightly improved following the introduction of AAC.

The impact of articulation work for children with motor speech impairments is another under-researched area. There are few data available to guide speech and language therapists as to whether they should direct their efforts towards direct work on speech or towards introducing and teaching augmentative systems of communication. Past clinical experience, the high number of adults with learning and physical disabilities who have had years of articulation work with little benefit for speech production, and the increasing number of competent augmented communicators, would suggest that there may be good neurological reasons for directing intervention towards functional outcomes using a total communication approach. Children with learning disabilities and additional motor speech impairments run a high risk of having very limited speech, with a significant gap between comprehension and expressive skills. As part of a communication management programme aimed at the development of effective social communication, the early introduction of AAC systems, as either temporary or permanent adjuncts to oral communication, is strongly recommended. Children with learning disabilities may require a range of communication methods for different situations and partners. A child with a severe learning disability may have some intelligible speech, but rely heavily on signing for functional communication with people who understand and use signing. He or she may use symbols for accessing the school curriculum and producing written work on the computer, and use a VOCA to participate in games and shared reading activities.

Chapter Twenty Six

Financial help for families with disabled children

26

Justin Simon

SUMMARY

Financial help is available for disabled children and their parents, but it is difficult to know what it is, who pays it and who is entitled to claim. The main sources of support are from the Department for Work and Pensions, and the government-funded charity the Family Fund. Other help may be available from local social services departments and Primary Care Trusts. Many barriers exist that make it hard for families to know what they are eligible to claim, and it is the responsibility of professionals to assist them in overcoming this.

PRACTICE POINTS

- One of the greatest barriers that prevent benefits being claimed is ignorance of their existence.
- Independent advice on completing benefit claims can be sought from local Citizens Advice Bureaux.
- Most benefits are payable from the time when the application form was requested, but payments may not be backdated.
- Applications for most Department for Work and Pensions benefits may be made online or by telephoning the Benefits Enquiry Line.

INTRODUCTION

This chapter describes only the main areas of financial help available, as it is not possible to cover all sources. The focus is on the most common ones, those most frequently overlooked, and those over which clinicians may have a direct influence, for example by being asked to write a letter of support. It is also important to appreciate the barriers that stop parents, carers and young people themselves from requesting help.

Financial help comes from the following main sources:

- the Department for Work and Pensions (DWP)
- social services
- charities.

The DWP was established in April 2001 and took over from the Department of Social Security. Some of the benefits to be claimed need the input of expert advice, so it is better to refer applicants to their local benefits office or Citizens Advice Bureau for independent advice, rather than to try to work it all out oneself. A number of national organizations may also be able to assist. This chapter covers England and Wales, and as there are some exceptions for Scotland, you will need to check whether the same rules apply.

Definitions of 'disabled' and 'disability' (Table 26.1) mean that there is potentially a very wide range of people who may consider themselves disabled, which makes it especially important to understand how the services define 'disabled' and what the criteria are when apportioning services.

FINANCIAL HELP FROM THE DWP

The main source of financial help for families with disabled children is the DWP.

DWP benefits for disabled children

The DWP benefits for children can be considered in chronological order (Table 26.2). If the child is entitled to any of the benefits listed in Table 26.2, then the child's parents may also be entitled to certain other benefits, depending on their circumstances. We will consider both sets of benefits in turn.

From birth: Attendance Allowance

Although not specifically relating to disabled children, Attendance Allowance is a benefit that may arise as a result of a terminal illness being diagnosed at birth, or at any other time.

'Terminally ill' is defined in the Social Security Contributions and Benefits Act 1992 as:[2]

> ...if at that time [you have] *a progressive disease and* [your] *death in consequence of that disease can reasonably be expected within 6 months.*[2]

Any person, child or adult, with terminal illness may qualify for this benefit if the conditions are met. This claim comes under Special Rules, and means that a family will be paid the highest rate for personal care and may be paid straight away without having to wait for the usual 3-month qualifying period. This claim requires a formal report from a doctor or specialist about the child's medical condition, which is the DS1500 Report. The DWP guidance notes state that the doctor does not have to see the child, and that the family will not have to pay for the report.[3]

Two main barriers prevent this financial help being claimed: lack of knowledge of its existence and the practical difficulty of completing the form at a time of great distress. The claim may not be backdated, so it is important that the family is encouraged to make the request for the claim pack at the earliest opportunity.

Table 26.1 Definitions

Term	Meaning
Financial help	Benefits that are not solely monetary payments
	If, for example, a child receives the high rate of the Mobility Component of the Disability Living Allowance, then the family can gain free Road Tax for a vehicle used to transport that child. This is not a payment as such but is of significant financial help
Child/children	Individuals aged 0–18 years
Disabled	Defined in the National Assistance Act 1948 and in The Children Act 1989:
	'A child is disabled if he is blind, deaf or dumb or suffers from mental disorder of any kind or is substantially and permanently handicapped by illness, injury or congenital deformity or such other disability as may be prescribed'.[1]
Disabled	Defined in the Disability Discrimination Act 1995:
	'A physical or mental impairment which has a substantial and long-term adverse effect on [an individual's] ability to carry out normal day-to-day activities.'[1]
Disability	Defined by Disabled People's International thus:
	'Disability is the loss or limitation of the ability to take part in the normal life of the community on an equal level with others, due to physical and social barriers.'[1]
	This widens the definition, and emphasizes that it is not the impairment itself that is disabling but the way in which society reacts, pathologizes and excludes people

From age 3 months: Disability Living Allowance – Care Component

There are two elements to the Disability Living Allowance (DLA), the Care Component and the Mobility Component. Children are not eligible to apply for the Mobility Component until they are 3 years old (see below).

The Care Component of the DLA is payable from when a child is 3 months old. As there is a 3-month qualifying period, a claim needs to be made as soon as a child is born in order that the payment can be made from 3 months of age. There is no upper age limit, but a further test for eligibility may be needed once a young person is over 16 years old.

The Care Component is financial assistance to help carers find someone to help children with their personal care needs; this is why it is identified as a benefit to the child rather than the parent, although, in practice, the payment goes to the parent. These personal care needs have to be substantially over and above what a child of a similar age would usually expect, and it is this detail that needs to be reflected in every part of the application form.

Numerous detailed questions must be answered before a child can qualify for the allowance. These are set out on the application form and are specific to the care needed during the day and night (Table 26.3).The questions cover what help the child needs in all aspects of daily living; for example, 'waking, getting up and going to bed, washing and bathing, getting dressed or undressed, help with toilet needs, communicating, when the child is in bed at night, and eating and drinking'.[4]

When filling out the DLA application forms, it is necessary to focus on how a child is less able than his non-disabled peers. Many parents find this very difficult, as they understandably want to think of the ways in which their child is the same as other children – not different. For the purposes of filling out these forms, it is, however, essential to concentrate single-mindedly on this difference, as the majority of decisions are based on the information provided on the forms.

Table 26.2 DWP benefits for children

Child's age	Benefit
0	Attendance Allowance (if the child is terminally ill)
3 months	Disability Living Allowance – Care Component (three rates)
3 years	Disability Living Allowance – Mobility Component – high rate
5 years	Disability Living Allowance – Mobility Component – low rate
16 years	Income Support
	Incapacity Benefit

Table 26.3 Benefit rates for Disability Living Allowance – Care Component (£16.50–£62.25 per week for the 2006–2007 financial year)

Rate	Care needed
Lower	The child will need care for a significant part of the day
Middle	The child will need substantial care during the day *or* the night
High	The child will need substantial care both day *and* night

Not knowing about these benefits is again one of the greatest barriers to obtaining them. Families often find out about benefits from contact with other families with disabled children or from professionals at child development centres, nurseries or schools. For families with very young babies or children, however, such contacts are much rarer, and parents may fall through the net. Similarly, families with poor literacy or who have English as a second language may not receive the right information, and leaflets alone may be insufficient. Some families think that they are not eligible to receive help because of the level of their earnings or savings, but earnings and savings do not affect any of the DLA payments. It is worth noting that these payments can be substantial, so families should be advised to apply for them, even though they may not be awarded.

From age 3 years: Disability Living Allowance – Mobility Component – high rate

The claim needs to be made 3 months before the child's third birthday so that it can be awarded when the child is 3 years old. This payment is for children who cannot walk or who have severe difficulty walking. Various tests are used to determine this, but it is possible to claim even if a child is physically able to walk.

From age 5 years: Disability Living Allowance – Mobility Component – low rate

This claim needs to be made 3 months before the child's fifth birthday in order for it to be paid when the child is 5 years old. DLA advice explains that this benefit is claimable:[5]

- if the child can walk, but needs someone with them to make sure they are safe
- if the child can walk, but needs someone with them to help find their way around in places they do not know well.

The leaflet also emphasizes that all children may need some supervision when outside, but that children being claimed for must need more help or supervision than their peers.

From age 16 years: Income Support

Income Support can be claimed by a disabled person aged 16, 17 or 18 years, even if still at school. The test is that such individuals would be unlikely to get a job if they left school and were available for work. Again, this focuses on what young people are not able to do, and on how they differ from non-disabled individuals of the same age.

From age 16 years: Incapacity Benefit

This benefit replaced the Severe Disablement Allowance in 2001.

Incapacity Benefit can be claimed from 16 years of age. It cannot usually be claimed by non-disabled young people in full-time education, but a young person who is receiving the high rate of DLA, is registered blind or has severe learning difficulty may qualify. Income Support and Incapacity Benefit may be claimed at the same time, but the level of Income Support is higher than that of Incapacity Benefit for the first year, and only the higher benefit is payable. If either is claimed, Child Benefit is not payable to the parent.

Making the claim

For all the above benefits, a report from the child's doctor or specialist will probably be requested, either by the parents or by a professional assisting the parents to complete the forms. It can take at least 2 hours for the forms to be filled in thoroughly, but as the benefit awarded is usually based on the information on the forms, this is time well spent. It is, however, also essential that any report from a doctor or specialist comments not only on the impairment, but also on its effects on the child. Without the latter, it may be assumed that there is no significant impact.

It becomes clear, as the definitions, rules and tests appear, how very complicated it can be to make a claim. The first steps for families are simply knowing that these benefits exist, having some details on how to find more information and possibly receiving help filling in the application forms. This is especially important for families for whom English is a second language or in whom literacy is an issue. Helping a family to complete a form can also sometimes be used as a way of offering support on a wider practical and emotional level.

DWP benefits for the parents/carers of disabled children

A narrower range of benefits is available for parents and carers, although they are usually nominated as the appointee and are in receipt of most of the above benefits.

Carer's Allowance (formerly known as Invalid Care Allowance)

This benefit (£46.95 per week for the 2006-2007 financial year) is payable to a person who spends over 35 hours a week caring for a disabled person and who earns less than £85 net per week. The disabled person must be in receipt of the DLA Care Component high or middle rate for the claimant to be eligible. There are also many other rules involved, and claimants must seek advice about whether or not it is in their interest to claim this benefit, based on their income and circumstances.

Because the person they are looking after, by definition, receives the DLA, carers may also be able to claim the Disability Premium, the Disabled Child Premium and Council Tax reduction, as well as the Carer Premium. If the high rate of the DLA Care Component is received, the Enhanced Disability Premium may be applied for. Other premiums, such as those for a family or a pensioner, are available, but these are not specific to disabled children.

Additional benefits available to claimants of the DLA – Mobility Component – high rate

- The Blue Badge Scheme (which replaced Orange Badges in April 2000) allows badge holders to park in disabled parking bays, on single and double yellow lines for set periods, and at parking meters for no charge. Applications can be made for any disabled child over 2 years old. If the child receives the high rate of the DLA Mobility Component or is registered blind, he or she is eligible. Application forms are available from local authorities. Badge holders may be exempt from Central London Congestion Charging for an initial £10 administration fee, by applying to the Congestion Charging Office.
- Exemption from Road Tax for one car may be claimed.
- Vehicles with an exempt 'disabled' class tax disc are automatically exempt if the vehicle is registered with the DVLA, Swansea.
- Parents can apply to Motability to join its hire or hire-purchase scheme to obtain a car. Motability is a charity, and different rules apply according to whether a new or a used car is to be bought.

113

It can thus be seen that the permutations are endless, which is why specific advice is necessary. Thousands of pounds worth of benefits are unclaimed each year, so a little knowledge can go a very long way.

SOCIAL SERVICES DEPARTMENTS

Chronically Sick and Disabled Persons Act 1970

This Act allows local authorities to provide aids and equipment to disabled children, following an assessment, usually undertaken by an occupational therapist. As Primary Care Trusts also employ occupational therapists and supply health aids, it can, however, be very confusing for parents to know where to go, and many families do not realize that aids may be provided free. Examples of such aids range from special cutlery, hand-rails and bath seats, to larger items such as hoists and special chairs. Other support to families with disabled children, which may be provided under this Act, include holidays and telephone installation.

Carers and Disabled Children Act 2000

Social services departments do not generally provide financial help to families, although they occasionally provide food or food vouchers for families in crisis, and they may give specific financial help to children who are looked after. Under the Carers and Disabled Children Act 2000, local authorities do, however, have the power to offer, after an assessment, direct payments to young disabled people aged 16 and 17 years in order to allow them to purchase services that meet their needs. Direct payments may also be made to the parents of disabled children after an assessment, rather than their having to rely solely on the services provided by their local authority.

Carers (Equal Opportunities) Act 2004

If an assessment is being carried out on a disabled child or young person, then an assessment may be undertaken to address what support the carer may need.

Disabled Facilities Grant

Disabled children may be eligible for a Disabled Facilities Grant if they are, or could be, registered as disabled with their social services department. The local housing department administers the grant, but the starting place for most assessments is via a social services occupational therapist. The maximum grant that can be paid is £25,000 in England, and £30,000 in Wales. Examples of possible adaptations are making the entrance to the home accessible, providing an accessible lavatory, installing a lift and building an additional room. There is no means test when the application is for a disabled child or young person under 19 years of age.

PRIMARY CARE TRUSTS (PCTS)

Equipment is also available from PCTs, although, as with social service departments, the service may vary from area to area. Most, for example, give support to people who are incontinent, including advice, incontinence pads and treatment. Medical or nursing equipment usually heralds from here.

If a disabled child has serious walking difficulties and needs permanently to use a wheelchair or pushchair, the child must be assessed to decide what is most suitable. A referral will be made to the local wheelchair centre, via an occupational therapist in either the social services department or the PCT. Age restrictions may apply.

CHARITIES

Hundreds of charities can be approached to assist families with disabled children. The majority focus on specific impairments, examples being Scope, which assists children and adults with cerebral palsy, and ASBAH, for people with spina bifida and hydrocephalus. The larger charities such as these often have regional offices to provide local support. Many can give help with holidays or own holiday caravans. Contact a Family provides parents and professionals with help to find a local or national support group related to the child's impairment.

The main charity that provides financial help specifically for disabled children is the Family Fund, which is fully funded by the government. Its purpose is to ease the stress on families who care for very severely disabled children under 16 years old, by providing grants and information related to the care of the child.[6] The Family Fund helps families who are living in the UK, whose income is not much more than £23,000 a year and who have savings of under about £18,000. It will not help when the child resides in local authority care.

Help provided by the Family Fund includes: holidays and leisure breaks; the provision of a washing machine or tumble dryer because of constant bed wetting; driving lessons; a computer and play equipment. Application forms are available direct from the Family Fund. Even though the government funds the charity, many families are resistant to applying because they do not see themselves as needing 'charity'.

The fund also publishes very helpful information leaflets on welfare benefits, help with holidays, transport, adaptations, bedding and clothing, and a booklet on transition to adulthood, of which all are free to parents.

CONCLUSIONS

A wide range of financial help is available to the parents of disabled children, and medical professionals may be the first to inform families of their existence. Applications may not be backdated, so a late application could mean that a financial benefit is lost. There are, however, also many barriers that prevent families making a claim, and professionals have a responsibility to help families to find ways of overcoming these.

In many cases, a report from the child's doctor or specialist is needed; in other cases, he or she may be in the best position to provide the 'statement from someone who knows the child'. Whether it is a requirement or a request, it is important that information is provided about the impairment and its impact on the child. Without this, it will be harder for the validity of the claim to be assessed.

Prioritizing care in a resource-limited health service

Sian Griffiths • Tony Jewell

SUMMARY

Resources for healthcare will always be limited, and difficult choices need to be made about how they are used. While government policy prioritizes children's health, particularly the need to focus on reducing inequalities and promoting healthy lifestyles, local health systems face the dilemmas of balancing central priorities with local freedoms. Dilemmas between population versus individual needs, prevention rather than treatment, consideration of patient choice, and the impact of unstable systems and continual policy changes all affect choices about care.

In response to such tensions we describe a model for local decision-making, the Priorities Forum established in Oxford-shire. The forum created an ethical framework for decision-making that utilized the values of effectiveness, efficiency and patient choice, and engaged key stakeholders in the difficult process of allocating scarce resources.

INTRODUCTION

The UK health service is a tax-based funding system which offers prevention, treatment and care, free at the point of need, across the whole range of health services. When it was established Nye Bevan, the first Minister of Health, told the profession:

...my job is to give you all the facilities, resources and help I can and then leave you alone as professional men and women to use your skill and judgement without hindrance.

The initial post-war optimism assumed that, with enough cash to treat a backlog of disease, costs would start to go down as the population became healthier. This was, as we now know, misplaced optimism. The cost of healthcare has continued to rise inexorably, not only in UK but across the world. The problem of meeting needs and balancing supply and demand within existing resources challenges all governments and societies. Whatever the model – tax funded, private or insurance based – dilemmas about affordable treatments persist in the face of technological advance, increasing longevity and more informed and articulate patients.

In his 2002 report, Wanless[1] identified:

...the need for a very substantial increase in resources for health and social care ... there will also need to be an increase in the number of doctors and nurses over that already planned.

Despite the subsequent UK cash infusion to redress the substantial underfunding identified by Wanless and bring spending to levels comparative to other similar economies, there is still a gap between demand and supply, and the NHS continues to face deficits and cuts.

The cost drivers of increasing numbers of older people living longer, of changing health needs, particularly the growing burden of chronic non-communicable diseases, of existing service commitments, the advances in medical technology and treatments, and of changing public/patient expectations, will not disappear. Limited resources will need to be spent efficiently and effectively to give best value to the population.

WHAT ARE THE HEALTH PRIORITIES FOR CHILDREN?

Governments across the UK have prioritized the health of children. In setting targets in the National Service Frameworks and through performance management strategies to tackle the major killers of cancer, heart disease and diabetes, the importance of the upstream approach to prevention is recognized explicitly. For example, children have been identified as a priority in England's *Choosing Health*,[2] in which improving the health of children is an explicit priority for all government departments. Other initiatives and policies that highlight the need to break the cycle of deprivation and give children from deprived backgrounds greater opportunities to be healthier, educated and economically secure include Sure Start[3] and the *National Service Framework For Children*.[4] Taking a life-course approach, these initiatives prioritize promoting the health of pregnant mothers by encouraging breastfeeding, and the provision of good support and care not only through the healthcare sector but also through education and enhanced social opportunity. Childhood initiatives, such as practice payments for childhood surveillance, and targets that reward GP practices for high immunization rates also help prioritize children's health. Initiatives such as the government funded Healthy Schools Programme[5] highlight the importance of investment in prevention – aiming to encourage healthy behaviours and reduce inequalities. Successive health ministers have reiterated the unacceptability of the 9-year gap in life expectancy of a boy born in the deprived north of England compared with his counterpart born in the affluent south-east. Even within Wales there is a 4-year gap in life expectancy for a boy born in the south Wales valleys compared with the affluent farming country to the west. Devolved governments set their own priorities, incuding childhood accidents as an inequalities target in Wales,[6] and breastfeeding has been included as a priority in Scotland.[7]

BALANCING THE BOOKS

While governments can produce longer term strategies, and the media comment with foreboding on the growing health threats of junk food, inactive obese adolescents and consumer society, healthcare providers and professionals are struggling with the day-to-day problems of making best use of available resources. They continue to face the need to balance:

- central priorities versus local freedoms
- population versus individual needs
- prevention versus treatment
- patient choice versus other wishes and needs.

Central priorities versus local freedoms

National service frameworks with explicit standards to be met and evidence-based clinical guidance have been put in place across the UK. However, there is also an expectation that local flexibility will tailor implementation to meet the needs of the local population. As such, the top-down agenda needs to be balanced with local needs and circumstances, and this sometimes produces conflicting priorities.

Local freedoms in England have been increased by the changes in primary care. Primary care commissioning has been strengthened (e.g. through Choose and Book in which GPs and their patients can 'shop around' for the best and most suitable care). The opportunity to choose from a range of public and private providers increases this freedom. Guidance from the Department of Health emphasizes local freedoms and gives encouragement for local innovation, but at the same time reinforces the need to deliver national programmes within a cost envelope. Thus all local choices take place within a managerial framework that has inherent tension.

At the national level, the Department of Health establishes high level standards, and the Healthcare Commission[8] establishes the regulatory framework and process within which the performance of local services can be judged. In addition, the National Institute for Health and Clinical Excellence (NICE)[9] appraises treatments for their effectiveness, often using measures such as quality-adjusted life-years (QALYs) and numbers needed to treat (NNT), and makes recommendations about what patients can expect their local primary care trusts (PCTs) to commission and their local services to provide. Politicians make clear to the public their expectations of national bodies such as NICE, anticipating that advice will be implemented universally and that resources should be found from within local financial allocations. At the local level, PCTs try to exert their independence, address their role in improving health to meet these expectations and at the same time balance their books.

Population versus individual needs

The dilemma about whether to invest in an expensive treatment for one individual or to use the same scarce resources on a programme benefiting a larger group of patients is an ongoing dilemma in priority setting. The case of Child B in Cambridgeshire[10] highlighted the pressures that local providers can be put

under to provide expensive treatment, particularly in tragic end-of-life circumstances. The moral dilemma to be faced is whether the chance of saving that one life outweighs the benefits of providing a service to a larger number, perhaps help in reducing childhood obesity, within the same available resources. Should resources be committed to giving an expensive but unproven cancer drug to a child who may only gain a few months more of life at the expense of investing in a smoking-cessation programme for teenagers, which might save more lives but its impact not become obvious for many years?

Gains that are substantial at a population level may have only limited benefit for an individual, and vice versa. For example, improving nutrition through promoting healthier foods or reducing exposure to tobacco smoke by banning smoking in public places may help a population, but treatment to reduce hypertension will help an individual directly.

Prevention versus treatment

While the case for investment in prioritizing prevention has been eloquently made by Wanless,[1] more often than not the shorter term rewards of curing illness take precedence. Treatment can bring observable benefits and is more tangible.

Using the example of raised blood cholesterol,[11] if 15–20% of people in the UK have raised blood cholesterol levels and are thus at increased risk, should treatment be targeted at the small proportion (5%) of people at highest risk? Or should everybody in the population be encouraged to make changes in their lifestyle so that the average level of blood cholesterol is lowered and every person's risk is lowered by a small amount?

Patient choice

Another major strand of policy has been the emphasis on patient, and to some extent public, involvement in decisions, and the increasing emphasis on patient choice. The government's intention is to empower both local people and local clinicians to become more involved in shaping and running their local health services. However, engaging the public in the debate about the best use of resources can starkly highlight the difficulties in balancing local wishes, such as keeping a community hospital open, with the need to deliver on national priorities such as waiting-list targets. The Child B case[10] highlighted a particular aspect of patient choice: the need to consider the child's views, not just those of the parents who, amongst other parties, play a role in balancing such decisions this poses.

UNSTABLE SYSTEMS AND CONTINUAL POLICY CHANGES

An additional complication to decision-making is the continual structural change to the NHS. The reforms introduced in *Shifting the Balance of Power*[12] gave decision-making power to PCTs to improve the health of their population, to secure the provision of services, and to integrate health and social care at a local level. No sooner was this arrangement introduced than structural change was reintroduced with reforms to the English system, at the same time as rules for commissioning change and hospitals had changed to create foundation trusts (hospitals with greater degrees of independence). Each change means new organizations coming into being, with new staff, new boards and new relationships to be established within the commissioning–providing process. The steep learning curve embarked on is not assisted by the spectre of continual change, the pressure to develop new models of care, and changing roles within the work forces of both health and social services.

Individual clinicians and their patients might well be forgiven for feelings of confusion. On the one hand, they are encouraged to make their own local decisions, but, on the other hand, they have to meet the top-down agenda with its emphasis on performance management and meeting targets. Difficult decisions, about defining boundaries and rationing care, continue to need to be made. The King's Fund[13] identified the main questions as:

- What range of services should be in the healthcare rationing debate?
- What is the range of ethically defensible criteria for deciding between competing claims and resources?
- Whose values should be taken into account?
- Who should undertake rationing?
- How will they be held accountable?
- How explicit should rationing principles be?
- What information would be needed to make rationing more explicit and to hold decision-makers more accountable?

The debate on the NHS continues to be ambivalent about the balance between prevention and acute care, between individual choice and public good, on what the NHS can be expected to deliver at the margins of care, and how the core of the NHS business can be defined. Revisiting the work of Ivan Illich, Moynihan and Smith[14] ask questions about the boundaries of healthcare from economic, ethical and international perspectives. It can be argued that there are vested interests in medicalizing life's problems, and in continuing to battle with the realities of death, pain and sickness, while at the same time ignoring the undoubted benefits that could arise from improving living standards and public health services (e.g. those increasing immunization uptake in developing countries). Within the UK there is a general belief in the NHS, but the belief has ragged boundaries. Balancing the needs and wishes of all parties – politicians, public, providing clinicians, GPs and patients – is a complex task. This is clearly demonstrated by our experience in setting local priorities, which is described in the remainder of this chapter.

THE OXFORDSHIRE EXPERIENCE

We describe here the experience of priority setting in Oxfordshire, when the county was a single health authority before splitting into three PCTs in 2002, only to recombine in 2006. As described elsewhere,[15] the model has been adapted and has influenced other healthcare organizations, such as the Cambridge and Peterborough public health network, who have developed their own frameworks.

The need to balance healthcare choices in an open and explicit way within limited resources led the health authority to create a forum, which openly discussed issues of prioritization. Starting in the time of the internal market, and initially dealing with cases of individual patients who requested treatment not included within the contracts set in the purchaser–provider discussions, the Priorities Forum (PF) was established by the health authority to enable open discussion at the margins of the NHS. The process that developed enabled Case Law to be established through systematic and open decision-making. The initial focus on individual cases soon raised the question of consistency and the justification of decisions.[16] To underpin the decision-making process, an ethical framework was agreed, the purpose of which was to support decision-making.

The ethical framework

The purpose of the PF's ethical framework was three-fold:

- It provided a coherent structure for discussion, ensuring that all important aspects of each issue were considered.
- It ensured consistency in decision-making over time and between different clinical topics.
- It gave the PF a means of expressing the reasons behind the decisions made, which was particularly important for the appeals procedure and for being open with the public about the rationing decisions that were being made.

The ethical framework had three main values:

- effectiveness
- equity
- patient choice.

Effectiveness

Effectiveness is the extent to which a healthcare intervention (a treatment, procedure or service) achieves an improvement for patients. The PF considers the evidence of effectiveness from research findings whenever it makes a decision or recommendation. The evidence falls broadly into three categories:

- If there is good evidence that a treatment is ineffective, then clearly it should not be funded.
- If there is good evidence that an intervention is effective, then it may or may not be funded, depending on other criteria such as value in terms of relative benefit compared with other interventions.
- In many cases, there is little firm evidence to conclude whether an intervention is effective or not. Interventions that fall into this category may or may not be funded. Here the PF has to make a judgement about the likely effectiveness without the benefit of good-quality evidence.

Equity

PF decisions are also formulated on the basis of equity (fairness), the core principle of which is that people in similar situations should be treated similarly. There should be no discrimination on the grounds of employment status, family circumstances, lifestyle, learning difficulty, age, race, sex, social position, financial status, religion or place of abode. Healthcare should be allocated justly and fairly on the basis of need, and in terms of maximizing the welfare of patients within the budget available. The PF tries to balance these approaches using a two-step process: first considering the cost-effectiveness of the intervention (e.g. using QALYs); and second, if the intervention is less cost-effective than interventions normally funded, it considers whether there are, nevertheless, reasons for funding it. Such reasons would include:

- urgent need (e.g. life-saving treatment)
- treatment for those whose quality of life is severely affected by chronic illness (e.g. patients with multiple sclerosis)

justification for a treatment of high expense due to characteristics of the patient (e.g. the same level of dental care should be offered to people with learning disabilities as the rest of the population, even if it is less cost-effective because more specialized services are needed).

Patient choice

Patient choice is considered by the PF to be important in reaching decisions about priorities for healthcare. The collective views of patient groups and those of individual patients are taken into account in the decision-making process. The PF recognizes that people need access to relevant information to help them make choices. The value of patient choice has three implications for the work of the PF:

- In assessing research on the effectiveness of interventions, it is important to look at outcome measures that matter to patients.
- Within those healthcare interventions that are purchased, patients should be enabled to make their own choices about which they want.
- Each patient is unique. The PF recognizes that some people may have a better chance than others of benefiting from a particular treatment.

However, patient choice is not the only criterion, and restricted resources mean that the PF often has to refuse access to treatment. The authority will not make an exception simply because a patient chooses it, since this would deny another patient access to more effective treatment. The PF, therefore, has to carefully balance the components of its ethical framework.

Application of the ethical framework

The ethical framework was used for all discussions in the PF, which worked on the basis of monthly meetings and wide representation from clinicians, managers, public health and the public. Each meeting would consider issues raised by clinicians and managers using the criteria of the framework. With the introduction of NICE, the process was adapted to explore the local implementation of its guidance. In addition, the PF continued to consider individual cases that clinicians thought should be exceptions to the agreed commissioning arrangements, or those not included either because their condition was rare and expensive or because it was new and as yet not included within existing services. Decisions were made public through a variety of mechanisms and the ethical values highlighted within this process. The output from the PF was in the form of clinical advice, not commitment of resources, and was fed into the commissioning discussions – most recently those around the service and financial frameworks. Although advice from the PF influenced decisions, it was not always taken in the final analysis due to other pressures on the system.

Some examples of the issues discussed which are relevant to paediatrics were:

- whether or not to fund sign-language counselling for deaf children (supported)
- whether to change policy to support universal BCG in schools (not a priority for resources at the present time – reconsider in light of forthcoming TB strategy)
- whether a specialist paediatric gastroenterology service, linked to university research work, should be funded by PCTs (lack of support, despite growth of clinical work)

- whether or not to support postnatal psychiatric services (supported by the PF but funding not made available by management)
- referral to specialist centre out of county (not supported on grounds of lack of evidence of effectiveness/equity for other patients).

These examples demonstrate the range of issues that the PF discussed, from preventive to specialist services.

The current changes to the structure of the NHS will once again create the need to review the work of the PF, particularly how PCTs will make such decisions. For Oxfordshire, the challenge will be whether it can once more work as a single system for the population of the county. Other challenges to be faced include:

- accommodating changing NHS structures
- being transparent about the relationship between clinical advice and financial decision-making
- defining the choices for perspectives of professionals and patients
- making decisions explicit and transparent
- handling expectations of the public about the limits of patient choice
- balancing top-down and bottom-up needs and demands.

Changing structures

The continual reorganization of the NHS redefines the powers of decision-making with each new policy and structure. The PF was initially established at the time of the purchaser–provider split, when there was often a confrontational relationship between the purchasers (health authorities), who were allocated funding, and the providers of services, who delivered to contract. A key principle of the PF was to bring clinicians, purchasers and provider managers together to discuss difficult decision-making. With the shift towards a health systems approach, the approach of the PF is now well accepted. However, the delegation of commissioning to primary care has changed the decision-making process, with more direct engagement of GPs, as well as new management and accountability structures. There is a natural tendency to discard the past, and to wish to do things differently. There is a risk of losing the shared understanding of the role of values and the ethical framework in making difficult choices, and there are anxieties about fragmentation, lack of understanding of specialist services by PCTs, and potential harm from failing to invest in less common conditions. Without local networking, there is an even greater potential risk of 'post-code prescribing' for smaller geographical areas.

Relationship between clinical advice and financial decision-making

Clinical engagement was a key feature of the process of decision-making, with clinicians presenting their case using standard guidelines. These guidelines emphasized the need to consider epidemiology, evidence of effectiveness, estimation of cost and quantification of health gain. They also highlighted the need to consider whether a treatment was replacing another less-effective or less important treatment, and whether there were other less-effective treatments in other specialties from which resources could be shifted. In practice, the latter was not a popular discussion point but the principle of substitution could be used to effect disinvestment.

One of the criticisms levelled at the PF over the years has been of raising clinical expectations and cutting across the financial decision-making processes. The myth that discussion implied commitment of resources had to be dispelled by close involvement of management. Within the climate of more PCTs and the government emphasis on frontline clinician involvement, there will be a bigger challenge to balance clinical aspirations with limited resources. The challenge will be most difficult when it comes to clinical innovation and the interface with research.

Defining the choices

One of the issues raised by the PF process is which decisions are subjected to the rigorous evaluation and discussion. In general, the discussions had been focused on NICE guidelines, on local hot issues or on desired innovations related to research. What was not addressed was the relative investments, for example between prevention or care, or between the different national service framework (NSF) programmes. Individual issues within NSFs were debated, as was the NICE guidance, but the PF failed to grasp the complex issues of justifying expenditure in one area, such as acute care, rather than another, such as support in the community. Consequently, the rigorous process of evaluating evidence of effectiveness, ensuring equity and balancing patient choice has only been applied to some elements of the allocation of resources.

Making decisions explicit

Explicit decision-making assumes a framework and set of values, which are owned by those involved in making these decisions. At the outset, the PF values were discussed by the health authority, who formally adopted them. Any new arrangements will need reclarification and ownership of values. The explicit values of the NHS plan are concordant with those of the PF's decision-making.

Expectations of the public about choice

Within Oxfordshire there were several strategies for involving the public in the process of the PF. The first was representation at the meetings through the presence of the local consumer representatives and non-executive board members. The second was by being open about decisions and making papers available via the website and board papers. Thirdly, there was an appeals process. In addition, there were seminars and workshops arranged on an ad hoc basis. However, it was a continual aspiration to increase awareness of the debates and of the issues involved in making these difficult choices that the PF was faced with – a challenge that PCTs will need to pick up.

CONCLUSION

Making choices about how to make best use of limited resources is not easy when expectations and demands exceed availability of resources. Although there will be evidence of effectiveness for some treatments, it may not be as robust as for others, which may be innovative or may focus on prevention and deliver health gain over a longer time period. Experience from the PF in Oxfordshire led to recognition that measurements such as QALYs are useful decision aids, but that the most important element of decision-making is open debate within an explicit ethical framework and with due process. The decisions made were best judgements informed by consideration of effectiveness, equity and patient preference, taking into account the views of all stakeholders. The new structures in England mean new ways of making decisions, perhaps based on the lessons from the past, but the biggest challenge remains to shape local decision-making to reflect local priorities and not just respond to the national political imperatives.

Chapter Twenty Eight

How do we choose which life to save? Equality of access or a fair go?

Julian Savulescu

SUMMARY

This chapter examines the ethics of distributing limited resources when demand exceeds supply. I examine two ethical theories, egalitarianism and utilitarianism, applied to an example of allocating hearts to children who have cardiac failure. I examine the strengths and weaknesses of these approaches. I argue that we must include some concern for equality of access (equal treatment for equal need). But this should occur within a context of first evaluating the impact of a medical intervention on how long an individual will live, his or her quality of life and the probability of the intervention succeeding. I propose a third more plausible approach: 'a fair go'. I also examine whether the cost of treatment, the existence of dependants and responsibility for illness should play a part in the allocation of limited resources. Finally, I briefly discuss the role of patients and their families in making these decisions.

PRACTICE POINTS

- All resources involved in the delivery of healthcare are finite, and questions of how fairly to allocate limited resources are inescapable.
- According to egalitarianism, limited resources should be distributed according to a principle of equality of access: equal treatment for equal need. Failure to treat people equally may constitute illegal discrimination.
- According to utilitarianism, resources should be distributed to bring about the greatest good to the greatest number. Utilitarians give priority to the person who stands to gain the longest prolongation of life, or the greatest improvement in quality of life, or who has the best chance of achieving a successful outcome from treatment.
- A practical compromise between egalitarianism and utilitarianism is the notion of 'a fair go', in which healthcare is delivered in such a way as to satisfy as many people's legitimate claims to healthcare as possible. A legitimate claim to healthcare exists when a person has a reasonable chance of reasonable extension of life and/or a reasonable improvement in its quality.
- Cost of healthcare in monetary terms of treating individuals is relevant in determining whether the maximum number of claims is satisfied.
- In practice, it is difficult to include considerations of responsibility for illness or injury or benefit to dependants in a fair way.

INTRODUCTION

All resources are limited. Resources in healthcare include expenditure on health, pharmaceuticals, medical procedures and investigations. But they also include human resources, such as numbers of doctors and the amount of time each of these has to spend on healthcare delivery. Very often, demand exceeds supply. We then face decisions about how to distribute limited resources among a population.

One example is the shortage of organs for transplantation. About one-third of children die on heart transplant waiting lists while waiting for an organ. Consider the hypothetical case of six children who are 16 years old (Box 28.1). Each has cardiac failure. Each requires a heart transplant. There are four hearts available. Who should receive a transplant?

There are two broad approaches to the distribution of limited resources: egalitarianism and utilitarianism.

EGALITARIANISM

Egalitarians claim that limited resources should be distributed according to a principle of equality of access: equal treatment for equal need. This is one of the founding principles of the NHS. It was recently affirmed by the Report of the Independent Inquiries into Paediatric Cardiac Services at the Royal Brompton Hospital and Harefield Hospital (the Brompton Report).[1] The Brompton Report investigated allegations that children with Down syndrome were discriminated against at the Royal Brompton Hospital. It was alleged that children were inappropriately 'steered away' from surgery to correct heart defects because they had Down syndrome. The Report recommended that:

> The Trust's policies confirm clearly that people with a disability are entitled to, and will be accorded in all departments and at every level, the same rights of access to services as those without a disability; and that consultants should take the lead in implementing policies and influencing attitudes regarding equality of access. (Section 110 of the Brompton Report[1])

BOX 28.1

Six children needing a heart transplant

- David has severe intellectual disability from Down syndrome. He lives in an institution. His parents visit him on weekends.

- Christina has cystic fibrosis and requires a heart–lung transplant.

- Luke has cardiac failure, which resulted from drugs used to treat leukaemia. His leukaemia has been in remission for 2 years.

- Victor has viral cardiomyopathy.

- Anne has heart failure secondary to severe anorexia nervosa.

- Simon has viral cardiomyopathy. Prior to developing cardiomyopathy, he expressed a desire to donate one of his kidneys to his brother who has renal failure. He is a compatible donor with his sibling. No cadaveric organ donor can be found for his brother. He hopes to donate a kidney after he has had a heart transplant.

Equality of access is required by law. The European Convention on Human Rights states that:

Everyone's right to life shall be protected by law ... No one shall be deprived of his right to life intentionally save in the execution of a sentence of a court following his conviction for a crime for which this penalty is provided by law. (Section 27.13 of the Brompton Report[1])

and

The enjoyment of the rights and freedoms set forth in this Convention shall be secured without discrimination on any ground such as sex, race, colour or other status. (Section 27.13 of the Brompton Report[1])

Denying a person medical treatment on grounds of disability would be unlawful discrimination under this Convention and the UK Disability Discrimination Act 1995.

Egalitarianism has many versions. The most sophisticated egalitarian theory is that advanced by Rawls.[2] Daniels has applied this to healthcare.[3] A key feature of this approach is that distributors of health resources should give priority to those who are worst off. How we decide who is worst off is a difficult issue. In the context of cardiac transplantation, this is often interpreted as being the person who is most likely to die without treatment or who will die soonest.

In the case of the children in Box 28.1, let us assume that each child needs a heart transplant equally (each is equally likely to die soon without it). According to a principle of equality of access, we should draw lots to decide which of the six children will receive one of the four hearts. Or choose some other random procedure such as 'first come, first served'. The idea behind egalitarianism is that each of us has a life of equal value, and arbitrary factors such as disability should not be considered in determining our eligibility for treatment. John Harris claims that each rational person wants at least three things from healthcare: (1) the maximum possible life expectancy for him or her; (2) the best quality of life for him or her; and (3) the best opportunity or chance for him or her of

getting both (1) and (2).[4] Treating people as equals requires giving equal consideration to each person's claim.

Equality of access thus instructs us to ignore all considerations of: (1) length of life; (2) quality of life; and (3) the probability of achieving these. The Brompton Report recognized this when it was critical of cardiologists including considerations of length and quality of life in calculating whether surgery was in the child's best interests. It was also critical of 'value judgements – for example, related to factors such as limited lifespan, inability to get the most out of life, or not being a burden upon others or upon society' playing a part in clinical decision-making.

But ignoring considerations of quantity and quality of life, and probability of success, is problematic. Only considering clinical need will result in some children with very good prognoses being denied treatment. Imagine that Luke's leukaemia relapses and he is given 1 year to live. His heart failure deteriorates. He needs a heart transplant if he is to live another year. If we transplant Luke, one of the other five children will necessarily die. It would be wrong to allow Victor to die if he could gain another 20 years of life from a heart transplant. In this case, we should give Victor priority over Luke.

It is also wrong to ignore quality of life considerations altogether. Let us assume David's intellectual disability is very profound, and he cannot recognize his parents or engage with the world around him. It would be wrong to transplant him and allow Victor to die. Or, take a more extreme example. Children born with trisomy 18 have profound intellectual disability and usually die soon after birth. But some survive. Some of these require a heart transplant if they are to continue to live. On a strict reading of equality, these children with trisomy 18 should have the same chance of receiving a heart transplant as a child with no intellectual disability and a normal life expectancy. This is wrong. Indeed, cardiac transplantation is not performed on children with trisomy 18, even when they need it.

Equality of access also urges us to ignore the probability of survival. Imagine that the administration of immunosuppressive drugs to Luke will increase the probability of his leukaemia relapsing. He has only a 40% chance of surviving 10 years. Imagine that Victor has a 90% chance of surviving 10 years. Equality of access requires that we toss a coin. Indeed, we should toss a coin even if Luke's chances are very small, around 1%. This is wrong. We should give preference to Victor over Luke, if his chances of survival are significantly greater.

When resources are limited and demand outstrips supply, equality of access will have the result that fewer people will live, and those who do live will live for shorter periods and lead worse quality lives.

UTILITARIANISM

Utilitarianism requires that resources be distributed to bring about the greatest good to the greatest number, as the father of utilitarianism, Jeremy Bentham, put it. Utilitarians give priority to the person who stands to gain the longest prolongation of life, or the greatest improvement in quality of life, or who has the best chance of achieving a successful outcome from treatment. For utilitarians, the intellectual disability of David detracts from the overall value of saving his life. This is a reason against treating him.

Health economists have attempted to combine all these factors into the quality-adjusted life-year (QALY) approach to allocating health resources. A QALY is a year of life adjusted by its quality:

The essence of a QALY is that it takes a year of healthy life expectancy to be worth 1, but regards a year of unhealthy life expectancy as worth less than 1. Its precise value is lower the worse the quality of life of the unhealthy person (which is what the quality adjusted bit is all about).[5]

While public rhetoric on distributive justice is generally egalitarian, courts have appealed to quality of life considerations to justify withholding or withdrawing life-prolonging medical treatments, such as artificial feeding, at least in cases of permanent unconsciousness or severe cognitive impairment.[6]

Courts are also attracted to explicit utilitarian reasoning. An example is the case of Jaymee Bowen. She had leukaemia and received one bone marrow transplant, but her leukaemia relapsed. She was refused a second bone marrow transplant. This was expected to cost £75,000 (in 1995). Sir Thomas Bingham, Master of the Rolls, said:

Difficult and agonizing judgments have to be made as to how a limited budget is best allocated to the maximum advantage of the maximum number of patients. That is not a judgment the court can make.[7]

Indeed, the General Medical Council apparently has some utilitarian sympathies. Recent guidance states that:

...the clinical team in determining priorities and the utilization of the resources made available to them by the NHS is entitled to take into account the likely success of the treatment proposed. It would be appropriate ... In assessing priorities for ... transplantation to take into account co-morbidities.[8]

Yet utilitarianism also leads to counterintuitive results. It seems to make too fine grained a distinction between the value of lives. For example, young people should have priority over older people on a utilitarian schema. The reason for this is that young people stand to benefit more from medical treatments that are life-saving or life-enhancing across a whole life because they will live longer on average. But it seems absurd to say we should give priority to someone who is 13 years old rather than someone who is 17 years old because, on average, he or she is expected to live longer. This feature of utilitarianism has been said to be 'ageist'.[9, 10]

Similarly, even small impairments in quality of life make someone a lower priority for treatment according utilitarians. Imagine that Anne's life is worse because of her obsession with body image and food. According to utilitarians, the value of saving her life is less because it will be of slightly lower quality than, say, that of Victor. Harris[11] has claimed that this constitutes 'double jeopardy', disadvantaging further those who are already disadvantaged.

Utilitarianism and health economics may also pay insufficient attention to need. For example, imagine that Victor could be managed on medications alone, but would suffer a serious decrement in his quality of life. A heart transplant would significantly improve his quality of life. Christina will die without a cardiac transplant. If Victor would live significantly longer than Christina with a transplant, a utilitarian approach might favour treating him. This would be so if the transplant was only life-enhancing and not life-saving. Many people would believe that Christina, in this situation, needs a transplant more, as she needs it to live. So she should have priority in this version of the case.

A RIGHT TO A FAIR GO

Egalitarianism gives insufficient weight to length of life, quality of life and probability of successful outcome. But utilitarianism gives too much weight to these, and no attention to need. Is there another way? John Mackie, a famous Australian philosopher, once said that distributive justice is about 'the right to a fair go.' But what is 'a fair go'? I believe getting a fair go is having a fair chance of receiving medical treatment that has a reasonable chance of providing a reasonable extension of one's life and/or a reasonable improvement in its quality. I have summarized the key elements of a fair go in Box 28.2.

BOX 28.2

A fair go (in lexical priority)

1. Each person has a legitimate claim to medical care when that care provides that person with a reasonable chance of a reasonable extension of life and/or a reasonable improvement in its quality.

2. Comparable legitimate claims are those referring to similar needs.

3. As many comparable legitimate claims should be satisfied as possible.

4. Provided as many comparable legitimate claims are being satisfied as possible, there should be equality of access to medical care, and no allocation on the basis of irrelevant factors such as socioeconomic status, race, gender, etc.

What constitutes 'reasonable' is determined in part by the scarcity of the resource. A reasonable prolongation of life in paediatric cardiac transplantation would be years, not months. It would be wrong to transplant children with severe intellectual disability with the result that children with much better intellectual functioning die. However, there is also great variation in the quality of people's lives with disability, and with Down syndrome in particular. It is true that Down syndrome is associated with intellectual disability, infertility, reduced opportunities for independent living and employment, shorter life span, and early onset Alzheimer disease. But a person with Down syndrome can have a good life. That might be enough to justify a claim on scarce community resources in a particular case, depending on the level of disability.

A decent theory of distributive justice would also prevent 'queue jumping'. People who clearly need a procedure less should not jump the queue in front of those who need it more. The plausible element of egalitarianism is that people must have reasonably comparable needs to be a candidate for treatment. Needs should be determined by comparing what will happen with and without the procedure, and how likely and soon these events are to occur.

Which four of the six children should be transplanted? It is not possible to say from the details provided. It will depend on what the alternatives are, how long each stands to live after transplantation and what their quality of life will be like, and how likely heart transplantation is to be successful. If there are significant differences in these factors, prioritization is justified. If there are not significant differences, everyone should have an equal chance.

OTHER FACTORS

Cost

Cost in monetary terms of treating individuals is relevant in determining whether the maximum number of claims are satisfied. For example, if providing care in a non-specialist centre is twice as expensive as providing it in a specialist centre, then only half the people who could be treated would be treated if care was solely provided in non-specialist centres. Respecting people as persons requires, I believe, satisfying as many legitimate claims that people have as possible.

In the context of the example of the six children, providing Christina with a heart transplant also requires providing her with a lung transplant. If this results in another child or adult not receiving a lung transplant, this is an indirect additional cost of transplanting her. It would be a reason against treating her.

Responsibility

It is sometimes said that smokers or alcoholics should have a lower priority for receiving scarce treatments because they are responsible for their illness. It might be claimed that Anne should have a lower priority because she is responsible for her predicament.

There are a number of problems with allocating resources according to how responsible a person is for their illness.[12] First, responsibility for behaviour is difficult to assess. Upbringing, peer pressure, and perhaps genes predisposing to addictive behaviour may combine to make a particular individual more likely to act in a certain way.

Second, prioritizing health delivery according to responsibility has broader implications. It implies that those who practise unsafe sex and contract the human immunodeficiency virus (HIV) should not be treated. The obese and those who eat fatty, salty fast food should not have heart surgery. Those who engage in risky sports such as mountaineering or skiing should be given lower priority over the sedentary and docile. Drivers and motorcycle riders should have a lower priority than public transport users, since it is known that these entail higher risks of injury. It is doubtful whether we can accurately determine how responsible a person is for his or her illness.

But there are more sinister consequences of using responsibility to allocate resources. Liberalism is based on giving individuals freedom to live their lives as they choose. All activities in life (including those which are fun) entail some risk. To use responsibility for illness as a criterion for allocating medical resources would be to indirectly discourage people from engaging in activities that involve risk, which may severely constrict the range of possible lives people can lead.

Dependants (or social utility)

During the 1990s, the New Zealand Government set up the National Advisory Committee on Health and Disability to advise Ministers on developing priorities for the delivery of healthcare. It developed guidelines to rate the relative priority of individuals with a particular condition for treatment. These guidelines were formed after public consultation. The early guidelines explicitly gave weight to dependants in establishing priority. In the early guidelines on cataract removal, for example, 16 points could be gained through having dependants, out of a maximum total of 100 points. The National Waiting Times project was the ultimate policy emerging from the early pilots. The scoring mechanisms consist of Clinical Access Priority Criteria (CAPC), which are an attempt to establish clinical need. In ophthalmology, the CAPC include reference to the well-being of others insofar as the capacity of the patient to live independently and to care for others can score 5 points (out of a total of 50).

In the case of the six children, treating Simon will also benefit his brother to a significant degree. As in the case of responsibility, it is not clear which benefits to others should count (does an employer benefit his employees?) and how we should determine this in a fair and accurate way in practice.

WHO DECIDES? THE ROLE OF FAMILY

Who decides what is 'reasonable'? There is no obvious answer. Those who decide that the length, probability or quality of life is unreasonable must be prepared to defend their decision. That defence should occur in comparative terms, taking due consideration of the other people they have in their care, and the impact of treatment on their relative in terms of the length, quality and probability of survival.

In response to my editorial on a similar topic,[13] Professor Brian Neville states:

There is nowhere in the argument a place for the views of families or people with Down's syndrome. Most paediatricians experience and respect the ways in which families and friends contribute to difficult decision-making. It would be a great mistake to assume that this is an adversarial situation.[14]

I agree with Professor Neville that the views of families are important in determining whether children are given life-prolonging medical treatment. However, if we take seriously the claims to equality of access made in the Brompton Report and current law, there is no place for such views.

Consider the following three points:

- It is in the best interests of (almost all) children with disability such as Down syndrome to live. Thus, it is in the interests of children with Down syndrome to receive cardiac surgery (Brompton Report) or other life-prolonging treatments (heart transplantation).
- The Disability Discrimination Act states that no one can be discriminated against because of disability (no matter how severe), including the provision of health (equality of access).
- Doctors have a legal obligation to do what is in a child's best interests, regardless of what his or her parents want. Thus they are required to give lifesaving blood transfusions to children of Jehovah's Witnesses, even if their parents object.

If we accept all these points, we should conclude that doctors must place all children with disability (no matter how severe) on waiting lists for heart, lung and kidney transplants, even if the parents do not want them placed on such transplant lists. The only possible exception would be disabilities so severe as to make life not worth living. This conclusion is hard to accept and would radically change clinical practice.

Public officials (doctors, or administrators, or politicians, or other public servants) must decide which treatments will be offered and to what extent. It is a simple consequence of demand outstripping supply of limited resources that not everyone who might benefit from medical treatment will be offered it. Families and individuals seeking treatment have important information to provide on the value of extending the candidate's life and on his or her quality of life. This will help doctors (or the relevant public decision-maker) to decide whether there will be a reasonable prolongation of life or a reasonable quality in a particular case. But, at least in public medicine, families and patients have only the choice to accept or reject treatment if it is offered to them. They have no right to demand what is not their fair share.

ANOTHER ALTERNATIVE?

I have previously argued that there is a better alternative.[13] We could change our attitudes to organ donation to increase supply. Then, hopefully, all those who have the prospect of a reasonably good life could have the chance to lead that life. The terrible constraint that forces us to decide between people would be removed.

But this is only a partial (although important) solution. Even if there were enough hearts to provide for all the children who need them, there will be other resources that cannot be provided to everyone who needs them. We could increase the amount we spend on health but, eventually, we will be able to spend no more. Questions of distributive justice are inescapable. Acknowledging the reality of our finite world of resources is the first and most important step in arriving at a plausible theory of distributive justice.

Chapter Twenty Nine

Withholding and withdrawing neonatal intensive care

29

Victor F. Larcher • Michael F. Hird

SUMMARY

Provision of intensive care enables the lives of small babies to be sustained or extended in circumstances previously regarded as impossible. However, such care may confer burdens that may have long-term consequences for infants and families, and the nature of these consequences is becoming increasingly recognized. A significant number of deaths in neonatal units follow decisions to withdraw, withhold or limit intensive care. The process of decision-making in such circumstances is stressful for both staff and parents alike. Individual team members can and do have strong views as to whether intensive care should be continued, withdrawn, limited or withheld. Parents do not want guidance that might imply that the lives of their children are less valued than others. Others may hold strong beliefs in the sanctity of life and the duty to preserve it in all circumstances if it is technically possible to do so. In this chapter the ethical and legal basis of professional decision-making is reviewed, and some practical guidance is given on how the process of withdrawing intensive care and its aftermath may be managed.

INTRODUCTION

Provision of intensive care enables the lives of small babies to be sustained or extended in circumstances previously regarded as impossible. Intensive care includes artificial ventilation, other forms of organ support and artificial nutrition delivered by invasive means and may follow cardiopulmonary resuscitation. However, as well as benefits, such care may confer burdens that may have long-term consequences for infants and families, and the nature of these consequences is becoming increasingly recognized.[1] Indeed, a significant number of deaths in neonatal units follow decisions to withdraw, withhold or limit intensive care.[2] Such decisions, whether in newborns or older infants, are difficult, emotive and poignant, and attract public interest and sympathy as well as controversy. Despite the publication of documents setting out the ethical and legal framework within which such decisions should be made,[3, 4] the process of decision-making is stressful for both staff and parents alike. Intensive care is delivered by teams of professionals; individual team members can and do have strong views as to whether intensive care should be continued, with-drawn, limited or withheld. It is therefore important that all members of the team are included in the decision-making process. Although such professional guidance is helpful, it cannot abolish controversy and ambiguity nor capture the complexity of competing moral claims. Clinicians require guidance that is practical and reasonably specific, but not prescriptive.[5] Parents of children with disabilities do not want guidance that might encourage stigmatization of disability, or imply that the lives of their children are less valued than others. Others may hold strong beliefs in the sanctity of life and the duty to preserve it in all circumstances if it is technically possible to do so. In this chapter we review the ethical and legal basis of professional decision-making and offer some practical guidance as to how the process of withdrawing intensive care and its aftermath may be managed.

TO WITHHOLD OR WITHDRAW?

Most authorities draw no ethical or legal distinction between withholding and withdrawing intensive care.[3, 4, 6] In contrast, professionals may make emotional and psychological distinctions; it may be easier not to start treatment than to withdraw it. But making such distinctions may prevent infants receiving treatment that might benefit them. It is therefore ethically acceptable to offer intensive care until a clearer view of the baby's prognosis and the wishes of the parents can be defined. Some guidelines can be interpreted as defining circumstances (e.g. extreme prematurity) in which intensive care should *not* be given. This may create tensions in circumstances where babies need to be transferred from one unit to another for intensive care, but the staff at the receiving unit do not feel such care to be appropriate.

BEST INTERESTS

A common and fundamental principle that underpins both ethical and legal decision-making is that the best interests of the child are paramount.[3, 4] Professionals have a duty to act in their patients' best interests, by offering treatments that are intended to sustain life and restore health to an acceptable standard.[7] This means using treatments whose clinical benefits outweigh their risks and burdens. There may be circumstances in which intensive care can sustain life, but without foreseeable benefits and at the expense of pain and suffering to the infant and his or her family. In these circumstances, intensive care may no longer be in the child's best interests.[3, 4]

Small babies, unlike adults, cannot determine what their own best interests are, and are thus reliant upon their parents and professionals acting in partnership on their behalf. Views of professionals and parents can, and do, sometimes conflict, and have been described as falling into one of four broad groups.[8] At one extreme there is the situation where a course of treatment is most strongly advised by clinicians but rejected by parents, with clinicians finding this attitude an affront to their professional conscience. In a second situation the clinicians hold similarly strong views as to the desirable course of action, but acknowledge there is something to be said for the parents' viewpoint. In a third situation, the clinician, whilst advising against treatment that the parents desire, is able nonetheless in good conscience to accede to their wishes. Finally, an impasse may exist where the clinician is unable to do what the parents wish in good conscience. The wider the scope of what constitutes a baby's best interests (in terms of parental beliefs, wishes and values) the greater is the potential for dispute. Such disputes may be extremely difficult to resolve, as all parties hold their views in good faith, and it is in such situations where ultimately the issue may be best resolved by the courts.

PARTNERSHIP

Healthcare professionals and parents have a duty to act in partnership to serve the best interests of the neonate. Any medical intervention, including initiation and withholding or withdrawal of neonatal intensive care, requires valid consent from parents. To be valid, consent must be sufficiently informed, given by a person able to understand what is involved, and freely obtained without coercion.[9] It may be practically difficult to satisfy these conditions in neonatal intensive care. Assimilating information requires time. Sufficient information about the infant must be accumulated to enable a prognosis to be given in terms that the parents can understand. Parents, confronted with the serious illness of their new baby, may neither comprehend the information they are given nor its consequences for themselves and their child. Rapidity of change in the baby's clinical condition may impose time constraints on the decision-making process, thereby compromising its voluntariness. Parents who have given written consent to research projects involving sick babies may neither recall that they have done so nor understand the consequences of what they have consented to.[10] Therefore, in making decisions about withdrawing treatment, parents need sufficient information given in a form and at a pace that they can comprehend. It is ethical to continue treatment until these criteria are satisfied. Parents must have time and space for reflection and decision-making. They may conclude that they wish others to make the decisions on their behalf, and if this view is freely held there seems no convincing moral reason why professionals should not accede to it.

LEGAL CONSIDERATIONS

Since the late 1980s, the law concerning withholding and withdrawing intensive care in infants has been clarified. Common Law judgements have held that in some circumstances it is not unlawful to withhold or withdraw life-sustaining treatment. Although legal judgements strictly only apply to the circumstances of the cases to which they refer, the following general principles may be inferred:

- The best interests of the child are paramount (Children Act 1989).[11]
- It is a criminal offence to take any action with the intention of shortening of life, but action intended to relieve pain and suffering is legal, provided it conforms to recognized medical practice.
- There is no legal distinction between withholding and withdrawing life-sustaining treatment.[6]
- Treatment should be given unless a child's life is so demonstrably awful that no reasonable person would want to live it.[12]
- There is no obligation to provide life-sustaining treatment to infants who are imminently and irreversibly close to death.[13]
- There is no obligation to provide futile or burdensome treatment that may also be inhuman (Human Rights Act 1998).[14]
- There is no obligation to provide treatment if the outcome for an individual is such that it would be unreasonable to expect him or her to bear it. For example, treatment of a child with severe cerebral palsy who is blind and deaf and who has no chance of ever being able to take part in any self-directed activity.[14]
- The final responsibility for deciding what treatments are *clinically* indicated rests with the doctor. The views of those close to the patient, including parents, should be considered, but are not determinative. Doctors cannot be compelled to give treatments, which they do not believe to be in the child's best interests.[15] However, when disputes arise and cannot be resolved by other means, the ruling of the court should be obtained.[16]
- Artificial nutrition and hydration are medical treatments that can be withheld or withdrawn,[6] but legal review is necessary in the absence of case law that applies to infants.

All medical decisions must be transparent and justifiable; the process of decision-making should be carefully recorded, and be subject to scrutiny and review. A balance must be struck between the infant's right to life, respect for the family's religious beliefs and the obligation not to provide treatment that is futile, burdensome, cruel or inhuman.

Disagreement between professionals and parents should, if possible, be resolved by negotiation, conciliation and compromise, perhaps assisted by ethical review. In only rare circumstances will the law need to be involved (e.g. when disputes are intransigent or new legal principles are involved).

ECONOMIC CONSIDERATIONS

Financial considerations cannot be ignored, because finite healthcare resources create pressures to set some limits as to which babies receive intensive care and for how long they may do so. Most guidelines stress that a decision to withdraw treatment should be based on analysis of the benefits and burdens of treatment, rather than on purely economic constraints.[3, 4]

Yet the costs of providing intensive care and the lifetime costs of providing for survivors are not inconsiderable, especially in the provision of medical or educational support.[1] In the UK considerable variations in practice and the costs of providing intensive care exist between units serving similar populations, and in the cost ratios of survivors to non-survivors. From this it can be inferred that some units withdraw intensive care more readily than others, while others spend a significant amount on babies who are not destined to survive. However, despite the importance of these economic considerations, they give little insight into the process of decision-making, which is arguably of much greater importance.[17]

PRACTICAL MANAGEMENT

Decisions to withhold or withdraw life support or intensive care from infants, whether from birth or following a period of treatment, have to be based on a careful assessment of the infant's clinical condition. While the long-term implications of certain clinical findings, such as bilateral cerebral intraparenchymal haemorrhages, diffuse periventricular leukomalacia and severe perinatal asphyxia with grade III hypoxic–ischaemic encephalopathy, are well established, the neurodevelopmental outlook in many other situations is often unclear.[1] Thus there is always potential for conflict and uncertainty, which is made more poignant by the seeming finality of the decision in hand. However, the way in which these issues are handled has been shown to have a significant impact on how parents and staff come to terms with the death of an infant. Partnership with parents is an integral part of neonatal care, and this should involve as much acceding to parental wishes as possible within the clinical best interests of the child. Regular, carefully documented discussions with parents are essential, and a consistent approach is important.

The individuals caring for the baby make up a large team; there may be considerable variation in levels of experience and expertise within the team, which may generate unease. This may be manifest in observed behaviour[18] or openly expressed opinions. To reduce potential conflicts, opportunity must be provided for all individuals to express their views as freely and as frankly as possible. This may be on the ward round, informally over coffee, at a regular psychosocial meeting, or by utilizing a third party to facilitate a formal discussion over a particularly difficult case. With the numbers of consultant staff on units now gradually increasing, it is essential that there is open discussion of cases where difficult decisions need to be made, and an 'in-house' second opinion where withdrawal of care is contemplated is good practice.

There is increasing recognition for some form of ethical support for those involved in making difficult decisions in which there are competing moral claims and where technology or scientific fact alone cannot determine what action should be taken. Such support may be provided by individuals or by clinical ethics committees. Both can provide ethical analysis of 'hot' cases, or the issues that they raise, as well as education and guidance.[19] They may provide a mechanism for mediation and conciliation in disputes over best interests, and where there are competing moral claims. Guidelines may not alter the final decision relating to withdrawal of intensive care that would otherwise have been made by senior staff. However, their existence does help to clarify and render more explicit the process to all concerned and may help to ensure consistency in discussion with parents. The authors have been involved in developing multidisciplinary guidelines to help professionals in managing the process of decision-making. Included in these is a checklist (Box 29.1), which it is hoped will prove helpful.

Personal experience suggests that there is often a role for the more experienced staff to clarify the degree of reversibility of some findings. A baby with Gram-negative sepsis may appear to be grossly oedematous, oliguric and moribund, with venous access becoming increasingly difficult, but those who have seen such infants respond can bear witness to the seemingly miraculous transformation in appearance and behaviour over time.

Honest and effective communication with parents is essential. In cases of babies being delivered extremely prematurely, much of the conflict that has been reported in the press appears to relate to ineffective communication. Clinicians need to be aware not just of

national outcome data for preterm babies, such as the EPICure Study,[20] but also of data pertinent to their own unit. Where in cases of extreme prematurity a decision is being made that resuscitation may not be initiated after birth, parents must be fully aware that their baby may be born alive and remain so for a period of time. The baby may have a definite heartbeat and make weak gasps. In such cases suitably senior staff should be present to, first, confirm the gestational age and state of the baby, and second, and above all, to provide support and reassurance to parents. In an antenatal discussion, one father visibly paled at the thought that his extremely preterm child might even gasp at birth. Yet, in the event, it was entirely natural and appropriate for him to hold his daughter in his arms, and both parents immensely valued that short period of close contact after birth and before death.

BOX 29.1

Checklist for decision-making
Individuals may find the following checklist helpful in formulating care plans and obtaining consent for them.

The child's clinical condition
- Are sufficient and adequate medical facts available to make a diagnosis and give accurate prognosis?
- Has a potentially treatable condition been excluded?
- Is a second medical opinion necessary/desirable?
- Is there a need for a psychiatric or psychological assessment of the child?
- What are the problems in providing nursing care in the current situation?
- What are the views of nursing staff about changing the goals for the child?
- What are the views of other therapists/professionals involved with the child?
- How has dissent in the team been handled?
- Is the child able to form a view about what he/she wants?
- Has he/she been consulted?

The family
- Is the family's understanding of their child's condition adequate?
- What are the family's relevant religious cultural beliefs and values?
- Has there been a psychosocial assessment of the family?
- What are the family's likely or actual views on changing the goals of treatment?
- Do the family need the help of an advocate?

The decision-making process
- How has uncertainty about the outcome been addressed?
- Has there been an ethical review of the case?
- Has there been a strategy meeting or psychosocial meeting?
- Have human rights issues been properly considered?
- Is there a proportionate justification for any infringement of human rights?
- Is there a need for a legal opinion?
- Is there a properly formulated care plan?
- Has informed consent for this care plan been obtained?
- Do the notes adequately reflect the process?
- How is the process to be maintained/audited?

The withdrawal process

Major issues that need to be considered relate to the timing of withdrawal of care, the need for privacy for the family and the continuing support for all those involved.

Good practice dictates that a consensus needs to be achieved without coercion, and frequently this may require repeated discussions with parents, allowing them time to assimilate the information provided and come to terms with events. 'Good medicine' may therefore entail continuing life-sustaining treatment for longer than a purely ethical approach might deem appropriate. Cultural and religious beliefs need to be accounted for, with time allowed for baptism or blessing of the child, and an opportunity offered, within reason, to allow distant family members to visit if desired.

It is necessary to discuss exactly how the withdrawal process is to be managed. Some parents (in our experience very few) wish their child to be allowed to die spontaneously while still 'on the ventilator'. However, the majority of parents accept the offer of having intensive care support withdrawn, and then spending their child's last minutes and hours in the privacy of a parents' room, unfettered by the trappings of technology, but always with an awareness of the immediate availability of unit staff. A very small number may wish their child to die at home; this can be achieved, but not without considerable logistical problems.[21]

It is also necessary to be aware of the impact of these events on parents of other babies on the unit. It is often worth spending time with them to discuss their feelings, and at the same time perhaps provide some reassurance regarding the progress of their own child. The proviso is that this must be done without compromising the confidentiality of the parents or the infant from whom intensive care is being withdrawn.

Sedation and paralysis

It is our belief that it is usual, and good practice, for an opiate to be administered prior to withdrawal of ventilatory support, in the normal dose used to provide analgesia or sedation. The intention is to alleviate pain or distress rather than to cause death (although some suppression of respiratory drive is foreseeable and acceptable, the so-called 'doctrine of double effect'), and this needs to be explained to the child's parents. The issue of paralysing agents is more complex. The Royal College of Paediatrics and Child Health guidelines permit the withdrawal of respiratory support if paralysing agents are concurrently in use, but such agents cannot be initiated prior to withdrawal. Continuation of paralysing agents during this process may cause discomfort amongst some members of the team; if they are to be used, the members of the team need to be quite clear as to why they are being continued. Some parents will express a wish for their cessation prior to stopping intensive care and this should be respected.

After withdrawal

Withdrawal of intensive care on the neonatal unit most commonly involves the cessation of ventilatory support, with the expectation that death will usually ensue. Recently published work by McHaffie et al. provides valuable insights into parental perceptions of treatment withdrawal and aspects of subsequent follow-up.[22, 23] It confirmed that parents wish to be involved in both the decision-making and the dying process. One specific area that generated distress was the time taken from the cessation of respiratory support to actual death. A swift demise appeared to confirm to the parents the appropriateness of the decision to withdraw, while delay raised doubts. This highlights the need to prepare parents adequately for the possibility that their child may not succumb at once, and to ensure that general supportive and palliative care for both infant *and* parents continues to be provided.

After the death families must feel at liberty to spend time with their child, and may often wish to be involved in bathing them, taking photographs, making hand- and footprints, etc., in accordance with the unit's usual practice.

It is also necessary to notify relevant primary healthcare professionals, including GPs, community paediatricians, health visitors and midwives, as soon as possible. Most units will have appropriate protocols for this.

Information needs to be provided about administrative matters relating to certification and funeral arrangements, and while preliminary discussions may on occasion have been held earlier about a post-mortem examination, this will need to be broached and consent sought, either at the time or on the following day.

Attitudes to post-mortem examination have recently been well explored, and the request may be acceded to or declined for a variety of reasons.[23]

Follow-up

This is a very important part of the whole process and significantly assists families in making progress through the normal grieving process. It is clear that contact needs to be made early, possibly within 2 weeks, and ideally within 2 months of death. Parents should be able to meet someone they are familiar with, and a truthful approach, concern over other family members' welfare and reiteration of details previously relayed to them all help to maintain trust and provide reassurance to the family.[24] Nursing staff in particular will often be represented at funerals and may maintain contact for a long time after, and this is much appreciated. An annual memorial service held by the unit has also been highlighted as good practice, and may provide parents with a sense that they are not alone in having lost a newborn infant. Withholding and withdrawing neonatal intensive care is very much a part of a neonatal unit's life, and its importance must not be underestimated. Discussions with parents about the possibility of withholding or withdrawing intensive care may have to commence before birth (in extreme preterm labour) and continue through life. It is essential to emphasize that, while *intensive* care may be withdrawn, care to preserve an infant's dignity will *not* be compromised. It is imperative that there is close senior staff involvement and that all involved strive to manage the process to the best of their abilities. At the end of the day, most parents take their newborn baby home. However, some parents will, sadly, only take home their memories.

Postscript

This article was completed before the publication of the document Critical Care Decisions in Fetal and Neonatal Medicine: Ethical Issues, which was published on 16 November 2006 by the Nuffield Council on Bioethics, London. Although the latter makes detailed recommendations concerning treatment choices, the ethical principles underpinning them remain very similar to those discussed in this chapter.

Chapter Thirty

The role of clinical ethics committees

Peter T. Rudd

SUMMARY

Clinical ethics committees (CECs) have been established in many hospitals in the USA and there are approximately 20 in the UK. Most are led by clinicians and have a number of different roles, including education of staff in ethical matters, ensuring policies that are sensitive to the needs and rights of patients, and providing expert advice for particularly difficult ethical problems. This chapter describes in detail the CEC at a large district general hospital in the west of England.

PRACTICE POINTS

- There are a small number of clinical ethics committees (CECs) in the UK.
- The CECs have evolved independently, so there is no single model.
- A CEC might be expected to support the development of policies where ethical issues are involved.
- An educational role is important.
- Some CECs provide individual ethics consultations.
- For success CECs require support from individuals with training in ethics and adequate administrative support.
- The effectiveness of CECs has yet to be evaluated.

INTRODUCTION

Clinical ethics committees (CECs) have been established in many hospitals in the UK. Most have been established by enthusiastic clinicians and ethicists, who have recognized a need for the discussion of ethical issues, no doubt fuelled by both medical advances and a shift from a paternalistic medical system to one that is more sympathetic to the autonomy of the patient.

Until relatively recently there was little or no education in ethics provided to the British medical student. Yet, the 'Hippocratic Oath', developed more than 2,500 years ago, was the basis of a number of declarations of the World Medical Association, which outlines the basic requirements for ethical practice.[1]

General ethical information is available to doctors through the publications of the General Medical Council (GMC), (e.g. *Good Medical Practice* and *Seeking Patients' Consents: The Ethical Considerations*). The professional bodies are also a source of information; the Ethics Advisory Committee of the Royal College of Paediatrics and Child Health (EAC-RCPCH) has published a report on the withholding or withdrawing of life-saving treatment in children.[2]

The first published data on clinical ethics committees came from the USA, and the Joint Commission on accreditation of Health Care Organizations requires hospitals to have a system for managing ethical issues of inpatient care, and it recommends a multidisciplinary ethics committee.[3] These committees fulfil a number of functions, including individual care consultations, either at the request of medical staff, or patients and family, developing guidelines of an ethical nature and education.

CLINICAL ETHICS COMMITTEES IN THE UK

The development of CECs in the UK has followed a similar pattern to those in North America, although individual case consultations are not available for most committees.[4]

Several publications describe in detail the work of CECs in both district general hospitals and tertiary centres.[5,6] One of these CECs was established in Nottingham in 1994 and has 20 members, who meet once monthly, but more urgently if required.[6] The terms of reference for the committee include the following:

- general ethical issues arising from established policies of treatment
- new initiatives in treatment
- individual patient issues
- advice on moral conflicts involving the clinician
- difficulties in relation to resources.

The committee membership of 20 encompasses a wide range of skills, including a paediatrician, a geriatrician, other physicians, surgeons, a ward sister, a nurse practitioner in oncology, a chaplain, a Public Health Director, GPs, lawyers and community health council representatives. Ethical issues discussed have included the inpatient hospital policy for 'do not resuscitate orders', disposal of fetal remains and consent. Individual case discussion has included advice on a neonate with inoperable bowel problems. Resource issues have included discussion of a case involving in vitro fertilization (IVF) required to prevent the transmission of a potentially fatal condition.

THE CLINICAL ETHICS COMMITTEE AT THE ROYAL UNITED HOSPITAL IN BATH

The author has personal experience of the CEC at the Royal United Hospital in Bath.[7] This is a district general hospital in the south-west of England with a catchment population of 450,000. The committee was set up in 1999, having the approval of the senior medical and nursing staff, following a hospital grand round in which two particularly difficult ethical problems were discussed. The Chief Executive and senior management within the hospital, influenced by the Department of Health White Paper on Clinical Governance, were keen that ethics be introduced into the framework of Clinical Governance,[8] and our committee both acts autonomously and reports via the Clinical Governance Committee to the Chief Executive.

We felt from an early stage that an ethicist should sit on the committee, not only to provide the necessary expertise, but also to be a source of training for committee members. The current membership includes an ethicist, four consultants (paediatrician (Chair), physician, surgeon and anaesthetist) a doctor in training, two senior nurses, a clinical psychologist, the hospital chaplain and a solicitor.

A salient feature of our practice is that members can be contacted at any time by any member of staff, at whatever level, who feel that the opinion of the group may help to resolve particular ethical difficulties. We do not take referrals from patients or their relatives. Unlike some other ethics committees, we have made it clear that referrals should relate to clinical ethical problems, and not to matters of competence or resource allocation, for which other mechanisms are available. Details of referrals are made anonymous by the referrer and entered on a proforma, as are the details of discussions. The roles of the committee are shown in Box 30.1.

BOX 30.1

Role of the clinical ethics committee

- To provide expert advice for particularly difficult ethical problems.
- To ensure that policies within the hospital are sensitive to the needs of patients.
- To provide education in ethics to those working in the hospital.

How the committee members approach referrals

The case referrals are the most challenging and difficult aspect of the work of the committee. For this reason, we would normally consult our ethicist as well as other members following a referral. We would hope to use a logical analytical approach to these. Members have had training from the Centre for Ethics in Medicine (University of Bristol) and the Oxford Centre for Ethics and Communication in Health Care Practice (Ethox).

Members were issued with a handbook of clinical ethics,[9] and have found the approach developed by Beauchamp and Childress particularly useful; i.e. consideration of autonomy, beneficence, non-maleficence and justice.[1, 10] Normally, discussion would involve phone calls, e-mails and sometimes a meeting with the clinicians involved.

Policy and guidelines

We have been anxious to avoid duplicating work already performed in drawing up guidelines. Thus, we have referred to the report produced by the Association of Anaesthetists in producing a document on the transfusion of children and adults who are Jehovah's Witnesses.[11] This has been agreed by the hospital Jehovah's Witnesses Group.

Guidelines are being drawn up for the management of sperm collection from dying patients, following a particular referral. We are already working with the hospital resuscitation committee and expect to implement a new 'do not attempt resuscitation' (DNAR) policy drawing on the British Medical Association (BMA)/Royal College of Nursing guidelines.[12]

Case referrals

This section describes a number of contrasting cases, all of which involve children. Other referrals in adults have included tube feeding after a stroke, drug treatment of a patient with a chronic psychosis against his will, and management of liver failure in alcoholic cirrhosis.

We were approached by one of the neonatologists who was unclear as to whether the porcine surfactant he had selected for babies with respiratory distress would be acceptable to Jewish and Muslim parents. We were able to consult with the Chief Rabbi and Muslim authorities, who were of the view that, because the products were not being ingested and were required for medical purposes, this was acceptable.

Another case involved a 15-year-old girl with secondaries from a relapsed solid tumour in which the prognosis was poor, even with further surgery and chemotherapy. A decision made by both the patient and her family to refuse this treatment was reluctantly agreed by the local paediatricians, specialist nurses and social worker after detailed discussion. However, this decision was challenged by a paediatric oncologist involved in the shared care, who discussed the case with the legal team in the tertiary centre. The legal team advised court action, and this was hastily referred to the CEC. The advice given at the CEC persuaded those in favour of legal action to respect the wishes of the patient and family. It was felt that legal action would have resulted in a breakdown of communication between the family and carers at a particularly crucial period of the illness. Although prediction of the outcome of any court case is difficult, application of the BMA/Law Society guidelines would have demonstrated full competence of the patient (Box 30.2).[13] I believe that, without the CEC, this particular case would have resulted in legal action likely to have caused distress to both the patient and family.

A challenging case to come before the committee involved a 14-year-old girl (Patient O) with a large ovarian cyst resulting in hydronephrosis of a kidney, who was refusing surgery. The patient consulted her GP in 1999 with abdominal pain. She had a large pelvic mass that was confirmed as an ovarian cyst on ultrasound. Patient O, an elective mute from the age of 5 years, has been under

BOX 30.2

Criteria for establishing competence (Law Society/ British Medical Association guidelines)

- Ability to understand that there is a choice, and choices have consequences.
- Willingness and ability to make a choice (including the option of choosing that someone else makes treatment decisions).
- Understanding of the nature and purpose of the proposed procedure.
- Understanding of the proposed procedures, risks and side-effects.
- Understanding of the alternatives to the procedure and the risks attached to them and the consequences of no treatment.
- Freedom from pressure.

the care of psychologists and psychiatrists. Surgery was recommended but, although she came to the ward for the operation and her parents signed the consent form, she refused to undress for the operation and returned home. At later consultations it was explained to her that damage might occur to her kidneys unless the cyst was removed, and she agreed to return to hospital. However, once again she refused a premedication, and the nursing and anaesthetic staff felt it would be inappropriate to use restraint. A subsequent renal tract ultrasound in mid-2000 showed right-sided hydronephrosis with obstructive atrophy.

The CEC was convened and it was agreed that an operation was in her best interest, and although her parents had consented to the surgery, the committee accepted the view of her doctors that forcible treatment might be seen as an assault. It was concluded that further preparation involving a psychologist should be arranged before legal advice was obtained. Patient O would not cooperate with the psychologist, so the CEC met the hospital legal team and discussed a number of issues as follows.

The law relating to consent to treatment in children under 16 years old was reviewed. This was set down in a House of Lords Judgement in the case of Gillick vs West Norfolk and Wisbech Health Authority, which concerned the prescribing of contraception to children under the age of 16 years without their parents' consent.[14] The term 'Gillick competent' is used to describe a child who has reached 'a sufficient understanding and intelligence to be capable of making up her own mind on the matter requiring decision'. If a child is judged Gillick competent, his or her consent to treatment is as valid as that of a competent adult. This does not apply to refusal of treatment.

A recent court ruling involved a 15-year-old girl (M) who could only survive with a heart transplant but was refusing surgery. Following interviews with the official solicitor, the judge was advised that M was too confused and upset to make an informed decision and was thus not competent to refuse surgery, which then proceeded.[15]

The law regarding refusal of treatment in children under the age of 18 years was laid down in the case of RW.[16] The patient had anorexia nervosa, and it was ruled that the refusal of a minor to undergo medical treatment could be overridden if the consent of her parents, or of the court, was obtained. What is more, this held even if the minor was judged to be competent to consent to treatment.

The same issues about competency to refuse treatment were considered in the case of Patient O, using the Law Society/British Medical Association guidelines.[13] The CEC agreed that Patient O had been unable to fulfil a number of the criteria because she was unable to communicate with her medical attendants and justify refusal to her parents, with whom she was able to communicate. It was agreed that there was no legal objection to surgery proceeding, but there was concern that the recently implemented Human Rights Act 1998 might have been sympathetic to her view. A number of options were considered:

1. To proceed with surgery without further legal representation on the basis of signed parental consent only, but with assurance from the legal team that staff were acting 'lawfully'.
2. To go to the High Court and before a judge ask for authorization of surgery, if it were considered that the parental consent would prejudice the parent–child relationship, or if the parents were to revoke their consent verbally on witnessing their child's protests or distress.
3. To notify the official solicitor (representing the patient) that surgery would proceed on a particular date; it was felt that this decision would probably not be challenged by the official solicitor and, if it were, then the case would go to the court.

Option 3 was adopted and surgery was arranged. The CEC expressed concern subsequently that, despite legal advice being obtained, Patient O might refuse to leave home on the morning of the surgery. To reduce the risk of failure, a specially briefed ambulance team and the ward sister who had been closely involved with Patient O were available for the transfer to hospital with her parents, and Patient O did not resist. An oral premedication was refused, as was the request for her to get undressed in theatre, but while distracted she was given an intramuscular injection of ketamine and surgery proceeded without complication. Both Patient O and her parents appeared happy with the outcome.

It could be argued that the same outcome would have been achieved in the absence of a CEC, but with direct referral to the hospital solicitor. However, we feel that the CEC helped in a number of ways; by providing an opinion as to the appropriate management of the patient without, at least initially, recourse to the legal process. This allowed a clearer view to be put to the solicitors. In addition, the committee members were able to make very practical suggestions about the supportive care around the time of the operation, and had a much fuller understanding of the ethical and legal aspects involved in this case.

THE FUTURE OF COMMITTEES

What is the future of CEC committees in the UK? Those already established are composed of enthusiasts, rather than individuals involved because of a statutory requirement under clinical governance, for instance. Certainly, to provide an ethical consultancy service requires the time of already hard-pressed individuals, as well as expertise from ethicists, of whom numbers are limited and who are confined to larger universities, or individuals with training in clinical ethics. Most CECs do not receive funding, but require at least adequate secretarial support. It is probable that some form of ethical committee will be required of institutions in the future, but almost certainly demanding attention only to guidelines, perhaps under the guise of clinical governance. Since, at the last count, there are relatively few CECs in the UK,[3] there are a number of uncertainties about the perceived needs for such committees, the systems used to make decisions and provide advice to clinicians, and the effectiveness of these organizations. A report produced by a working party of the Royal College of Physicians[17] suggested that those involved in healthcare should be able to access ethical advice at any time, and that healthcare institutions should review their existing arrangements for providing ethical support and consider how these needs could be met and in certain circumstances establish CECs. The recent establishment of the UK Clinical Ethics Network has provided an opportunity for members to meet and exchange expertise; there is a website providing details of ethics committees as well as information on ethical issues.[18]

Larcher et al.[19] investigated by interview the need for ethical support in two London children's hospitals. They found that staff expressed a need for a forum that could provide consultation on ethical issues, develop guidelines for good ethical practice and undertake teaching and training.

An audit of 600 internists involved in critical care and general medical specialities showed that 55% of physicians had asked for an ethics consultation.[20] Triggers to requesting a consultation included: (1) wanting help in resolving a conflict; (2) wanting assistance in interacting with a difficult family, patient or surrogate; (3) wanting help in making a decision on planning care; and (4) emotional triggers. End-of-life issues featured in 74% of consultations, with 57% of problems related to patient autonomy and 39% involving conflict (the figures add up to more than 100% because more than one category was allowed). It is not clear from this paper whether the ethicists or committees were perceived as successful.

In conclusion it is clear that ethics committees are an exciting development; they require enthusiasm and commitment from members, and I believe they will only thrive if allowed to act in an advisory capacity for difficult ethical decisions.

ACKNOWLEDGEMENTS

Thanks are due to Dr Anne Slowther (Ethox) and Professor Alastair Campbell (University of Bristol). The report on Case O appears in Rudd PT, *HEC Forum*.[7] The parents of O have given consent to publication.

Chapter Thirty One

Clinical ethics committees – a personal commentary

31

Martyn Evans

SUMMARY

In this cautionary response to a description of the remit of an actual clinical ethics committee (CEC), I suggest that the good that such committees can do may come at too high a price; if the CEC's reach extends into adjudication on individual clinical cases, it stands in danger of eroding the personal trust and commitment that ought to lie at the heart of the clinical relationship. The opportunity to discuss individual cases is vitally important to the clinician but, if formalized, such discussion risks being strait-jacketed by procedures and outlooks (such as the 'four principles' framework for medical ethics), which can be inappropriate in individual cases as well as mechanical. It is also unclear that a professional 'ethicist' has any special expertise in moral conduct or practice; the professionalization of what is, in reality, an extension of ordinary moral life is suspect and dangerous. Two of the three roles claimed for a CEC may be reasonable – a general educational resource on the content of policies, and a discussion forum on how these might in general terms be put into operation. However, the third, individual advice and adjudication on cases, risks displacing the moral commitment to the patient that ought to be held personally on the part of individual clinicians. This admittedly conservative view of professional clinical practice is defended in terms of the centrality, in clinical healthcare of the patient's experience, of sensitive personal communication, and of the patient's trust and commitment, which can be extended only towards individual clinicians taking personal responsibility for their own decisions – not towards committees.

INTRODUCTION

I am going to start with an apparently unrelated confession. While generally regretting the advent of mobile phones, mobile phone companies and mobile phone users, I notice, to my shame, that I too now carry one, switched on for much of the day. Years of heroic, not to say smug, self-denial came to an end when I realized that in only a month or so I had three times resorted to borrowing someone else's phone (in circumstances, I assure the reader, of the very greatest urgency). Plainly, my hypocrisy had become conspicuously worse than the embarrassment of owning one of the damned things myself. So I bought one.

This is an example of how modern living from time to time presents us with conveniences that can seem hugely useful on particular occasions, but nonetheless feel like a larger step in the wrong direction. I doubt whether the world is really safer or more convenient because of mobile phones. It is just noisier; and people are more careless of their own and others' interests because they think they can afford to be when help is only a keypad away. Such carelessness has its own implications for convenience and safety. It is harder to write or read on trains nowadays; ill-driven vehicles kill and maim, midconversation.

But new 'protections' can also be like this. To take a minor example, my previous university resolutely sealed off a gate used by many pedestrians and cyclists, because an exposed tree root on the other side of the fence presented a hazard to the unwary. I imagine they successfully avoided one source of litigation, but they made the journey into the university longer and more awkward for many.

Now, the advent of clinical ethics committees, while embodying praiseworthy intentions and enthusiasm, is at risk of generating another, potentially serious, example of the same sort of phenomenon – although for perhaps subtler reasons, which I will try to set out as best I can. In doing so, I am at risk of seeming to be a bit of a killjoy, or a representative of the 'never satisfied' section of public opinion. Dr Rudd, who clearly and persuasively articulated the merits of the CEC in the Royal United Hospital in Bath[1] (see also Chapter 30), might be thought particularly entitled to take that view. I ask him to extend patience towards a devil's advocate, during what follows.

My claim is that CECs can do much good, but at a price; my difficulty is that the price is quite hard to specify, or pin down. It has something to do with the slow erosion of the personal clinical relationship between practitioner and patient, especially as it concerns personal trust and commitment. This erosion is probably happening anyway, and CECs are not solely responsible for it. So the reader must decide whether that portion of the price that attaches to clinical ethical committees is really so expensive as all that. I think that it is, and I am nervous that it might be too expensive. So my response to Rudd consists mainly in trying to express this.

WHAT PATIENTS WANT

To begin with, I must acknowledge that I am not basing my remarks on a survey of popular opinion. However much one might distrust such expressions of opinion on particular occasions, we might think it would be helpful to find out what patients want in the matter of discussions and consultations on the ethically most taxing aspects of their management. In particular, much of the apparently endless biffing of the medical profession in the media seems to consist in castigating individual clinicians (occasionally, managers) for acting in isolation, and precisely for not consulting colleagues or for not submitting themselves to institutional scrutiny, or for not conforming to an existing code or protocol.

This certainly makes it look as if what patients want is more conformity and accountability on the part of errant individual clinicians, and a greater willingness from those clinicians to get clearance or approval for their actions from properly constituted bodies of their peers and other colleagues. CECs might then seem to fit the bill very nicely.

Be all this as it may, my own starting point can be neither surmise nor a report of some actually expressed vox pop. The fact is that, beyond what anyone can read in a newspaper, I as a philosopher all too plainly have no special access to expressions of popular opinion, nor any expertise in prompting or eliciting them. I can start only from thinking about what I might myself want my own clinicians to do. After all, if a vox pop survey on matters of this sort were ever to include me (and, at 49 years old, I have still to meet anyone who has actually taken part in a MORI or Gallup poll) then I would say to them just what I am going to say here.

PRELIMINARY RESERVATIONS

I want to start by standing four-square with Rudd in acknowledging the value of discussion in thinking about moral matters. Recognition of the need for ethical discussion is, according to Rudd, what lies behind the establishment of most CECs in the UK. But an argument for discussion is not the same as an argument for establishing a committee. The obvious alternatives include informal 'unburdenings' with friends, colleagues or family; or, more formally, at case conferences involving the clinicians directly engaged in the cases (or at least the kinds of cases) at stake. It can be helpful, of course, to discuss things with colleagues who are precisely not involved, and even to do this at regular agreed intervals, but this still does not require a formally constituted committee. Other opportunities range from tea breaks to journal clubs. Whatever the intrinsic advantages of a committee are, they need to be spelled out. Rudd implies two, namely that a committee embodies a wide range of expertise, and that it has an established status and visible presence, making it available (in principle) to all, and at any time. If it were only committees that could do this, then they would have two useful advantages.

But committees can suffer from the constraints of their own constitution and procedures; in the worst cases they become 'a cul-de-sac to which ideas are lured and then quietly strangled'.[2] This risk must seem remote to the enthusiasts who set them up, but I notice that the Bath CEC has adopted what I think can be a regrettably formulaic framework for medical ethics analysis, namely the 'four principles' approach,[3] which evolved and was pioneered in a context to which it is far better suited than our own, namely the individualistic societies of North America, where the four principles' relative neglect of the communitarian aspects of publicly funded healthcare is less apparent, and less of a problem. (The North American understanding of 'justice', typically the fourth of the four principles, has I think a discernibly different basis from the social solidarity which might be thought to underlie

the NHS.) In saying this, I accept that I am uncomfortably at odds with some of the most distinguished and admirable figures in medical ethics circles in the UK; I wish it were otherwise, but there it is.

Then there is the question of the special expertise that Rudd attributes to the 'ethicist' on the committee. I have a particularly bad conscience here, having served for some years on a local research ethics committee, to which I was recruited on the basis of my professional involvement in the study of philosophical problems in medicine and healthcare. While I steadfastly rejected the label 'ethicist', I think it was somehow assumed that I had 'ethical expertise'. But I was never clear – and I am still not clear – what 'ethical expertise' is supposed to consist in. Jonathan Miller once shrewdly remarked that 'We are all PhDs in morals', referring to a qualification obtainable only from the University of Life. Knowing a lot about moral theories entails absolutely nothing about being possessed of actual moral sensitivity or judgment. Indeed, the disjunction between the two can be frankly spectacular.

Moral life in general is, of course, finally inseparable from life as a whole. And there is nothing special in this regard about the clinical context. So 'medical ethics' (or, here, 'clinical ethics') should be considered as inseparable from ordinary moral life: it is discussion about ordinary moral concerns, but carried on in the special circumstances of the clinical context and clinical responsibility. Its ordinariness of course connects the concerns of the clinical professional with those of the other members of the ethics committee, and rightly so. But then we might feel entitled to wonder who the ethicist really is on the committee.

I would say that in this sense all are ethicists, if anyone is. Yet those who are not clinical professionals should be cautious when they say things that might carry clinical consequences. The role of being a declared ethicist is, for someone who never has to carry personal responsibility for those consequences, a perilous one.

WHICH ROLES FOR A CLINICAL ETHICS COMMITTEE?

Rudd reports three roles for the clinical ethics committee at the Bath Hospital: (1) to provide expert advice for particularly difficult ethical problems; (2) to ensure that policies within the hospital are sensitive to the needs of patients; and (3) to provide education in ethics to those working within the hospital. These are, I imagine, perfectly representative of the roles that might become typical for CECs.

I will approach these in reverse order. Unfortunately, Rudd says nothing about the third, 'education in ethics'. At first sight, providing education is a praiseworthy role, but it requires a little care in its specification. If ethical education means learning what this or that institution or society have agreed (or legislated) is acceptable in connection with a certain sort of situation, then this is obviously helpful in the hospital context.

Just as helpful would be finding some way of encouraging colleagues to put that agreement into practice habitually. Here the educational aim leads into the second of Rudd's envisaged roles, since it could mean something as straightforward as overseeing the dissemination of new guidelines, as they emerge or are published, to the relevant clinical staff within the institution concerned. Rudd mentions two excellent examples, the dissemination of existing guidelines on blood transfusion and the development of new ones for sperm collection. But if ethical education means learning to be a more ethical person, I doubt the committee can do this. At most, it might help one's self-education to have access to a forum for ethical debate, and the committee could be a resource of this kind.

In this spirit, one might approach a committee as a resource for discussing typical kinds of ethical problems in clinical practice – the sort of thing that could one day result in new guidelines. But the trouble now is that this shades into something else entirely, namely the substantive discussion of and advice on individual clinical cases. Rudd is very clear that this is the most challenging part of the CEC's work, although he is less clear about why a separate consultation with the ethicist is especially called for by individual cases, or what it is expected to achieve. Let me stress that, for all I know, this committee's ethicist, not identified in Rudd's paper, may be a truly outstanding individual. However, the key question, as outlined previously, is whether the ethicist's role has anything special to offer – particularly if the incumbent has no experience of what it is to carry clinical responsibility.

Rudd illustrates this aspect of the CEC's work with a most interesting case – the pressing need to treat an ovarian cyst in a particularly challenging and non-consenting young patient – and it is one that clearly raises difficult and urgent moral questions. I have nothing but sympathy and admiration for the clinicians and managers involved. Such a case, entailing as it does questions of law and procedure, certainly benefits from the range of advice available to a properly constituted committee.

Arguably, a good decision was reached. What is less clear is the authority of the CEC (against that of lawyers, for instance, in the event that the lawyers disagreed with the CEC). In the other case Rudd mentions (concerning a 15 year old with secondary cancer) the CEC seems to have prevailed against the decision of a 'legal team'. How, and why? How would the CEC's success here have fared in court? Again, the outcome sounds good – but was it fortuitous? We cannot tell because we do not know why their advice prevailed. If the committee has earned a measure of moral authority it would be good to know this, and to know its basis.

In fact, we need a more detailed exploration of both cases, and of the CEC's discussion, in order to judge what value the CEC offered to the clinicians involved. In the ovarian cyst case, Rudd mentions a benefit enjoyed by the committee, namely that they emerged with a 'much fuller understanding of the ethical and legal issues' involved. Good news, of course, but hardly the outcome for which the committee was established.

DISCUSSION

My chief anxiety about the notion of a CEC is that it might become more than a resource intended to support or inform the individual clinical commitment of the individual practitioner – it might start to replace an important part of the clinical relationship, namely the moral commitment of the practitioner towards the patient. This will occupy me for the rest of these remarks.

Now, an objector will reasonably want to know what this moral commitment comes to in practice; whether it is so hard as all that to achieve; why, if it is hard to achieve, it is so hard; and whether it is fair to expect such a difficult thing from the average hard-pressed practitioner in every case. In short, it appears I am relying on a somewhat heroic or romantic view of the practitioner–patient relationship, and advocating that we maintain it.

Well, I suppose I do have such a view in mind. Implicitly, I am supposing that there is something special in the practitioner–patient relationship, which we would not want a committee to supplant or to replace, either because we think it cannot be done properly by a committee, or because we fear that perhaps after all it can, but that it would be changed or attenuated or even debased that way – because we believe that it is somehow morally important that this 'special something' be provided by an individual, namely, the practitioner.

You might say that the importance of individual, non-shared, responsibility is that it requires a personal commitment towards the patient that is possible only on the part of a single human being acting responsibly by his or her own intention, and accepting such commitment towards another single human being (the patient, in any particular case) as part and parcel of the clinical role. As a patient, I feel that I want that. But is it reasonable for me to ask it of my clinicians?

I suppose I am adopting a kind of conservatism here. This notion of personal commitment is part of what clinical medicine historically professes. The importance of individual, non-shared responsibility is actually given, supplied, by the clinical relationship – this relationship has a special dimension to it, that is not found (nor expected) from other professionals like lawyers or accountants, although it is expected from clergy and from teachers. It embodies something we would call sacrosanct or even 'sacred'; but something which, it might be objected, simply has no place in modern technology-driven, high-throughput healthcare. There is no time for it. As W. H. Davies lamented, when life is "full of care" we indeed 'have no time to stand and stare'.

Yet staring with the ears and with the mind and with one's moral sense is, I should have thought, an indispensable part of committed clinical care. Many ethical problems arise initially because the patient senses that he is not able to communicate properly with his clinicians, nor they with him. This is often a direct consequence of having too little time to stand and stare. And it is a consequence that is really not dealt with by being passed onwards to a CEC: remote, impersonal, generalized, averaged, democratized, with an agenda of similar cases amongst which this one case is somewhere to be found as an item. The CEC has no special commitment to the individual patient beyond various trails of accountability as an advisory arm of the employing trust or health authority, perhaps. It is easy for personal commitment to become diluted or even to disappear entirely in such circumstances. At any rate, somebody owes us a well-worked account of how this dilution is to be overcome or avoided.

Furthermore, the CEC, through having to deal with perhaps a list of such cases, has still less time to stand and stare, still less opportunity to communicate with the individual patient – if indeed individual communication ever could be undertaken by a committee. And suppose that it could – would I as a patient plausibly wish that my need to be heard were met by a committee rather than an individual? And even if CECs somehow did manage to compensate for the lack of time for better developed clinical relationships (by more 'efficient' or 'authoritative' ethical decisions(?)) one might still see them as just that – a compensation, a poor kind of substitute; or, worse still, as making the consequences of 'too little time' invisible by masking them.

Why is it that such communication time is needed? This is the second aspect of my conjecture. I think the importance of this communication time is to do with the fact that experience is central to my understanding of my own clinical circumstances, and to my understanding of the healthcare interventions that are offered to me. The patient's experience has indeed a three-fold centrality – in the realization of something being 'wrong', sending him to the doctor in the first place; in his appreciation or otherwise of how he is dealt with, clinically speaking; and, most radically, in the wider story of his circumstances and how these influenced the way he fell ill.

In such an experience-rich context, the respective meanings that the patient and practitioner attach to the terms in which the patient's problems are presented are, notoriously, liable to differ.[4] This is partly a matter of the different vocabularies of descriptions that are often, perhaps typically, available to patients on the one hand and practitioners on the other. But partly it is a matter also of the different phenomena to which patients on the one hand, and physicians on the other, will be inclined to attend.[3, 4]

Let me praise CECs for what they can do well – namely, advising on the design and implementation of general clinical policies, and providing a valuable, often educational, forum in which all know that the issues thrown up by cases can be discussed. At the same time, let me sharpen my reservations regarding the role of clinical case 'jury'.

I have suggested that the core ethical troubles in troubling cases arise all too frequently from a breakdown in communication and trust between patient and practitioner. My fear is that resorting to a CEC will be seen as (or, worse, will become) a kind of retreat from the moral commitment that clinical medicine professes to the patient. If we lament, as we do, the breakdown of trust in the clinical relationship, then the question must arise as to how this is best re-established: through CECs or through re-engagement in a spontaneous, authentic and, above all, personal commitment to the patient?

I choose the latter, partly on emotional grounds but partly on grounds that are intellectual or, if you like, 'philosophical'. It is of course true that I could have more or less confidence in the likelihood that a committee will come to a given decision, but I do not see how I could trust the very same committee to do the very same thing, because 'trust' does not seem to apply to collective entities. Trust seems to be irreducibly a relationship of commitment between individuals. Could I meaningfully trust a corporation, or a school, or a state? I might have more or less confidence in getting what I expected from them. But when I trust someone, I myself make a commitment to them in trusting them, as well as relying on a commitment from them towards me. I do not see I can engage with a corporation or a school or a state in this way. Committees are a kind of algorithm, a sort of embodied process for working things out. But they are not personal entities, and as such I do not think they can attract my trust.

It might be, of course, that I could partly base my trust in an individual clinician on the thought that if she were stuck about how to proceed in my case, she might consult or discuss more widely. If she chose family or friends as her sounding board, I would want to trust her professional confidentiality and discretion. If she chose a CEC I would want to trust her to seek guidance from them, as a means to reaching her own authentic decision. But I do not think that my trust could be based on the thought that she adopted the decision of a committee unwillingly, still less mechanically: trust would require that she made that decision her own. And making it her own is just what she cannot ask the CEC to do; she has to do that for herself.

Chapter Thirty Two

Palliative care: moving forward

32

Richard D. W. Hain • Stefan J. Friedrichsdorf

SUMMARY

Children with life-limiting conditions cannot yet expect the same access to specialist palliative care services that are available to adults. At the same time, the paediatric approach to the care of patients already embodies much of what specialist palliative medicine can offer. Paediatric palliative care must, of course, develop from within paediatrics if we are to meet the needs of children. At the same time, we have much to learn from our colleagues in adult medicine, both corporately and individually. Adolescent palliative care, in particular, is an opportunity for collaboration.

Specialist palliative care in children needs to be delivered in many different clinical locations. To achieve this, the consultant must take on an advisory and coordinating role as well as giving specialist advice. The exact role of the consultant in paediatric palliative care will depend more on the individual child than on the model. This chapter considers the point we have reached, and where we are going in the development of this new subspecialty.

PRACTICE POINTS

- The more holistically one looks at children, the more different they are from adults.
- Children needing palliative care may be at home, at school, in a children's hospice or in hospital.
- Home is usually the preferred place of death for children, but children's hospices and even hospitals can provide a comfortable alternative for some.
- Cancer is the most common single diagnosis among children needing palliative care, but more children have non-malignant life limiting conditions.
- Most paediatricians will encounter dying children, but usually not often enough to feel comfortable with palliative care techniques.
- Techniques of symptom control in adults can often be adapted for children, and adult palliative medicine physicians can be an important resource if no paediatric specialist is available.
- Symptoms in children are often inadvertently undertreated because of unfounded fears of drug toxicity.
- Adolescents with life-limiting conditions have particular needs that are, on the whole, not well met.

INTRODUCTION AND DEFINITIONS

Since the early 1960s adult physicians, led by Dame Cicely Saunders, have recognized the particular needs of the patient with incurable disease, but it seems to have taken much longer for those needs to be recognized by paediatricians. Perhaps adult physicians have had to recapture a vision that paediatrics has never fully lost. Like all aspects of paediatrics, palliative care emphasizes an active and total approach to care that embraces physical, emotional, social and spiritual elements.[1] The need to work with other disciplines and professionals has always been recognized, as has the importance of delivering care to the child in many different clinical environments. The aim of palliative care is to preserve normality as far as possible; for the great majority of children, this means delivering care in the home, but there are many who will need support in the school, hospice or hospital ward.

Although the paediatric specialty is relatively young, there are ways in which we already anticipate our colleagues in adult medicine. The range of life-limiting conditions (LLCs) in children is wide, and although cancer is the single most common diagnosis, more children have non-malignant conditions.[2-4] The diversity of LLCs in children has been highlighted by the Royal College of Paediatrics and Child Health (RCPCH).[1] Working with the Association for Children's Palliative Care,[5] the RCPCH identified four groups of LLCs:

- Group 1: life-threatening conditions for which curative treatment may be feasible but can fail. Palliative care may be necessary during periods of prognostic uncertainty and when treatment fails (e.g. cancer, irreversible failure of heart or liver).
- Group 2: conditions where premature death is inevitable, where there may be long periods of intensive treatment aimed at prolonging life and allowing participation in normal childhood activities (e.g. cystic fibrosis, muscular dystrophy).
- Group 3: progressive conditions without curative treatment options, where treatment is exclusively palliative and may commonly extend over many years (e.g. Batten's disease, mucopolysaccharidosis).
- Group 4: conditions involving severe neurological disability that may cause weakness and susceptibility to health complications and may deteriorate unpredictably, but are not considered to be progressive (e.g. severe cerebral palsy).

The first edition of the ACT/RCPCH publication[1] in 1997 was highly significant in the development of paediatric palliative care (PPC) in the UK and many other countries. It established for the first time that children with LLCs have needs in common that mark them out from children with other illnesses. It acknowledged too that paediatricians have an important role to play in the care of such children but that they are only part of a team that includes family, professional and lay carers, doctors and nurses in the community, primary and secondary care as well as the increasing number of children's hospices. The document also describes the scope for specific palliative expertise among specialist paediatricians.

In summary, the ACT/RCPCH document showed that the need for palliative care in children was much greater than had previously been recognized, and described the role that paediatricians could play in providing it.

EPIDEMIOLOGY

By defining PPC, the RCPCH allowed meaningful epidemiological studies to be carried out. The annual mortality rate (AMR) for children aged 0–19 years with a LLC is 1.5–1.9 per 10,000, the prevalence of LLCs generally being higher, at least 12 per 10,000 for children in the same age group.[1, 6] Reliable data are available only for conditions for which there are national registers, and there is an urgent need to establish local-district-based data, particularly for non-malignant LLCs. Prevalence data are available for some specific conditions, including cancer (1.1 per 10,000), cystic fibrosis (3.9 per 10,000), mucopolysaccharidoses (0.2 per 10,000) and Duchenne muscular dystrophy (1.8 per 10,000). Among adolescents (13–24 years old), the mortality rate is 1.7 per 10,000.[7] These British figures mirror data from other countries. In Germany, the leading causes of children aged 0–15 years dying from LLCs were cancer (31%), followed by neurodegenerative/neuromuscular (20%), congenital/genetic (16%), cardiovascular (12%) and metabolic conditions (9%).[8]

THE NEEDS OF CHILDREN WITH LIFE-LIMITING CONDITIONS

The number of children dying is small compared with that of adults. Familial disorders often affect more than one family member, so genetic counselling is important. Palliative care should support family and community, ideally extending to siblings, school friends and involved teachers. Individual disorders are rare. While the entire course of some diseases occurs within childhood, others may persist into adulthood, and the need for palliative care may range from days to years or even decades. Throughout a child's illness, it is essential (and indeed a legal requirement) to provide appropriate education.

CONCEPTS OF DYING

One challenge of palliative care is the child's ever-changing level of physical, emotional and cognitive development, and its impact on the understanding of disease and death. Many researchers have sought to define the child's complex concept of death, Kane's nine components[9] often being quoted. The earliest component,

realization, is attained at around 3 years of age. This is followed by: separation and immobility (5 years); irrevocability, causality and dysfunctionality (6 years); universality (7 years); insensitivity (8 years); and appearance (12 years). Two other well-known constructs are those of Piaget[10] and Nagy.[11] Piaget observed that the younger the child, the more concrete were the thoughts surrounding death. Nagy suggested that 3–5 year olds think of death as a temporary sleep, neither definite nor irreversible, whereas 5–9 year olds personify death, seeing him as a shrouded or dark figure who can be avoided. Older children recognize that death is inevitable and begin to understand its biological mechanisms.

What these theories have in common is the recognition that a child learns first that death occurs, and then that it is both irreversible and inevitable, the child finally becoming concerned with details, such as physical changes. What the theories can obscure, however, is the impact of life events on development, including chronic illness itself. A cognitively aware child with an LLC will typically acquire a precocious understanding of illness and death.

SYMPTOM CONTROL

We may, as paediatricians, be the coordinating healthcare professionals in charge of the child in the 'palliative phase'. Whether this takes place on the hospital ward or in the child's home, a clear and precise plan of management for potential symptoms is vital. For the family who wishes their child to be at home, there should be a named key worker whose role is liaison and coordination among the multiprofessional team of carers.

As local paediatric community services vary with locality, it is important to individualize the child's package of care. Twenty-four-hour cover by experienced community nurses is often necessary, especially during the terminal stages of a child's illness. Prior to discharge from hospital, a multidisciplinary meeting of hospital and community staff (and, ideally, parents) is an excellent way of anticipating practical issues, such as special items of equipment that may need to be ordered in advance. It is also an opportunity to alert medical and nursing staff in the community to the child's current symptoms and how to anticipate what symptoms are likely to develop, as well to give advice on how to manage them effectively. Clear identification and documentation is appreciated by paediatricians and GPs, and should include a range of drug doses and possible routes of administration. The family, too, needs to be told of the probable course of the illness, including what symptoms are likely. The purpose of this is to reduce fear of the unknown; it has to be done sensitively in order to avoid increasing anxiety about events that are, in reality, unlikely.

The symptoms that should be anticipated will depend on the diagnosis, some common symptoms being listed in Table 32.1. The management often includes both pharmacological and non-pharmacological approaches. Management of pain, dyspnoea and excess airway secretions are considered below.

Pain

Pain, although one of the most common symptoms experienced by the child with an LLC, is often poorly managed. Regular pain assessment (the '5th vital sign') using validated and easy-to-use measurement tools is the key to managing pain from infancy to adolescence. Professional comprehensive paediatric pain management in the 21st century requires a combination of a pharmacological

Table 32.1 Common symptoms in paediatric palliative care

System	Symptom
Musculoskeletal	Pain, muscle spasm, fatigue
Respiratory	Dyspnoea, cough, excessive secretions, pain
Gastrointestinal	Nausea, vomiting, constipation, diarrhoea, anorexia
Oral	Mucositis, dysphagia, candidiasis
Skin	Itch, pressure ulcers, infection
Genitourinary	Urinary incontinence/retention, candidiasis
Central nervous system	Convulsions, cerebral irritation, thalamic pain
Neuropsychiatric	Anxiety, agitation, depression, confusion
Haematological	Haemorrhage, anaemia, bruising

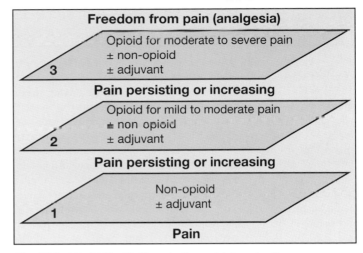

Fig. 32.1 World Health Organization guidelines for the management of pain in children.[12]

approach with integrative therapies such as cognitive–behavioural techniques (e.g. guided imagery, hypnosis, abdominal breathing, distraction, biofeedback) and physical methods (e.g. cuddle, massage, transcutaneous electrical nerve stimulation (TENS), comfort positioning, heat, cold).

The World Health Organization (WHO) analgesic ladder (Fig. 32.1) provides a systematic approach to effective pain management in children.[12, 13] The four WHO core principles include:

- 'By the WHO ladder' – strong pain requires strong opioids
- 'By the clock' – analgesia should always be prescribed regularly, and not just 'as needed'
- 'By the appropriate route' – using child-friendly routes such as oral, transdermal, intranasal, buccal (intramuscular application is obsolete)
- 'By the child' – regular pain assessment and adaptation of the management accordingly.

Adjuvant drugs include ketamine, amitriptyline and gabapentin for neuropathic pain, bisphosphonates for bone pain and baclofen for muscle spasm. Paediatricians still tend towards overcaution in prescribing opioids to children, despite the fact that the pharmacokinetics of these drugs are now quite well understood.[13–15] Children outside the neonatal period probably clear morphine more quickly than adults and often need higher doses than adults to achieve the same degree of analgesia.

Dyspnoea

It is again important to consider the underlying cause of the symptom, which may include pulmonary disease, such as an effusion of malignancy, cardiac failure, anaemia, ascites, pain, or existing medical problems, such as asthma. Anxiety and fear can also be direct causes of dyspnoea. Dyspnoea should only be treated if causing distress for the child and not simply on the basis of measurements, such as arterial blood gasses, oxygen saturation or breathing rate.

Practical measures (positioning the child with pillows and providing an open window or a fan) are often effective. The application of morphine (or other opioids) is the main pharmacological therapy recommended in managing dyspnoea; the starting dose is

usually half that for pain. Nebulized bronchodilators and sometimes oxygen may be useful and appropriate. Buccal or intravenous midazolam, a benzodiazepine that reduces both anxiety and the sensation of dyspnoea, is a useful drug, as is levomepromazine (Nozinan; formerly Methotrimeprazine in the UK), a phenothiazine with multiple actions including sedation but not anxiolysis. These two drugs are compatible with each other and with other drugs used in syringe drivers, including diamorphine and morphine.[16–19]

Excess secretions

A distressing symptom in the terminal stages is the 'death rattle' – an accumulation of airway secretions. The child him- or herself is usually unconscious and does not suffer from the death rattle. Hence an indication to treat may only be given if the child appears distressed or the family cannot tolerate the sometimes extremely noisy breathing. Preparing the parents and sibling about the potential symptoms a child might experience during his or her terminal phase is often beneficial. Anticholinergic drugs (transdermal hyoscine hydrobromide or glycopyrronium etc., p.o. or i.v.) to dry secretion, positioning and suctioning may be effective.

PRACTICAL AND CULTURAL ISSUES

Having to organize the funeral may be a major hurdle for grieving parents, and help from medical or nursing staff may be welcome, as may practical advice on registration of the death and prompt completion of the death certificate.

Healthcare providers should routinely inquire about spiritual belief systems in a family, and it often is advantageous to include an appropriate representative of the respective religion early in the holistic, multidisciplinary care of a child with an LLC. Awareness of religious rituals is paramount.[20] Hindu rituals, for example, include prayers, the reading of holy scripture, the tying of thread in blessing and the use of holy water in order to prepare the child for the next life. The Muslim family may wish the child's bed to be turned towards Mecca. The Hindu tradition, in all but the younger child, is for cremation, while Jewish and Muslim families will want the funeral to be carried out as soon as possible after death.

MODELS OF PAEDIATRIC PALLIATIVE CARE

In considering how to deliver palliative care, it is first necessary to consider where children are. Most are at home much of the time, and it is not surprising that the majority of families looking after a child with an LLC choose to remain there at the time of death.[21] Any model of palliative care must acknowledge and facilitate this. Another normal environment is school. Special schools are intimately involved with children with non-malignant LLCs, and the emotional needs of staff there are easy to overlook. For children with cancer, the challenge can be to accommodate the anxieties of school staff with regard to drug administration and storage. Children's hospices provide a 'home from home'. Most emphasize the provision of high-quality respite care, but some have developed considerable skill in symptom control and management of the terminal phase. For families who cannot face the death of a child at home, hospices can provide a valuable alternative.

Acute wards are ill equipped to deal with the needs of a dying child, as it is typically difficult to provide the physical and temporal space that families need. In addition, medical and nursing staff may be unfamiliar with practical issues of specialist symptom control. Death on the wards is nevertheless not uncommon, and puts great demands on staff.[22]

Several models have developed, largely independently of one another, to meet the needs of children in these environments,[23] and there are encouraging signs that a unifying framework is emerging. Rather than developing from a single vision, specialist PPC is evolving as a means of coordinating, complementing and supplementing models that are already in place. The role of the palliative care paediatrician is to evaluate the child's needs, identify those that existing services can already meet and become a focal point for coordinating them, while at the same time attempting to provide those that are missing. It is rare for the palliative care paediatrician to become the main consultant; most work alongside existing teams in a shared-care capacity.

Anticipating the concept of the managed clinical network, the RCPCH has proposed a network of tertiary specialists in PPC.[1] A relatively small number of such consultants should disseminate their skills through other paediatricians with a special interest in PPC, and then through the array of other professionals involved. The particular needs of adolescents and young people with an LLC have received special attention.[7] It is essential to acknowledge their distinctness from both children and adults. Issues of emerging autonomy and sexuality have a particular challenge and poignancy when they occur simultaneously with impending death. Adolescent palliative care is an opportunity for collaboration with adult colleagues.

WHAT'S NEW?

Ten years ago, the first consultant in PPC was appointed at Great Ormond Street in London, but it was 2000 before a second was appointed, in Cardiff. In 2006, there are still only four or five consultants in paediatric palliative medicine in the UK potentially able to offer specialist training. Worldwide, there are only four designated fellowship programmes (Cardiff; London; Boston, USA; Sydney, Australia). But many paediatricians, often from community or oncology backgrounds, are electing to make palliative care their major interest. Many more paediatric specialist registrars are tailoring their training to PPC. They are hampered by a lack of training opportunities, but even here there has been progress. There are specialist registrar rotations at Great Ormond Street and in Cardiff. There are established PPC conferences in Cardiff, as well as in Australia, Canada, Poland, Germany and the USA.

In addition to the umbrella organization ACT, there are interest groups for doctors (the British Society of Paediatric Palliative Medicine) and for nurses, which facilitate communication between professionals working in different environments.

Increasing interest among paediatricians in palliative care has resulted in an expansion of educational resources. For children's hospice doctors, most of whom are from a GP background, there is a training scheme in Oxford, and there is one postgraduate course in Cardiff specifically teaching palliative medicine in children. The Initiative for Pediatric Palliative Care (IPPC) provides downloadable teaching modules free of charge over the internet.[24] The first edition of the *Oxford Textbook of Palliative Care for Children*,[25] published in 2006, brings together the competence and knowledge of some leaders in the field of PPC.

CONCLUSION

Children with LLCs cannot yet expect the same access to specialist palliative care services as adults, but the paediatric approach to the care of patients already embodies much of what specialist palliative medicine can offer. PPC must, of course, develop from within paediatrics if we are to meet the needs of children. At the same time, we have much to learn from our colleagues in adult medicine, both corporately and individually, adolescent palliative care in particular being an opportunity for collaboration.

Specialist palliative care for children needs to be delivered in many different clinical locations, and to achieve this the consultant must take on an advisory and coordinating role as well as providing specialist advice. The exact role of the consultant in PPC will depend more on the individual child than on the model used. This is an exciting time in the development of this new subspecialty. Educational opportunities, including conferences, training and textbooks, are growing. An increasing number of trainees and established consultant paediatricians are taking on palliative care as their main or even only clinical interest, and there are expanding opportunities to exchange experience and views through the British Society of Paediatric Palliative Medicine. Children needing palliative care are, at last, particularly through the emergence of the ACT as an umbrella organization, beginning to find a voice.

Chapter Thirty Three

New medicines for children: who is protecting the rights of the child?

Richard Bowker • Terence Stephenson

SUMMARY

Children have the right to have research undertaken on the diseases that affect them and the drugs used to treat them. They also have the right to safeguards from that research and the researchers, the right to informed consent (or their parents' consent), 'human rights' and the right to research governance. Sometimes, superficially, these various rights appear to be in conflict, but this need not be so. This chapter explores the historical background to explain why there has been insufficient research into children's therapies, and suggests that continuing pressure is required to rectify this anomalous situation.

PRACTICE POINTS

Children have:
- the right to have research undertaken.
- the right to safeguards.
- the right to informed consent.
- 'human rights'.
- the right to research governance.

None of these observations gives grounds for complacency. Who then is protecting the rights of the child when new medicines are developed, from the very earliest pharmacokinetic and dose-ranging studies to a definitive multicentre randomized trial?

IS THERE ROOM FOR COMPLACENCY?

Prior to the mid-1960s, medical research was relatively unregulated. In 1967, Maurice Pappworth published a book entitled *Human Guinea Pigs: Experimentation on Man*.[1] Pappworth was one of the first to raise concerns that medical research was conducted without adequate consent and sometimes involved risk to the subject. He acknowledged the need for clinical research, but also the need for safeguards. In his book, some of his examples referred to research on children. For example, he reported a study investigating a new antibiotic treatment for acne. The 50 subjects were all either juvenile delinquents or young people with learning disabilities. After taking the drug for 2 weeks, 50% of the subjects had some evidence of liver damage. The drug administration was continued, with the expected result that 'these liver abnormalities became more marked and in two children jaundice occurred'. In eight of the children, subsequent liver biopsy showed severe liver damage and in four children liver biopsy was undertaken twice.[2] Eventually Pappworth's work and that of others, together with the impetus from the thalidomide tragedy,[3] led to the establishment of research ethics committees. Over 30 years later, anxieties about research fraud[4] and research governance remain, as the government and research sponsors have begun to ask whether we need to develop new ways of showing that research is being carried out and reported in a proper fashion.[5] The inquiries in Bristol[6] and Liverpool[7] have further undermined society's confidence in the medical profession, with consequences for medical research, and there have also been concerns about scientific fraud and cheating among medical students.[8, 9]

WHO IS PROTECTING THE RIGHTS OF THE CHILD?

The rights of the child can be considered in five different ways:

- the right to have research undertaken
- the right to safeguards
- the right to informed consent
- 'human rights'
- the right to research governance.

A new therapy is prohibitively expensive. It has been estimated that it costs US$350 million to bring a new drug to market, a process that currently takes on average 15 years from initial chemical synthesis of the molecule to marketing approval.[10] Much of this money goes to meet the regulatory requirements of various governments for the necessary clinical trials. Generally, only large pharmaceutical companies can afford the money and resources needed for clinical drug development. If one adds the particular ethical problems[11, 12] and litigation risks for research in children[13, 14] as perceived by the pharmaceutical industry, it is not surprising that there is far less research into new drugs for children than for adults. Following the thalidomide disaster, 'legislation was introduced to ensure that no new drug could be marketed until independent experts were agreed that it had been adequately tested and safe'.[3] Throughout the world, this goal has been achieved beyond all expectations, such that relatively few drugs come to market for children. The fact that new drugs cannot be marketed (i.e. promoted by the company that manufactures them) does not prevent doctors from prescribing them. Children's doctors must continue to act in the best interests of children and, as a consequence, prescribing outside the licence (a licence is the marketing authorization) is relatively common for hospitalized children.[15] In the neonatal intensive care unit, 90% of infants receive unlicensed or off-label drugs (drugs that have a licence but not for that age group or for that disease), and even in primary care 11–33% of prescriptions for children in Europe are unlicensed or off-label.[16, 17] In response to these problems, legislation in the USA has guaranteed companies who perform paediatric studies on drugs that may be appropriate for children an extra 6-month extension to the exclusive patent.[18]

Indeed, where the potential market is large (e.g. antibiotics) or the disease severity allows the company to charge a high price for each vial of drug (e.g. surfactant), companies do undertake highly ethical studies in children and successfully apply for licences for those drugs. This suggests that industry can overcome the apparent ethical, legal and logistical obstacles 'when the price is right'.

The guideline for the ethical conduct of medical research involving children, published by the Royal College of Paediatrics and Child Health Ethics Advisory Committee,[19] noted that research involving children is important for the benefit of all children and that children are not small adults. Children have unique features which mean that the necessary research into drugs for children cannot always be undertaken in human adults or young animals. In an accompanying commentary, Sir David Hull suggested that 'children, like adults, are capable of being generous and doing something worthwhile even if it means they experience discomfort'. Nevertheless, the guidelines also state that, for research into children to be worthwhile, each project must have 'an identifiable prospect of benefit to children'. Whilst this may be easy with hindsight, it is not so simple with foresight. It is arguable whether Mary Ellen Avery could have predicted, when she began to study hyaline membrane disease, that this would ultimately lead to surfactant therapy. The guidelines also state that 'research with children should only be undertaken if work with adults is clearly not feasible'. Again this requires a degree of foresight. Obviously surfactant therapy or sudden infant death syndrome can never be studied in adults. Who knows how events might have unfolded if, 30 years ago, a 'group of experts' had concluded that leukaemia in adults was essentially a similar disease to that in children. Over the last 30 years there have been over a dozen randomized trials of acute lymphoblastic leukaemia in children, associated with a dramatic fall in mortality from this disease, and yet chemotherapy for adults does not produce such good results. What a tragedy if this important work had been omitted because it was presumed that the research was clearly feasible in adults.

This 'presumption against child research' has been widespread. In 1991, the Department of Health stated that research proposals should only involve children when 'the information required cannot be obtained using adult subjects'. In 1991 the Medical Research Council stated, 'children should take part in research only if the relevant knowledge cannot be gained by research in adults'.[20] Whilst no one could argue with the sentiments of these statements, it is never explicit who will make the judgement as to whether the relevant knowledge can be obtained from adults. Furthermore, these 'experts' must predict that the relevant knowledge can be gained by research in adults in advance of any data being obtained from children. Finally, as a consequence of their judgement, no data would ever be obtained from children in the future, and therefore children may miss out on treatments that work for them but not adults.

Because researchers have been willing to embark on research in children, despite facing considerable ethical, legal and financial hurdles, there have been tangible benefits: there is now a 90% survival rate for infants receiving neonatal intensive care who are above 1,000 g; deaths from sudden infant death syndrome have been halved; and deaths from *Haemophilus influenza* type B have been almost abolished in the UK. Despite these successes, there is still a pressing need for more research to be undertaken in the childhood population. In a recent survey, Campbell et al.[21] noted that, over the last 15 years, only 249 randomized, controlled trials had been published in the *Archives of Disease in Childhood*, 43% funded by pharmaceutical companies and 50% with fewer than 40 recruits. Rudolph et al.,[22] in a subsequent survey of the evidence to support community paediatric practice, concluded that only 40% of their clinical work was supported by research evidence.

THE RIGHT TO SAFEGUARDS

Local research ethics committees (LRECs) and multicentre research ethics committees (MRECs) perform a very important role. The Central Office for Research Ethics Committees (COREC) was established in 2000 to improve the training of research ethics committees (RECs), to help standardize the process and to prepare for the implementation of the EU Clinical Trials Directive. As part of the Arm's Length Body Review in the summer of 2004, it was decided that the National Patient Safety Agency should 'take over responsibility for COREC' from April 2005.

The duties of LRECs include, in addition to considering any particular ethical concerns:

- To take advice from the 'experts' in children and in science – external peer review.
- To decide whether the study will answer a useful question.
- To address whether the study is designed in the best possible way.
- To ensure the study involves a statistically appropriate number of subjects (unless it is a pilot study).

The EU Clinical Trials Directive

Directive 2001/20/EC was implemented in May 2004. The Regulations implementing the Directive in the UK set a statutory framework for the conduct of clinical trials of medicinal products, both within and outside the NHS. The Directive required EU Member States (including the UK) to arrange for the establishment and operation of RECs for the purpose of review of clinical trials of medicinal products. The Regulations provide for a single UK-wide opinion for multicentre studies. To avoid the confusion that would result from having parallel but different operating systems, the UK Health Departments agreed to apply this approach also to all other (non-medicinal) research.

REPORT OF THE AD HOC ADVISORY GROUP ON THE OPERATION OF NHS RESEARCH ETHICS COMMITTEES

The *Report of the Ad Hoc Advisory Group on the Operation of NHS Research Ethics Committees* was published in 2005.[23] The evidence submitted revealed a common perception that the NHS Research Ethics Committee system is dominated by the review of clinical trials, and that the whole system is designed accordingly. While the changes in the operating system were driven by the need to comply with the EU Clinical Trials Directive, only some 15% of applications are for such trials and half of the committees do not review any trials at all. Some researchers felt that the committees did not understand their research or had preferences for certain clinical research methodologies. The report accepted that, while the criticism may be valid, it risks missing the point that RECs are not, and should not be, responsible for detailed scientific review.

At first sight, this seems at odds with the enquiry into clinical paediatric research in North Staffordshire,[24] which highlighted that if research is not scientifically sound, then by definition the research is not ethical. Do LRECs therefore have a duty to look at the science of the research as well as the ethics?

The report by the Ad Hoc Advisory Group stated that, because it is unethical to conduct scientifically inadequate research, the REC's role is to be reassured that there has been adequate scientific review of the design. For most applications, this review will have taken place before the application reaches the REC. The report's authors did not believe RECs should function as a secondary form of scientific review; indeed, to do so would have significant implications for REC membership. Where peer review has taken place, the RECs should accept this in all but exceptional cases; if it has not taken place, RECs should be able to refer the application, for scientific review purposes only, to a Scientific Officer based in COREC.

Children can also be safeguarded in drug research if those undertaking the research have had proper training.[25]

Common problems with clinical research are summarized in Box 33.1.

BOX 33.1

Common problems with clinical research

- The research is not peer reviewed.
- There has been an inadequate literature research and the research is duplication.
- The study is underpowered to answer the question.
- The research is never completed or published.
- There are multiple small local audits that never complete the audit cycle. A smaller number of well coordinated regional audits would be more useful.

THE RIGHT TO INFORMED CONSENT

Caroline Faulder has alleged that, in August 1981, an 83-year-old woman was entered into a randomized, controlled clinical trial of an anticancer drug without her consent. Two weeks later she died of what was an alleged drug side-effect. Apparently, at the inquest, it was noted that no fewer than 11 hospital ethical committees had accepted the trial and agreed that the informed consent of patients was not required.[26] While one would hope that this would not occur 20 years later, there will always be ethical dilemmas around the nature of consent for children.

In the case of Gillick versus West Norfolk and Wisbech Area Health Authority,[27] in which Mrs Gillick claimed that she should be informed by the GP if her daughter should seek contraceptives, the Law Lords concluded by a majority of three to two that this was not necessary. The majority were of the view that the criterion of capacity to consent *to treatment* in law is not a matter of age but of the ability of the person to understand what is involved. In contrast to treatment, there is no law governing the conduct of clinical trials. Ian Kennedy, Professor of Medical Law and Ethics (and subsequently chairman of the enquiry into children's heart surgery at the Bristol Royal Infirmary) implied in 1988 that the public does not understand risk or randomization but expects the benefits of research. Kennedy questioned whether genuinely informed consent really was feasible, and the issues are even more complex when applied to the young.[28]

An even more difficult problem arises when the drug or treatment being studied in childhood is for an emergency. In these circumstances, there is insufficient time or even no time to seek truly informed consent. Where there is insufficient time, assent has been used initially, rather than consent. Assent implies acquiescence, whereas consent implies positive, informed agreement. In the UK Oscillation Study (UKOS),[29] where infants were randomized to conventional ventilation or high-frequency oscillation shortly after birth, assent for randomization was obtained before delivery, as delivery was often imminent and the parents were often in a distressed state. The parents were then seen as soon as possible after birth. In a recent trial of buccal midazolam versus rectal diazepam for the termination of status epilecticus, there was literally no time to seek informed consent. Parents cannot be expected to discuss a research protocol for even a few minutes while their child is having a convulsion. For this trial, the weeks of the year were randomized so that during certain weeks children receive midazolam and during other weeks, diazepam. Families were approached after the conclusion of the emergency treatment and their child's recovery for informed consent for their child to continue in the trial. Clearly this is informed consent for follow-up and for the child's data to be used, but cannot be consent to treatment which has already been given.

HUMAN RIGHTS

The Human Rights Act 1998 became law in England and Wales on 2 October 2000 and allows UK citizens to seek a remedy for unlawful violation in the courts. Amongst rights potentially relevant to research are the right to equality and freedom from discrimination (Articles 1, 2 and 7).[30] Human rights concerns arise when populations are completely excluded from research that could benefit them. For example, pregnant women and children are frequently excluded from research. Furthermore, in many UK universities, prohibitively high insurance premiums for academic clinical research in pregnant women and children inhibit research. The 1998 Human Rights Act includes the right to life, which can be interpreted as a right to receive medical services essential to maintain life or health. If a population is excluded from research that could benefit them, this discrimination could result in a lack of effective treatments being developed for them. Therefore, while the Human Rights Act is generally thought of as guaranteeing 'liberty rights', and perhaps protecting children from being unwittingly forced to participate in research, as potentially important as these 'freedom rights' are 'entitlement rights', which exert positive claims to services.

There are many safeguards and quality checks involved in controlled trials. It is perhaps not surprising, therefore, that a systematic review of 15 studies comparing patients treated in the context of controlled trials with apparently similar patients treated outside a trial protocol showed that, on average, the outcomes of patients in trials were better.[31] Further evidence to support a more inclusive approach to participation in randomized, controlled trials comes from trials of leukaemia care in the UK.[32] There is also some evidence that children enrolled into trials have better outcomes, irrespective of the arm of the trial to which they are randomized.[33] On the other hand, there are concerns that not all commercially funded trials are necessary. In a review of 136 randomized trials of myeloma in adults, 64% of commercially funded trials favoured the tested treatment over the control treatment, whereas in only 53% of trials funded by the government or non-profit organizations was the new treatment superior.[34] In perfect equipoise, half of the trials should favour the new treatment. Different results for industry- and non-industry-sponsored studies have also been reported for third-generation oral contraceptives and the risk of venous thrombosis, for calcium channel antagonists and for non-steroidal anti-inflammatory drugs.[35-37] This discrepancy may arise, in part, because the trials are required for drug regulatory authorities.

ENCOURAGING MORE RESEARCH IN CHILDREN

New EU legislation to encourage more medicines research in children, following the example set by the USA, is unlikely to become law before 2006. The key measures included in the draft European paediatric regulation are:

- New medicines:
  - a requirement at the time a company seeks a licence for a new medicine for a plan, if the medicine could be of benefit in children, on how and when data on the use of the medicine in children will be acquired
  - a system of waivers from the requirement for medicines unlikely to benefit children
  - a system of deferrals of the requirement to ensure medicines are tested in children only when it is safe to do so and to prevent the requirements delaying the authorization of medicines for adults.
  - a mixed reward and incentive for compliance with the requirement in the form of, in effect, a 6-month patent extension on the active moiety
  - for orphan medicines, a mixed reward and incentive for compliance with the requirement in the form of an additional 2 years of market exclusivity added to the existing 10 years awarded under the EU orphan regulations.
- Old medicines:
  - a new type of marketing authorization, the Paediatric Use Marketing Authorization (PUMA), which allows 10 years of data protection for existing medicines where new data relevant to children have been generated
  - a reference to an EU paediatric study programme, Medicines Investigation for the Children of Europe (MICE), to fund

research leading to the development and authorization of off-patent medicine for children.

THE RIGHT TO RESEARCH GOVERNANCE

Public concern in the UK about issues related to children's healthcare have been at the heart of recent enquiries into the events in Bristol, Alder Hey and North Staffordshire.[6, 7, 24] The latter particularly highlighted the need for research to be conducted with transparency and to the highest ethical and scientific standards with fully informed consent.[38] The government has now implemented proposals for research governance[5] (see Boxes 33.2 to 33.4).

BOX 33.2

Research governance

- Sets standards.
- Describes monitoring arrangements.
- Safeguards the public.
- Includes non-clinical and clinical research, if that research relates to the responsibilities of the Secretary of State for Health (i.e. Public Health, Department of Health, NHS, Social Care Services).
- Includes 'all those involved in research with human participants (therefore, both patients and healthy volunteers), their organs, tissue or data'.

BOX 33.3

What does research governance involve?

- Assessment of the quality of research.
- Assessment of the research environment, including equipment facilities and safety.
- Assessment of the experience or expertise of the researchers.
- Ensuring arrangements are in place to review significant developments as the research proceeds (data monitoring committees and 'stopping rules') and to approve modifications to study design.
- Ensuring research is conducted according to the protocol approved by the ethics committee.
- Random checks.

BOX 33.4

Responsibilities of the research sponsor

- To ensure the scientific quality of the proposed research.
- To ensure ethics committee approval is obtained.
- To ensure that the research is managed and monitored.

The dangers of increasing research governance for children are that there could be even greater perceived obstacles to research in this neglected group,[39] and that research in children could become prohibitively expensive. It is ironic that doctors 'need permission to give a drug to half their patients but not to give it to them all'.[40]

CONCLUSION

Following the thalidomide disaster of 1962, it was stated that 'the thalidomide tragedy wonderfully concentrated the minds of the pharmaceutical industry under the various agencies responsible for licensee drugs'.[3] If adults were asked, or if government asked the electorate, 'Would you prefer to take a licensed drug (i.e. one scrutinized for safety, quality and efficacy) or an unlicensed drug?', then the answer would be obvious. The fact that children have no voice, no money and no vote means that they continue to be a group whose preferences are ignored, and who have no option but to receive unlicensed or off-label drugs from their well-meaning carers, since to do otherwise is to deprive them of any treatment at all. Those who prescribe for children should continue to choose the medicine that offers the best prospect of benefit for that child.[39] Provided that prescription is in accordance with current practice in the British Isles,[41] the prescriber will be protected by the Bolam judgement of 1957: 'a doctor is not guilty of negligence if he has acted in accordance with the practice accepted as proper by a responsible body of medical men skilled in that particular art'.[42]

Children certainly have the right to be protected from unethical, unscientific and dangerous research, but they also have the right to have their diseases and the drugs required for them studied in the same depth and to the same standards as for adults. Since such studies are expensive, and the better they are conducted the more expensive they are, steps must be taken to work with the pharmaceutical industry jointly for the good of children, capitalizing on the expertise of both children's doctors and nurses and a very successful UK industry. Ultimately, the solution probably lies with Europe rather than the UK, as there are 75 million children in Europe, which represents a very attractive financial market to the industry.

The May 2004 report *Safer and Better Medicines for Children*, from the RCPCH,[43] which was commissioned by the Department of Health, the Medical Research Council and the Association of British Pharmaceutical Industry, established the state of play in children's research and outlined areas for development in the UK. Children's medicine is one of the first areas to be developed under the umbrella of the new UK Clinical Research Collaboration (UKCRC), which will provide infrastructure and networks to enable studies in children of both old and new drugs.

The UK Government's decision to invest new money in this priority area of research on medicines for children is, therefore, timely and welcome. It is crucial that this money is well used, utilizing the expertise of primary care, district general hospitals and academic centres. It is equally important that the resources produce tangible benefits for children, and this is most likely if the data are published in peer-reviewed outputs where they can be subject to scrutiny and properly assessed.

Chapter Thirty Four

Coping with distressed and aggressive parents

Mike Shooter

SUMMARY

Illness is distressing, not only for the sick child, but also for parents worried simultaneously about their child's prognosis and the hospital system they are caught up in. Staff may become just as distressed as those in their care. When badly handled, such distress is easily turned into distrust, anger and blame, in parents who feel their complaints are unheard, who feel they have no one close to turn to, who feel kept in the dark or assaulted by bad news insensitively given, who feel left out of the care of their child and decisions about the future, and who feel discriminated against. The challenge for the paediatrician is to get beyond the defensive stereotypes, to try to understand why the parents of a child have become so angry, and to learn from the experience. Three archetypal 'cases' are offered for discussion.

PRACTICE POINTS

- Illness is distressing for everyone, patients, parents and staff alike. Everyone needs support.
- 'Heart-sink' situations occur where the demands of parents exceed the ability of staff to satisfy them.
- Where distress is badly handled, it can easily turn to anger. Individuals may become unfairly blamed.
- Parents should be told how to complain about bad practice. Where complaints are about resources, parents can be useful allies.
- Continuity is important. Parents need to feel that they have a key person they can trust in the process of their child's illness.
- Information should be given freely, sensitively, and in packages that patients and parents are capable of taking in.
- Beware of inventing certainty where none exists. Parents may never trust you once they have become disillusioned.
- Parents should feel that they have a role in their child's care. Major decisions are best taken by parents and staff together.
- It is easy unconsciously to discriminate against the most vulnerable groups, whatever the best intentions.
- Practice improves by understanding the origins of difficulties, not by retreating into stereotypes of angry patients and defensive doctors.

INTRODUCTION

Doctors are aloof, arrogant and autocratic. Parents are angry, abusive and thoroughly annoying, are they not? Well, no. While all of us will have had experience of some people who fit the description, these are stereotypes that must be abandoned if doctors and parents are to work in partnership for the good of the children in their care. Perhaps this chapter should not be about how staff can 'cope' with angry parents, but how they can 'understand' how their anger has arisen in the first place. The following three scenarios are fraught with conflict.

How does conflict arise in such archetypal scenarios? How can we better understand the anger of parents? How can we prevent it from surfacing so often? How can we handle it more sensitively when it does?

GENERAL FACTORS

Every doctor–patient–parent relationship must be set against the backdrop of the general dynamics of illness and its treatment, and the emotions painted large upon it.

The inevitable stress of illness

Being ill is painful, in all senses of the word; being in hospital adds to the distress. Whether the illness is acute or chronic, sick child-

ren and their carers go through agonies of hope and anxiety, elation and misery, insight and confusion. We know that the stress involved in an illness like that of Leanne can take individual and family relationships to the limit, and beyond, and exactly the same emotions may be carried by staff who have grown close to them over the years. Everyone sharing the agony of decisions that have to be made in intensive care, with children like Rhys, may be scarred by the process in time.

Patients, parents and staff alike need supportive outlets for their emotions, and there is good evidence of modelling at work here. Where staff can be seen to be supportive of each other on the ward, patients and their carers are more likely to be more openly supportive of each other too. Where staff remain imprisoned in an old-style 'professionalism', patients and carers are more likely to be aloof from each other, and feelings, unexpressed, build up to boiling point. But the situation is still more complex.

Case illustration 43.1

Rhys: a neonate

Rhys was born 3 weeks prematurely after a problem pregnancy in which his mother paid little attention to antenatal advice. Rhys is admitted to the paediatric intensive care unit with multiple organ failure. The outlook is bleak.

The natural parents had only a passing relationship. The mother is just 18 years old, has spent most of her life in local authority care, has little family support, but desperately wants her son to be saved at all costs. The much older father has a long-term partner by whom he already has three children. He does not feel that Rhys should be treated.

Despite heroic initial efforts, Rhys' condition worsens and the decision is taken not to proceed to further surgery. His mother is distraught, accusing the staff of letting her baby die because she is a teenage mother and nobody listens to people like that. The staff are split.

Case illustration 43.2

Kirsty: 8 years old

Kirsty has been admitted to the paediatric ward with a 2-month history of sore throat, intermittent pyrexia, lethargy, low mood and flitting aches and pains. She is described as a girl with an anxious personality, who often sleeps in her parents' bed, and worries about school, even though she is a high achiever. There has been a cluster of traumatic events in the family's life over the last few years, including the father's illness, business worries and the mother's miscarriage, none of which has been openly talked about.

After a difficult pregnancy, Kirsty's mother has given birth to a son at 26 weeks' gestation who needed 3 months' care in the neonatal unit. Kirsty visited him every day. She became ill as soon as her mother brought the baby home from the hospital.

All investigations have proved negative, except for one brief episode of proteinuria, but Kirsty's condition seems to be worsening and she is now bed bound. The consultant suggests bringing in a child psychiatrist, but the parents react angrily, saying that their daughter is ill, 'not mad'. They demand a transfer to another hospital.

Case illustration 43.3

Leanne: 14 years old

Leanne has been in and out of the paediatric ward for most of her life, with acute exacerbations of cystic fibrosis. The family has been through a switchback of despair and hope as the disease has relapsed and remitted. Several of her fellow patients have died during the course of her own illness.

In the process, Leanne and her family became very close to their female consultant, who has recently retired. Heart–lung transplantation has been considered but never actively sought because of the parents' fear of the consequences.

Leanne is currently well enough to be back at school and out socializing with her friends at weekends. She has become an attractive adolescent and is the apple of her father's eye. The new, young, male consultant has persuaded Leanne to reconsider transplantation. The father demands to see him, complaining, belligerently, that it was unethical to talk to Leanne about treatment without her parents being there, that Leanne cannot agree to transplantation without their agreement and that the consultant should be 'struck off' for his incompetence.

The vulnerable relationship

All children are vulnerable, by virtue of being ill and needing treatment. All parents are vulnerable, by virtue of having to call upon expert help when their skills as parents are not enough. All doctors are vulnerable, by virtue of having to provide that expertise. The sometimes fragile trust in which that triangle of vulnerabilities is held is easily shattered. Such trust relies on a 'fit' between the personal qualities of patients, parents and staff; and between the expectations of the patients and parents and the ability of staff to satisfy them. If that fit is disrupted, the ordinary distress of illness is magnified on all sides. In Kirsty's case, the expectations implicit in her illness, although expressed in physical need, are much more to do with family dynamics. The parents are unwilling to see that and the consultant is damned for doing so – the truly 'heart-sink' situation.

The power of projection

In such circumstances, the diffuse emotions inside the patient and parents can easily be translated into aggression and focused on a single professional, a staff group or a hospital that can be attacked and blamed – as in Kirsty's and Leanne's cases. Their 'failings' can be more comfortably addressed than the more painful imponderables of illness and its refusal to be cured. Even more confusingly, the internal conflicts within individual patients and within family relationships around them, like those unspoken traumas in the life of Kirsty's family, or the different vested interests of Rhys' parents, can be projected out onto staff that try to help them. Not only may staff feel unfairly attacked from outside, but they may begin to play out those conflicts between themselves. The temptation to get angry back, to retreat into defensiveness, or to absorb the anger to the destruction of normal team working, may be overwhelming. Again, this is an argument for regular support to the ward staff and the insights of a 'facilitator' close enough to paediatric practice to earn its trust, but sufficiently distant to be able to spot what is happening within the team and help it towards a resolution of its conflicts. The team may then be able to live with the anger of patients and parents long enough to help them with it, rather than reinforcing it in their own relationships.

SPECIFIC FACTORS

Within this context, of course, the distress of patients and parents may result from very much more specific issues.

Standards of care: 'What's the use of complaining? ... You lot always stick together'

Paediatrics, like any other branch of medicine, still struggles to come to terms with the legitimate complaints of parents against individual or corporate standards of care. The vague assertions of patients' charters and the more specific details of complaint procedures, pinned to the clinic wall or not, have failed to give patients or parents sufficient power to voice their misgivings – while the system trundles over them towards individual patient disaster or massed calamities such as those at Bristol or Alder Hey. While the government, the General Medical Council and the royal colleges vie with each other to create ever more systems of inspection and appraisal, the individual doctor and team can only keep on auditing their practice and accepting that parents can be angry about real deficiencies as well as the 'unfairness' of illness in their child, and point them to the complaints procedures where necessary. Indeed, where those deficiencies are ones of resources rather than skills, parents and professionals can become useful allies. It may be argued, of course, that parents have a reciprocal duty to care, and that an employing health trust has a responsibility to back up its staff against the 'vexatious complainant'.

Availability of staff: 'Every time I ask to speak to someone, they give me someone different'

It is small wonder that in the monolithic structure of most medical services it is the regular, face-to-face contact with an individual paediatrician, nurse or key worker that patients and parents value most – and being handed on like a relay baton makes them most angry. Despite the relentless retreat into management, medicine is almost unique among the caring professions in not promoting its practitioners away from contact with the consumer. But just as services have to be rationed, so the time of the staff is not infinitely expandable. Such an asset needs to be properly managed. Parents need to feel a sense of continuity in which a key person or group of people is felt to stick with them through all the vicissitudes of

an illness such as cystic fibrosis, and from whom they are able to draw advice and support – personal and private contact rather than the public embarrassment of a ward round, however sensitively handled. The corollaries of such closeness are many. It puts a heavy onus on the key worker, whether a member of care staff or a consultant, carrying the load of the parents' emotions, while balancing the twin necessities of confidentiality and the team's need for information. Roles within the team must be flexible enough for the key worker to 'become' whatever is required of him or her by parents at any one moment – from practical aid to grief counsellor – in total honesty. The end of the relationship, by the retirement of Leanne's consultant or junior staff moving on, needs to be managed carefully lest parents, like those of Leanne, feel let down again. The ultimate transition, from paediatric to adult services, is becoming an increasing problem as survival rates improve in even the most seriously ill children.

The empowerment of knowledge: 'No one ever tells me anything round here'

In transactional analysis, the four-paned 'Johari window' represents the life of a person in which the upper-left quadrant is that area in which other people know more about 'me' than I know about 'myself'; the upper-right quadrant is what 'I' and others both know about 'myself'; the lower-right quadrant is what neither 'I' nor others know about 'myself'; and the lower-left quadrant is what 'I' know about 'myself' that others do not know. It would seem that paediatric practice has moved around that circle in the last few decades, from the old paternalism of professionals knowing more about a child's illness than they were prepared to share. Staff have had to learn the art (and attitude) of open communication – now on the curriculum of even the most conservative of medical schools. There can be little excuse now for even bad news being withheld, or broken insensitively in hasty, jargon-riddled asides at the end of a busy clinic or ward round, with no privacy, to a lone parent left with the burden of it to get home as best as they can. Yet that will still occur, and parents will be rightfully distressed, and angry, about information kept back, grudgingly given or delivered in one-off chunks that they were unable to take in at the time. The upper-right quadrant of patient–parent–professional partnership relies on a true equality of information and the empowerment that it gives. It hardly feels as if the mother of Rhys was drawn into the decision-making process as an equal partner. An 18 year old in the midst of complicated technology could easily find that she is treated like a child herself.

Living with uncertainties: 'If you don't know, say so – don't beat around the bush'

Knowledge, however, has its limits. Individual consultants and their teams, despite being kept up to date by the exercise of continuous professional development, can never know everything. They must learn to accede to parents' request for a second opinion before it becomes an angry demand, and hand over to more specific expertise with dignity, in the interests of the patient rather than their own pride. But medicine, as the one-time Secretary of State, Mr Milburn, was apt to say before the Health Select Committee of the House of Commons, is not an exact science. Doctors, patients and their carers have to learn to live with successive layers of uncertainty – of Rhys' prognosis, of the nature of Kirsty's illness or of the outcome of Leanne's transplantation. The temptation for doctors, faced with parental questions they cannot answer, is to 'invent' a certainty, the falsehood of which will undermine the trust that parents have in them once exposed. Perhaps it is better to admit, as in that lower-right quadrant of the Johari window, that this is an area in which none of us knows the answer, but we will work together to find it out. There are times too, of course, where sick children or their parents may know more about their condition than their doctor – the bottom left-hand quadrant. It is not uncommon for parents, in their day-to-day care of their child, to sense something wrong long before it shows up in overt signs or symptoms. It is a skilled doctor who has learnt to listen to such experiences, to trust in it and bear it in mind rather than fob it off for lack of investigatory proof. Having their parental opinion dismissed by doctors makes parents just as angry as having to ferret out information from doctors in a climate of suspicion.

Reinforcing the parental role: 'I don't know how I can help my child anymore'

It is easy for parents to feel deskilled by white-coated experts being better 'parents' to their sick child, to lose all sense of what role they might play in their child's life, and to feel shut out, alienated and angry in the process. The risk of this can be diminished by involving the parents in the day-to-day care of their child on the hospital ward, and reinforcing the fact that they remain the parents whatever the expert help that is needed. This is not just an attitudinal problem but a logistical one too – for chronic illness may often end up with a split family in which the mother remains close to the child in hospital while the father and siblings develop a separate existence at home. It can be very difficult for such families to revert to 'normality' if and when the sickness is over.

Parents need to be fully involved, too, in the major decisions about their child's treatment. It is no good being included in knowledge about their child's condition if they are not given a share in acting upon it. But some decisions, of the life or death of Rhys, for example, are almost too painful to bear – and certainly too great a responsibility for one parent or consultant to take alone. Medicine in the USA has retreated to the law to decide on issues such as the withholding or withdrawal of treatment, while in the UK we have preferred to rely on general guidelines or on case precedent. At worst, this can be a mishmash of conflicting trends, and at best a licence for parents and staff teams, acting together, to use their discretion in the 'best interest' of a child. Where parents disagree with each other, or staff are split about what to do, as in Rhys' case, it may require the advice of bodies such as clinical ethics committees to achieve a resolution. Adolescents, of course, will demand a say in their own life or death, and the law may give them power to

have it, protected from the trespass of their parents. It will require enormous tact on the part of Leanne's new consultant to allow a Gillick-competent 14 year old to opt into treatment, against the wishes of a father who is feeling displaced by a man who appears to be sharing closer confidences than he is with his own daughter.

Aspects of discrimination: 'You don't understand where I am coming from, do you?'

Finally, the paediatric team needs to be vigilant about elements of discrimination that can otherwise creep unnoticed into practice. They need to be able to see things from their patients' and their parents' way of life, in a non-judgemental way, rather than imposing upon them their own values. They need to be able to assess the 'meaning' of their own actions for such patients and parents, rather than rely on their own best 'intentions'. Rhys' mother may be right to complain that an 18-year-old, single, 'girl' from local authority care is all too easily dismissed as an 'inadequate mother' whose voice is barely listened to, and that the baby of such a mother, born in such circumstances, may be seen as less 'viable' than a baby with similar handicaps from a middle-class, professional home. Patients and parents from ethnic minorities may need advocates and interpreters before they can even get to the point where they feel confident enough to be angry with an alien system. Whatever the rationality behind it, the 'reframing' of Kirsty's illness as psychological by the blunt introduction of a psychiatrist, was bound to provoke an angry reaction in her parents – and destroy any remit that a psychiatrist might then have. How much better it might have been to express relief that investigations had shown that Kirsty did not have a serious illness and to involve the parents in thinking how we might get her slowly back to as normal a life as possible, despite her undoubted, validated physical problems.

CONCLUSION

The main lesson to be learnt from all this is that lessons can be learnt. We can never prevent illness from being distressful. We can never wholly prevent the parents of sick children from becoming angry. Anger is an emotion intrinsic to the stress of illness and its treatment. But by trying to understand, in each case, what lies behind that anger, the individual consultant and ward team may act upon it to lessen the chances of it recurring, or to handle it more sensitively when it does. Such attitudes, in general, and the more specific skills required with patients like Rhys, Kirsty and Leanne, can and must be taught.

Chapter Thirty Five

Understanding and coping with complaints

David J. Scott

SUMMARY

Dealing with complaints is becoming a necessary and increasing part of everyday life. To minimize the stress that they cause requires a constructive systematic approach. This chapter describes the feelings of clinicians when faced with a complaint, puts complaints into context, and recommends how to deal with them and prevent them, highlighting suggestions for good practice.

INTRODUCTION

Clinicians, like all true professionals, like to think that they are doing or have done a good job. When someone complains, it is therefore natural that they feel annoyed, angry and indignant; they are also often scared and worried. These are natural feelings; no one likes criticism and the perception that one's future career might be damaged is obviously worrying. It is therefore understandable that most clinicians, when faced with a complaint are defensive.

Complaints are almost always a result of failed expectations and, by implication, the clinician's failure to communicate with the patient or relative as to what they should expect. It is therefore important to reflect on why complaints occur, what can be done to prevent them and, most importantly, what lessons can be learned to prevent them happening again.

Parents and patients are anxious and increasingly expect perfection. Anything short of that leads to failed expectations and may cause them to complain. Complaints are inevitable, so learning to cope with them is a necessity.

All most complainants want is an apology and an assurance that what happened to them will not happen to anyone else. The complaints process aims to meet these expectations, and clinicians

PRACTICE POINTS

- Quality matters – complaints are a salutatory reminder that this is indeed the case.
- Healthcare is a service industry, and it is worth remembering that 'the customer is always right'.
- Dealing with complaints should be an integral part of the business and not a subsidiary that merits scant attention or respect.

must therefore be prepared to acknowledge that things may have gone wrong and not seek to justify their actions, when it is clear to everyone that things could have been done differently and, in many cases, better.

CLINICAL GOVERNANCE

Complaints are an integral part of clinical governance and the risk management process, and should be viewed as incidents or concerns about clinical practice. It should not matter whether a concern is raised by a patient, another member of staff, or by clinicians themselves. The message is the same: practice needs to be reviewed and, if necessary, lessons need to be learned and changes made in order to prevent a recurrence.

PRACTICE POINT

- Organizations should have a process in place that ensures that all complaints are properly and appropriately investigated, so that complainants can have confidence in the system and be assured that their concerns are properly addressed.

WHO GETS MOST COMPLAINTS?

Paediatricians are fortunate in that they generate fewer complaints than average. An analysis of complaints over a 4-year period in my hospital, taking into account workload, has shown that by far the largest number of complaints occurred in the orthopaedic and accident and emergency (A&E) departments (Fig. 35.1). A&E departments tend to treat some of the sickest patients in the hospital and are staffed by some of the most junior doctors. It is therefore perhaps not surprising that a significant number of complaints arise from this area. In the orthopaedic and A&E departments there were significantly more complaints than average about the standard and organization of care, and attitude and waiting times than in other departments.

In contrast, as expected, the service departments (pathology, anaesthetics and radiology), where there is less direct patient contact, had fewer complaints. The numbers of complaints in medicine, surgery and psychiatry were similar.

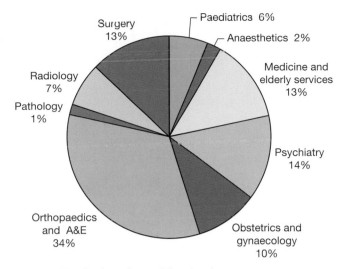

Fig. 35.1 Distribution of complaints by department.

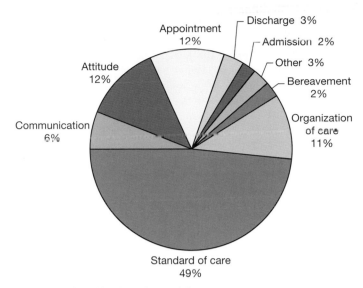

Fig. 35.2 Classification of complaints.

CATEGORIES OF COMPLAINT

It is worth reflecting that complaints not only come from patients, but can also come from one's colleagues and other members of staff. However, it is patient complaints that are the most upsetting and cause clinicians the most distress. Complaints from colleagues are usually about management matters and are rarely about patient care. Having said that, constructive criticism from one's colleagues may prevent future patient complaints. One would therefore do well to listen to friendly advice and suggestions from one's fellow team members. Consultant colleagues, junior doctors and nursing colleagues may all be sources of useful advice about how to change one's clinical practice.

When dealing with complaints it is worth reflecting on whether the complaints are personal or about the team and the team's modus operandi. Complaints about services, and team complaints, merit a team approach to any response, and should be the catalyst for a service review and possible change in working practice.

Personal complaints are always upsetting. These days, due to the pressure on time and the drive for greater throughput, many patients are denied appropriate information and are left in the dark about what is going to happen to them. The internet and the media have led to patients being better informed and, as such, they and their relatives come with certain expectations. If these are not fulfilled they feel let down and may feel the need to express their dissatisfaction.

An analysis of the different types of complaint at the Conquest Hospital over a 4-year period from November 1988 to November 2002 is shown in Fig. 35.2.

All categories of complaint include an element of failure of communication on the part of the healthcare professional, who was either too busy, or who failed to take the time to ensure that the patient or relative really did understand their proposed treatment, or how the treatment was progressing.

Unwell patients are anxious, and it is important to check that they have understood fully what has been proposed for them. In the past, nurses have fulfilled a vital role: checking with the patient in outpatients and on the ward that they really have understood what the doctor has just told them. Bad news is not received well, and many patients 'switch off' when being given bad news and genu-

inely do not hear what is being said to them. At the time, the doctor is convinced that he or she has given the patient all the information required. The reality is that the patient has not heard it.

Paediatric complaints follow a similar pattern. The parents and carers of children with disability have high expectations and, as such, their reactions when things do not 'go right' mirror those of bereaved relatives. A breakdown of paediatric complaints is shown in Fig. 35.3.

PRACTICE POINT

Consistently high categories of complaint relate to:
- communication
- attitude
- waiting times
- organization of service
- medical care
- nursing care.

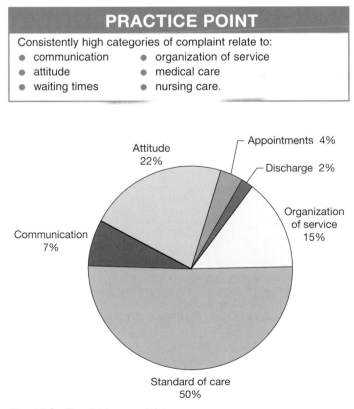

Fig. 35.3 Paediatric complaints.

THE COMPLAINTS PROCESS

The NHS Plan[1] proposed the setting up of the Patient Advocacy Liaison Service (PALS); this is now well established in many areas, and has been very successful in dealing with patient concerns at an informal level. Many consultants do not understand why patients and their relatives find it difficult to voice their concerns, and why patients are genuinely fearful of appearing to criticize their doctor, fearing that their future treatment will be compromised.

Consultants often resent the fact that patients do not come and discuss their fears and concerns. They would do well to reflect on why this is the case. In many instances it is easier, and as a consequence more productive, for a patient or their relative to discuss their concerns with someone who is independent; hence the success of the PALS.

Informal enquiries

Wherever possible, patients and their relatives should have access to a senior member of the team and be able to discuss their concerns in a timely and unhurried manner. This applies to both inpatients and outpatients; all clinicians are, therefore, encouraged to make time to see patients and their relatives to address their concerns.

PRACTICE POINTS

- Many formal complaints could be prevented if clinicians made themselves more available and spoke to patients and their relatives using appropriate language.
- Avoid the use of 'medical jargon' when communicating with children and their parents.
- Check with patients and their relatives that they have understood what they are being told.

Formal complaints

The NHS Complaints Procedure[2] sets out the mechanism for dealing with complaints. All complainants should receive an acknowledgement of their complaint within 3 working days and a written response within 20 working days. A member of the health trust management team usually investigates the circumstances of the complaint, and the clinician involved should receive a copy of the complaint and provide a written response. This response may either be sent to the complainant verbatim or will be used to construct the official reply. Similar processes exist in Scotland,[3, 4] Wales and Northern Ireland.

PRACTICE POINTS

- Wherever possible, clinicians are encouraged to meet complainants at an early stage in the complaints process, unless there are good reasons for not doing so.
- An apology and an assurance that 'things will change, to prevent the problem happening again to someone else', will go a long way to ensuring that a complaint is resolved at an early stage.

Local resolution

Sadly, for a variety of reasons, not all complaints can be resolved. Common reasons for this are entrenched positions, a failure to apologize for mistakes that have obviously been made, and a failure to see the situation from the other side. Humility is a real asset under these circumstances, as is honesty and an admission that 'the customer is right'. Many complaints that should have been resolved locally are not, because these simple rules are not followed. Wherever possible every attempt must be made to try and ensure that complaints are investigated and handled at a local level.

Independent Complaints Advocacy Services (ICAS)

The ICAS is a statutory service that was established in September 2003.[5] It provides information, support and guidance to complainants. Such support may include drafting letters and attending meetings. The aim of ICAS is to 'help clients find a solution as close as possible to the point of the service that has caused dissatisfaction'. The Citizen's Advice Bureau, the Carer's Federation and other organizations provide the service.

The Healthcare Commission

In some circumstances, it will not be possible to resolve an issue at a local level. In England the complainant may then ask the Healthcare Commission to review their complaint.[6]

The Health Service Ombudsman

Complaints that are unresolved may be referred to the Health Service Ombudsman, whose duty it is to investigate both the original complaint and the procedure used for dealing with it. The Ombudsman's findings are often made public, and it behoves all, wherever possible, to ensure that complaints are resolved without recourse to the Ombudsman.[7]

The General Medical Council

The other avenue open to complainants is a referral to the General Medical Council (GMC). This is when complainants judge that a doctor is guilty of serious professional misconduct and is in breach of the standards laid out in *Good Medical Practice*.[8] Complaints are dealt with by the GMC under their fitness to practise procedures,[9] and recent guidance has been published by the GMC to assist medical managers.[10]

RESPONDING TO COMPLAINTS

Replies to complaints should be factual, objective and constructive and, if possible, should reflect empathy and concern. If a complaint does highlight a significant clinical incident, this merits discussion before putting pen to paper. Where there is an error, acknowledge it and offer an apology. If remedial action is required, include this in your report. If the complaint is not justified most Chief Executives will defend their staff, but do be prepared to defend your response if there is a review by the Healthcare Commission or the Ombudsman decides to take on the case.

In many cases, when complaints escalate, it is worth reflecting on what is behind the complaint. Many complainants are motivated to complain by the fact that they do not want what happened to them to happen to anyone else. Others are motivated by money, the wish to see staff punished and subjected to disciplinary action, or they may have personal agendas, which may not be clear at the time. Getting behind the real motivation for the complaint is the key to early resolution. As far as possible this is about giving the customer what they expect; this may not be the same as what they want.

> **PRACTICE POINT**
>
> When answering complaints, the complainant usually wants:
> - an explanation
> - an apology
> - an assurance that what happened to them will not happen to anyone else.

Complaints in paediatrics

Complaints in paediatrics are, in many respects, similar to bereavement complaints. The loss of the perfect child, the stress of coping with a child with disability, and the real demands of coping with children with behavioural problems all lead to a higher incidence of child abuse in these groups and a 'cry for help'. Whilst their complaints are often directed against an individual, many parents of children with special needs complain out of frustration over lack of support and because their expectations are not fulfilled, rather than because they are upset with individuals. When investigating such complaints it is worth reviewing the support offered to parents, as well as individual practice.

Child protection

Several recent high-profile cases[11, 12] and a number of other cases[13] have highlighted the problems and risks facing doctors who undertake child-protection work. A survey by the Royal College of Paediatrics and Child Health has documented these.[14] Of the 3,879 practicing or recently retired paediatricians who have been involved in child protection, 13.0% (550) reported that they had been subject to complaints related to child protection. Of these 536 paediatricians, 533 reported a total of 786 child-protection complaints. Overall, 79% of complaints were dealt with exclusively locally; 8% went for independent review and 11% were referred to the GMC. Of those doctors who responded to the survey, 29% were affected in terms of their willingness to become involved in potential child-protection cases subsequently. As such, paediatricians working in this field must seek help and support when dealing with child-protection cases, and are advised not to deal with complex and difficult cases on their own.

Professor Neil McIntosh has highlighted, what he calls 'savaging by the media' and the tendency, in a large proportion of cases, for the media and family to go public before a judgement has been given.[14] Paediatricians in these instances have no way of defending themselves against the charges made. As Professor McIntosh says; 'If you've not battered your baby, you are certainly angry to be accused. If you have battered your baby, you are both scared and angry that you've been found out'. Those dealing with such cases need to be aware of this reaction and be prepared for it.

Bereavement complaints

Bereavement complaints are particularly difficult because, in many cases, the bereaved feel their loved ones are immortal and that when they die someone must be to blame. Childhood deaths are relatively rare and, if not due to accidents, are frequently expected. Bereavement complaints are therefore much less common in paediatric practice.

PREVENTION AND DAMAGE LIMITATION

As has been highlighted earlier, most complaints are, at least in part, due to poor communication. Either the clinician has misunderstood the child or parent's needs and wishes, or has failed to explain the treatment in a way that they can understand. Medical jargon is poorly understood, and is best avoided when communicating with children and their parents. It is therefore worth asking the question: Is there good communication between clinical staff, reception staff and the public? Inform and update patients about delays and problems with their treatment. Always document any untoward incidents – it is much easier to do this when the events are fresh in your mind, and may pay dividends if the patient subsequently complains.

Consent

A patient must consent to the release of confidential information about them. This is particularly tricky when relatives complain on behalf of a patient, and it is good practice to obtain written consent from a patient before releasing information to a third party. Failure to do so may result in another complaint and could result in an appearance before the GMC. It is not unusual for a relative to complain, even when the patient is relatively satisfied with their treatment.

CONCLUSION

Think of responding to complaints as an educational process whereby important lessons can be learned. All NHS staff should receive training in communication, the breaking of bad news and customer care. These issues should be addressed as part of the appraisal process. To avoid complaints, manage patient expectation and ensure good communication.

> **PRACTICE POINT**
>
> Most complaints occur as a result of:
> - poor communication
> - raised and unfulfilled expectations
> - different perceptions.

36

Chapter Thirty Six

The post-mortem consent process: ethical and legal issues

Stephen J. Gould • Mary Y. Anthony

SUMMARY

The past few years have seen considerable focus on post-mortem practice. This largely follows two inquiry reports from the Bristol Royal Infirmary and Royal Liverpool Children's Hospital and the associated public reaction. In response, there have been numerous further publications, culminating in the Human Tissues Act (2004) and the establishment of the Human Tissues Authority, which has produced a number of Codes of Practice. It might be supposed that these changes will affect only pathologists, but it is the process of consent that is at the centre of many of these recommendations. Paediatricians now need far more knowledge of the issues around the post-mortem examination than formerly, although the limits of discussions, that may be needed before post-mortem consent might be considered appropriate, remain flexible. This chapter reviews aspects of usual post-mortem practice and some of the issues raised by the various recent reports. Emphasis is placed on the concerns of parents revealed in recent years.

PRACTICE POINTS

- To give appropriate consent for post-mortem examination, parents will need more information than in the past and more time to consider the issues.
- Paediatricians taking consent for post-mortem will need to ensure that they are familiar with all aspects of the post-mortem.
- Information provided to parents will include a knowledge of what tissue samples may be taken, why they are taken and what may happen to them afterwards.
- Clinicians and parents need to be aware of what long-term information may be lost without a full post-mortem examination.

INTRODUCTION

The last few years have seen major convulsions throughout pathology practice from the 'disclosure' that tissue and organ retention was a routine part of a post-mortem examination. This has been felt particularly in paediatric practice, where the emotional impact on many parents has been understandably considerable. Some parents have been outraged, while others have indicated that they can accept that some part of their baby or child may have been used for research. A significant proportion have indicated that they would willingly have granted consent for organs to have been kept for research had they been asked.

Tissue and organ retention has always been a standard part and, indeed, an essential part of a thorough post-mortem, where it is important not only to examine the obvious but to search for and document or exclude the rare and unexpected. Pathologists have been bewildered[1] at events, disappointed at episodes of misrepresentation and concerned at the obvious distress caused to parents.

Since the issue was first aired in 2001 at the public enquiry into cardiac services at the Bristol Royal Infirmary, there have been various reports from England and Scotland.[2–4] Guidance has been issued by the Royal College of Pathologists,[5] and interim guidance by the British Medical Association.[6] The Department of Health

document *Families and Post Mortems: A Code of Practice relating to Families and Post Mortems*[7] was particularly critical in pointing the way forward in this field. This has now been superceded by a series of Codes of Practice issued by the Human Tissues Authority (HTA) and approved by Parliament in July 2006. Finally, the HTA was established in 2005 as a result of the Human Tissues Act, which received Royal Assent in November 2004.

The UK approach to post-mortem examinations has not been, in any way, out of step with that in other countries,[8] and similar inquiry has occurred in Australia and Ireland. However, similar post-mortem protocols and levels of consent on mainland Europe appear to have caused little reaction.

While much of the opprobrium has been directed towards pathologists, the source of such misunderstanding neither sits within this specialty in isolation nor, certainly, any solution to future practice. Indeed, in the recent report about organ retention in Scotland, it was recorded that:

> The evidence received by the Review Group suggests that there is more cause for concern about the quality of information provided about the possible removal, retention and use of tissues or organs than there is about the post-mortem examination itself.[4]

The ethical dilemma rests with what is the appropriate level of information that should be provided to parents to obtain valid consent. Furthermore, what can be gained from a complete post-mortem examination with organ retention versus what may be lost without it? This falls to the paediatrician.

The Human Tissues Act (2004) and the Human Tissues Authority Code of Practice on Consent[9] now forms the statutory background for the consent process, and so will be considered briefly. This chapter considers those issues that might need discussion with parents, such that their consent, if given for post-mortem, might be considered valid. This chapter cannot be prescriptive, and it will fall to each paediatrician to decide individually the nature and extent of the information that they bring into discussion in the light of recent experience. Some of the more philosophical aspects of tissue retention are not considered here.[10]

WHY ASK FOR A POST-MORTEM EXAMINATION?

Autopsy rates have fallen, even the traditionally high rates of neonatal autopsy. Rates above 70% were common in the early 1980s when the post-mortem examination more clearly fulfilled multiple functions. It provided diagnostic information, audit data, facilitated education and contributed to clinical research projects, such as the use and accuracy of cerebral ultrasound. The most recent figures from the Confidential Enquiry into Maternal and Child Health (CEMACH)[11] show a relatively constant neonatal autopsy rate of 30% in the 3 years 2000–2002. While there will be differences due to background population, autopsy rates are probably far more determined by the nature of the interest of the clinician and, in some areas, the availability of specialist perinatal services. A similar picture is present in the USA.[12]

Post-mortem examinations provide information on normal and abnormal tissues and structures. They can provide diagnoses and the cause of death, contribute to audit and research, and provide a resource for teaching. Very rarely will the post-mortem findings change the fundamental diagnosis if the definitive, 'gold-standard' test has been conducted before death (e.g. demonstration of chromosomal abnormality). The most recent study in the UK showed that new information was obtained in 25% of neonatal autopsies (autopsy rate approximately 60%).[13] Two studies of neonatal autopsies in Australia and the USA showed remarkably similar results. In both, the autopsy rate was just below 50%, and major discordancies were found in some 10–12% of those cases autopsied.[14,15] Lesser discordance was found in 17–32% of cases.

'Target' autopsy rates[16] are probably no longer appropriate. However, one potential barrier to autopsy request arises if there is a perception that the only post-mortem of value is one that reveals new or unexpected information. It is curious that confirmation of clinical diagnosis should now generally be regarded as a negative rather than a positive outcome of a post-mortem.

THE POST-MORTEM EXAMINATION

The various components of the post-mortem need to be fully understood by whoever is involved with the consent process so that an informed discussion can take place.

Photography and radiography

Photographs are commonly made of abnormal facies of dysmorphic infants, structural abnormality, or other unusual, acquired pathology. These form part of the medical record of the post-mortem. Inevitably, anonymized photographs can be valuable as a teaching aid. Especially where dysmorphism is concerned, the photographs would constitute a permanent part of the family medical record. Radiographs complement and help to direct the post-mortem examination by demonstrating some pathology better than the physical examination. Both forms of image may contribute to diagnoses becoming possible within the family some years later.

During the recent controversy, there has been considerable disquiet amongst parents regarding images, and many have required their return. In addition, there is debate over the ownership of such records. The General Medical Council[17] has produced guidelines on the use of images and recordings in medicine, including the autopsy. No separate permission is required to take photographs of microscope slides or internal organs. Permission is required if images and recordings may be identifiable or are for use in publicly accessible media such as medical journals.

External and internal examination

Past practice has usually been not to detail this part of the post-mortem examination when taking consent. Initial incisions will usually be a full-length central incision from neck to pubis, or it may be more T-shaped to allow better access to the neck. An incision from behind the ears over the back of the head (approximately at the level of or just anterior to the posterior fontanelle) permits examination of the brain. At the end of the post-mortem the incisions are sutured, and they should be invisible when the baby is appropriately dressed. During the post-mortem examination, all organs will be removed from the body cavities before more detailed dissection and weighing. Organ weights and their comparison with normal tables of weights for age or weight are a valuable, relatively objective, if sometimes non-specific, indication of pathology. In the immature baby, organ weights can assist in the assessment of gestational age, and in the very early neonatal death relative organ weights can give an indication of intrauterine chronic stress or other disease processes.

Histology

Microscopic examination of tissues is critical. Indeed, with the possible exception of some structural abnormalities, in the absence of tissue histology, diagnosis is only achievable with microscopic examination. Histology sampling is wide and will involve tissues not obviously from the site of pathology. While this might seem obvious to doctors, for parents the concept that tissues other than the main site of pathology may contribute to the understanding of the death requires explanation. Furthermore, histology provides a means of confirming and permanently documenting the post-mortem examination findings.

Most initial tissue samples that are taken are fairly small, the maximum size being some 20 mm × 15 mm × 5 mm, although these pieces of tissue may be 'trimmed' further to provide smaller blocks for histology. Many pathologists now place thinner samples straight into the cassettes for processing. Even from the larger organs these samples may be little more than 10 mm × 10 mm × 3 mm in size, although this may represent a significant proportion of the organs of very small babies. The sections cut from these tissue 'blocks' for slides are generally in the region of 4 μm (i.e. 4/1000 of a millimetre) thick. Traditionally, tissue blocks and slides and wide sampling have constituted a substantial archive of material. Review may occur because questions not apparent at the time of post-mortem arise in subsequent weeks, or new techniques are developed many years later that may need the use of further tissue sections.

Despite the small size of these tissue samples, their significance should not be underestimated. For many parents, they have proved to carry considerable emotional status, and return of blocks and slides with subsequent interment or cremation has been commonplace.

Organ retention

This has been the most contentious aspect of past practice. Retention generally occurs because the tissue is not in an ideal state for examination at the time of autopsy, and information may be lost if examination is conducted too early. It also allows a second expert, specialist opinion to be obtained. The brain, which is soft, especially when immature or when affected by pathology such as ischaemia or haemorrhage, is the most likely organ to be retained. Fixation in formalin is required to make the tissue more firm before neuropathological examination. Traditionally, fixation has required weeks before examination, but sometimes it can occur much quicker, even within a few days, depending on factors such as brain size. Discussion with the pathologist and knowing local practice and options is critical here.

The heart might also need to be retained, usually in the context of congenital heart disease, especially after surgery. The fixed heart can be easier to examine (often within a day or two) and it also provides an opportunity for detailed examination by an expert pathologist or discussion with paediatric cardiologists and surgeons. Again, discussion with the pathologist about an individual case is vital. Valuable teaching collections have been generated in some centres from hearts with complex congenital malformation, especially if surgically corrected.

Limited or full autopsy

The full autopsy involves investigation of all body cavities. While omission of a body-cavity investigation will seem reasonable if no pathology is expected, it inevitably removes the possibility of identifying an unexpected finding and information will be less complete. Care needs to be taken to ensure that clinical and parental expectations are appropriate to any limited procedure.

ORGANS AND TISSUES AFTER THE AUTOPSY

Almost universally, pathology departments have archived diagnostic blocks and slides. In common with surgical tissue used for diagnosis, this material has always been regarded as part of the medical record, and it was understood that there was an obligation to keep the tissue for possible review. Besides diagnostic review, these archives have also provided a teaching and research resource, and their value should not be underestimated.

The long-term retention of organs has always been a more variable occurrence. In many centres, the routine involved disposal following the diagnostic examination. Other organs were kept in archive for research and teaching, or for display in medical school museums, although the latter has decreased significantly in recent years.

Since the existence of organ collections has become widely known, some parents have demanded the return of organs and new

guidelines for 'disposal' have been developed. More surprising to many has been the demand for return of blocks and slides, despite the relatively miniscule amounts of tissue involved. The demand for return has tended to be higher when organs have also been retained, possibly due to the greater symbolic significance that these small pieces of tissue then acquired.

If consent for retention of organs or tissue in block and slides is not granted, then tissue has to be either reunited with the body before the funeral (which will introduce a delay) or will need to be disposed of 'lawfully and respectfully'. There are likely to be local solutions for disposal, to account for relatively permanent materials such as glass and the health and safety issues raised by tissues that have been fixed in formalin. The appropriate mechanisms of tissue disposal are still evolving, and further guidance from the HTA is awaited (see below).

THE HUMAN TISSUES ACT (2004)[18, 19]

Rosie Winterton, Minister of Health, when introducing the second reading of the parliamentary bill stated that the origins of this legislation arose from the '... distress ... felt by families when they discovered that the organs of their deceased loved ones had been retained without consent'. The 2004 Act replaces a number of previous Acts that were inadequate. It covers not only human tissue storage and use (including genetic studies) resulting from autopsies, but also surgical specimens and organs for transplantation, and other areas not relevant to this article. It received Royal Assent in November 2004 and came into force in 2006.

The Act now provides the statutory framework for much of the hospital autopsy consent process. It covers the storage of any human material and the requirements for *appropriate consent* that will allow material to be stored legally. It is worth noting that the only aspect of 'appropriate consent' the Act specifies is *who* may give consent. In the paediatric field this will include:

- A 'Gillick-competent' minor (further guidance on this is likely to be forthcoming, e.g. on proving a minor is Gillick competent).
- The person with parental responsibility:
  - mother
  - father, married to the mother at the time of birth
  - others who have acquired parental responsibility.

The Act itself is all but incomprehensible to the casual reader – a point of concern, given that one of its intentions was to clarify the law. Furthermore, it provides the framework but not the practical detail necessary for its implementation. For this, the Act provides for the formation of the HTA to oversee the introduction and implementation of the Act: its members were appointed in April 2005. The major advantage of this approach is that, rather than the need to change primary legislation in the future, the HTA's guidance is more easily modified as medicine advances or new challenges arise. The HTA's functions in relation to the autopsy will be to:

- Maintain a statement of general principles relating to the removal, retention and use of human bodies and their parts.
- Provide general oversight and guidance.
- Monitor activities covered by the Act.
- Develop Codes of Practice. The most relevant Codes of Practice to this chapter published in July 2006 are No. 1 on Consent and No. 3 on Post-mortem Examination. These Codes outline, amongst other aspects, the required communication with the

family in relation to the conduct of the post mortem examination and the use of tissue for scheduled purposes (e.g. research or teaching).

A critical component of the change in the law is that storage of human material (and this could amount to just a few cells) from a deceased person without the appropriate consent may constitute a criminal offence. If, at any time, the validity of the consent for autopsy is questioned by the family, the burden of proof will lie with the professional; the consent form may be evidence, but does not in itself constitute proof that the consent obtained was 'appropriate'. A record in the notes of the discussion about consent may be wise.

THE CONSENT PROCESS

The Bristol Royal Infirmary Inquiry Interim Report[2] (Paragraph 50) suggests that consent should be seen as a process, a view supported by the interim British Medical Association guidelines.[6] The phrase implies more than just a brief form-filling exercise, but one that allows time to reflect after the appropriate information had been given. In the past, the information given to parents when consent was sought for post-mortem was limited. This has since been labelled an inappropriate 'paternalistic' approach. The Royal Liverpool Children's Hospital Inquiry (RLCH),[3] quoting the *Concise Oxford Dictionary*, defined paternalism as 'the policy of restricting the freedom and responsibilities of one's dependants in their supposed best interest'.

Beyond the generally agreed principle that parents should have more information about the post-mortem process, the early reports were inconsistent on how much information this should be. The RLCH inquiry suggests (Chap. 11[3]) that, for consent to be valid, information given to parents should be 'comprehensive'. For instance, discussions should include descriptions of organ removal and other facets of the post-mortem procedure 'no matter how distasteful the giving of this information might be to the clinician concerned ... [nevertheless] ... their responsibility cannot be avoided.' A test for fully informed consent would be whether the omission of a significant detail might have led to a different decision by parents.

However, the Royal College of Pathologists post-mortem guidelines and information leaflet of May 2000[5] were subject to comment by the Bristol Royal Infirmary Interim Report when it stated that:

The information in the proposed 'Information Leaflet' is helpful not least because it is detailed and specific. But, by being so, we recognize that it will be painful to some parents, already reeling from the loss of their child, while other parents will find it of assistance. We cannot square this particular circle. There is a price to be paid for being informed.

The HTA Code of Practice 3 – Post Mortem[9] acknowledges that there will be variation in the level of information required, and Paragraph 73 states:

When discussing the post-mortem, some people will want to know in considerable detail about what will be done to the body. In such cases the procedure should be sensitively, but honestly and fully, explained. Others will not want so much or even any detail. This should be respected.

That this view was justified was supported in the judgement on the Nationwide Organ Group Litigation. Lord Justice Gage in his judgement, March 2004, stated:

I accept that there may be some circumstances in which a clinician might have been justified in giving no details to parents of a post-mortem examination. I also accept that in all cases the question of how much information should have been given to parents will be a matter of judgement for the clinician [20]

Whatever the detail given or offered, it is clear that those taking consent will need a much greater knowledge of both the post-mortem process and the options available to parents after the post-mortem has been completed. In particular, paediatricians should have some knowledge of:

- the incisions that are normally made and what happens after the autopsy
- the general process of the autopsy (i.e. organ removal and dissection)
- the extent of histology sampling and what is meant by blocks and slides
- how the pathology department disposes of residual tissue (if there is any)
- what specimens might be needed for other, non-histological investigation
- what organs might need to be retained in any particular case and for how long
- the alternatives to the post-mortem examination and their limitations
- when results might be available.

It is not that all parents will want to discuss this information in detail. However, the clinician should have explored the issues sufficiently that parents are not under any illusion about what the autopsy will entail. The autopsy does not involve a keyhole incision with a 'peek inside', a not uncommon past perception of some parents. While the paediatrician should be able to discuss this reasonably knowledgeably with parents, it is entirely appropriate that the pathologist is involved before post-mortem examination is broached with parents so that any discussion will be more informed. If feasible, many paediatric pathologists are more than willing to take part in such discussions, although patterns of referral may preclude this for many centres.

The obvious essential features of the changes are about being prepared to give very explicit details about post-mortems and ensuring free and open dialogue between all involved parties: family, physician and pathologist. Clear and full documentation of all discussions is advisable, as is maintaining easy channels of communications between all parties during the consent process and post-mortem so that any queries or unforeseen difficulties may be addressed. An exchange of contact telephone numbers can avoid much confusion and misunderstanding, yet even in the best regulated and intended of practices it is recognized how difficult this process can be.

Of course, to avoid these dilemmas and a difficult discussion, one solution is not to ask for a post-mortem. This approach is also not without the potential for paternalism, as it effectively removes parental choice. Even if the major diagnosis is relatively certain, perhaps some parents would like the opportunity to contribute to research or education. Consent for long-term organ donation (the preferred term to organ retention) has been substantially reduced.

However, it is clear from some studies[21] that a high proportion of parents are willing to donate and allow brain retention, for instance, if appropriate information is given.

An important aspect of informed consent is knowing and understanding what the consequences are if a procedure (surgical treatment or post-mortem) is not carried out. For a post-mortem, this could include unknown valuable information, or possible storage of tissues that might yet help at a later date.

The recent debate is a marker of a new era. A few years ago, the role of the post-mortem and the pathologist was relatively straightforward. 'Good pathology' required the post-mortem to be conducted in such a way as to document, in detail, the presence or absence of pathology. This allowed the cause of death to be identified (usually), provided information about the effects of treatments, and allowed for documenting and learning about sometimes rare, unexpected occurrences or associations. New observations inevitably provided material for research. It also meant that further evaluation, possible as part of a research project, could occur on retrospective case review, often many years later.

Recent events have challenged that underlying philosophy, and virtually every aspect of the post-mortem process has been questioned. For pathologists this has required detailed explanations about past pathology practice in the context of previous consent procedures, and even the vagaries of the coroner's system, sometimes over 40 years. Alternatives to a full autopsy, such as magnetic resonance imaging, are being promoted, although full evaluation has yet to occur. There is increasing pressure, by limiting the scope of post-mortem examination, to search only for the obvious and not to seek or exclude the less likely possibilities. However, it is in the unexpected finding that the real value of the post-mortem often lies.

THE CORONER'S POST-MORTEM

Paediatricians will inevitably be involved at some stage in deaths that come under the jurisdiction of the coroner. Notifying the coroner is usually clear in sudden unexpected deaths or deaths during surgery. Sometimes, a requirement for the coroner's involvement is less obvious, but the clinician should be cautious if there are any doubts regarding death certification. Any doubts should be discussed with the coroner. One position to avoid absolutely is referring a case to the coroner because the death certificate cannot be completed after the parents have refused consent for a hospital consent post-mortem examination. It may appear as if a post-mortem is being obtained by whatever means is available, and against the parents' wishes. Caution might also be exercised if there has been a medical error prior to death, even if it is considered by the clinician to be irrelevant to the death.

For many parents (and indeed for many medical staff as well), the coroner's system is confusing. Especially in community-based deaths, it is very easy for explanations to be inadequate if, for instance, they are left to the coroner's officers. One of the surprising outcomes of organ retention enquiries was the number of parents who were not aware of the coroner's involvement, that a post-mortem had been conducted on their child, or did not know the results of the autopsy. This is clearly unacceptable, and both clinicians and pathologists should have a role in ensuring that appropriate levels of communication and feedback are in place.

Parents do not have a choice about whether or not a coroner's post-mortem is conducted, but there are aspects of the process where their consent may be needed. The first concerns any investigation performed on a baby after death (e.g. suprapubic aspiration for metabolic investigation of urine) and whose death is likely to be reported to the coroner. In this circumstance, the body comes under the jurisdiction of the coroner immediately after death. The coroner's view on such tests should be obtained, and it may be prudent to obtain written parental consent before proceeding. *Any* tissue samples taken after death can only be taken on appropriately licensed premises, a process directed by the HTA. Hospital mortuaries will be licensed, but clinicians should be aware that other hospital locations where this sampling might occur (e.g. accident and emergency departments) also need to be covered.

The second situation arises after the coroner's post-mortem examination. Changes to the coroner's rules (from 1 June 2005) mean that tissue blocks and slides cannot be kept on the coroner's authority after the coroner's 'function' has been fulfilled. This will usually be at the point at which the cause of death has been given or at the end of an inquest. Retention of blocks and slides and any other tissues therefore requires the consent of the parents. Most pathologists would regard this as important, especially if there are further deaths in the family. The statutory duty to determine the parents' wishes is the coroner's (and will, therefore, usually fall to the coroner's officer). However, the clinician may wish to be involved in this process, or be in a position to explain the reasons why retention of tissue blocks and slides may be helpful to the family in the long-term.

CONCLUSION

Recent changes in the consent process for autopsy have involved more information being passed on to parents and further detail offered. Information does not have to be comprehensive for consent to be appropriate but, equally, parents should not be misled about the post-mortem examination by withholding unpalatable detail. It will mean the consent process will require more time, more knowledge of the post-mortem examination and of the options available, and an understanding by clinicians and parents of what might be lost without a full post-mortem.

Chapter Thirty Seven

Informed consent for neonatal research

A. Bryan Gill

SUMMARY

Research is the cornerstone of progress in medicine. Neonatal research, both basic science and the randomized controlled trials (RCTs), have demonstrated the positive and negative aspects of new treatments. The RCT is recognized as the gold standard for determining the effectiveness of new treatments. Informed consent is central to any research taking place, but in neonatal research this presents a number of problems.

By the nature of the subjects, the consent is 'proxy consent'. In addition, the timing of the consent is often shortly after birth and/or at times of severe emotional distress. Recent research has shown that the quality of the informed consent falls below the requirements expected of it. This appears greatest for research where consent is required urgently and/or the study is considered to have significant risks. While research ethics committees place great store on the value of the parent information leaflet, in their decision-making parents appear to rely more on their communication with the doctor who is obtaining the informed consent.

Improvements to the obtaining and the validity of informed consent for neonatal research are possible through improved understanding of the role of all those involved. The meeting with parent(s) to obtain informed consent should be viewed as the first stage of continual involvement of the parents and their baby(s) in a research project.

PRACTICE POINTS

- Fully valid informed consent requires that the person(s) giving consent:
  — is competent to do so
  — receives all the necessary information
  — understands the information
  — acts voluntarily.
- Neonatal research projects may present problems in obtaining fully valid informed consent.
- Appropriate communication with parent(s) is the key to improving the validity of informed consent.

Areas for research

- Examine the validity and acceptability of staged consent for urgent and/or high-risk neonatal research.
- How do we educate the public on the importance of neonatal research?
- Having implemented an improved process for obtaining informed consent, has this worked?

INTRODUCTION

Since the 1940s consent has been seen as central to any medical research on human subjects. This is reflected in the Declaration of Helsinki, which states:

> ... each potential subject must be adequately informed of the aims, methods, anticipated benefits and potential hazards of the study and the discomfort it may entail ... where the subject is a minor, permission from a responsible relative replaces that of the subject in accordance with national legislation. (Declaration of Helsinki, revised 1975, 1983, 1989 and 1996)

Progress in medicine, and in particular in neonatal care, requires clinicians to deliver the best available care. It is hoped that the 'best available' care is evidenced based and that the evidence has been acquired from randomized controlled trials (RCTs). The RCT is commonly stated as the gold standard for research, and there are many examples of neonatal RCTs that have changed neonatal practice.[1–3]

Fully valid informed consent from the parent(s) or guardian(s) is legally necessary in the UK, and some commentators view it as ethically justified for the majority of RCTs in neonatal care.[4, 5] Informed consent for neonatal research, however, presents a number of difficulties to the researcher obtaining consent before the informed consent can be considered 'fully valid'.

The problems associated with obtaining informed consent in neonatal research, including the views of parents, have only recently become clearer.[6] In addition, publicity around the randomized trial of continuous negative extrathoracic pressure (CNEP) ventilation[7] in a Department of Health report[8] called into question issues around the validity of the consent process. Although the researchers were exonerated and commentators have questioned the report's findings[9] the issue of consent within this trial was a major factor in the parents' concerns regarding the trial. Many of these issues appeared to relate to problems with communication by doctors obtaining consent, and the possible failure to recognize the difficulties with making the consent fully informed.

In the light of these problems, this chapter discusses in detail why informed consent may be problematic in neonatal research, and the present role of research ethics committees (RECs). It outlines the reasons why the validity of informed consent for neonatal research has been questioned, and guides the reader on ways that may improve the validity of the consent process for those involved in neonatal research.

WHAT IS INFORMED CONSENT?

Fully valid informed consent for research (and treatment) is not simply a signature on a consent form. Consent has four components: competence, information, understanding and voluntariness. For consent to be considered 'informed', the following requirements are necessary against these component criteria of consent:[10, 11]

- *Competence*: person(s) giving consent must be deemed mentally competent to do so. In the case of neonatal research, the researcher has responsibility for determining whether or not the person(s) are in a fit state of mind to give consent.
- *Information*: sufficient information must be given for the person(s) to make an informed choice. It is through communication and the information leaflet that the level of information provided is determined. The information leaflet, prepared by the researcher, is assessed by the REC, although there are few guidelines as to a minimum standard of content.
- *Understanding*: the person(s) giving consent must be considered capable of making a reasoned choice. The researcher obtaining consent must judge the level of understanding of the parent(s).
- *Voluntariness*: the person giving the consent must do so voluntarily and must recognize that withdrawal from the study is possible at any time without this affecting (in this case the baby) care.

In practice, as the majority of clinicians who have taken informed consent for research know, the level to which perfection is achieved against these criteria will vary from study to study and from researcher to researcher. Recent research has provided an insight into the validity of informed consent for neonatal RCTs.[6]

PROBLEMS WITH CONSENT FOR NEONATAL RESEARCH

By default, it is not possible to obtain consent from the subjects directly involved in the RCT. Therefore, consent is necessary from a 'proxy', which is normally a parent(s). Ethicists argue that this can never be 'fully valid' informed consent, as the person giving consent must do so from the subject's point of view rather than their own. As the neonate does not have values, it could be argued that the parents are not able to infer what these would be. This is relevant when considering the validity of consent against the criteria above, as the degree of perfection of the consent will always be less than absolute.

Recruitment into neonatal RCTs can be before or shortly after birth (ventilation trials). The condition of the infant may be life-threatening[3] and/or the mother may have had an emergency caesarean section. Some treatments (e.g. hypothermia for intrapartum asphyxia) are considered to be elective only if started within a few hours after the insult, while others could be considered high risk (e.g. extracorporeal membrane oxygenation (ECMO)). By using

the ECMO trial[3] as an example of a neonatal RCT likely to present problems with valid informed consent, and discussing each of the components of consent in turn, the problems with trying to obtain fully informed consent can be immediately seen.

- Competence – by virtue of the baby's condition, the parents were approached within a short time after birth after discovering that their baby had developed a potentially fatal condition.
- Information and understanding – the parents had to receive a full explanation of this new treatment on top of an explanation about their baby's life-threatening condition. They would have had to understand that ECMO is a complex treatment requiring the movement of their baby to another centre, assuming their baby was randomized to receive ECMO. Parents needed to understand that they were consenting to a randomization process rather than ECMO per se.
- Voluntariness – parents invariably faced very little time in which to decide. They were also informed that ECMO was not available outside of the trial. By the nature of the trial it was not possible to withdraw from the actual treatment once it had been started, although it was possible to withdraw from follow-up.

These problems encapsulate the difficulties with consent in the 'real world' of clinical medicine. However, the trial clearly demonstrated a benefit of ECMO, for certain conditions, over conventional treatment, and ECMO an important component of the armamentarium used for term infants with respiratory failure. It is interesting to note that in Ireland statute decrees that there must be a period of 6 days from obtaining consent before entry into a trial.[12] This statute has prevented any meaningful participation in early intervention trials in newborn infants in that country.

It is important, in order for informed consent to be obtained, that the researcher, or anyone who is taking consent, understands the impact of their particular study on the potential problems with the validity of the informed consent process.

THE ROLE OF RESEARCH ETHICS COMMITTEES IN THE CONSENT PROCESS

As clinicians are aware, all protocols for any research on human subjects within the NHS in the UK (and the majority of Europe) must be submitted to an appropriate local or regional REC. Significant attention is given to the acceptability of the parent information sheet, although regulation as to its content is generally left to individual RECs.[13] Interestingly, the law in France[13] stipulates that every information sheet for research must include the following information as a minimum:

- the research aim
- that the trial involves randomization
- whether a placebo is being used
- the expected benefits
- the foreseeable risks
- any likely discomforts to the baby
- any measures to reduce discomfort
- the freedom to withdraw from the trial
- the REC's opinion of the trial.

In the UK the opinion of RECs is not included on the parent information leaflet as there is concern that this represents a degree of coercion to take part. This French template for the information sheet has significant merit for all researchers embarking on designing a parent information leaflet.

When obtaining consent it is considered mandatory for a parent(s) to sign a consent form. Occasionally, oral consent can be used, although this must always be followed by written consent within a short time window. The majority of European Union (EU) countries permit consent from one parent, although notably France, Germany and Greece require consent from both parents (except in exceptional circumstances) before entry into a trial. This has implications for multicentre European neonatal research.[12]

RECs stipulate that the lead researcher or responsible clinician should obtain consent. It seems surprising in the present clinical governance environment that there is very little checking on the taking of consent for research (not just neonatal), although a recent Department of Health directive outlined the first steps of an audit trail.[14]

VALIDITY OF INFORMED CONSENT IN NEONATAL RESEARCH

The research by the Euricon Study Group[6] was one of the first studies to examine the validity of consent obtained for neonatal RCTs throughout nine EU countries. The main focus of the project involved face-to-face semi-structured interviews with parents of 200 infants, who were approached for entry into many different neonatal RCTs. Interviews were taken within 1 year of the approach for consent. In addition, 107 neonatologists were interviewed regarding their understanding and their approach to obtaining consent.

The major important clinical findings were:

- Less than 30% of the informed consent obtained from parents for neonatal RCTs could be considered fully valid against the criteria for informed consent.
- The greater the perceived risk of the research and the shorter the time window for obtaining informed consent, the less valid the informed consent, although even those studies in which there was a significant time in which to decide there were still problems with the validity of the consent obtained.
- The majority of parents valued the requirement that it was necessary for them to give informed consent, although many considered it a burden.
- Parents considered it their right to be asked for consent. They believed that it was one of the ways in which they could take part in their baby's care.
- The majority of parents relied on the level of communication from the person obtaining consent, backed up by an information leaflet in some cases, when arriving at a decision. This contrasts with many clinicians' views that the information leaflet was at least as important as communication. For those who have been involved in running an RCT, it is in stark contrast with the attention RECs devote to the parent information leaflet.
- The majority of clinicians received no training in the legal and ethical requirements for informed consent or in the communication skills necessary.
- On many occasions when consent was declined, it was commonly the approach of the researcher that put the parents off giving consent. Many parents referred to the 'trust' between clinician and parent(s) as a factor in their decision-making.

This study appears to have highlighted for the first time the key areas in which problems exist. Improved awareness of these problems provides an insight into finding appropriate solutions and improving the validity of consent for neonatal research.

HOW CAN THE VALIDITY OF CONSENT BE IMPROVED?

I make the assumption that neonatal research in the form of RCTs will continue to require informed consent, although some authors have suggested that it should not always be necessary.[15]

The findings of the Euricon study have raised the question as to how the validity of the consent can be improved. The Royal College of Paediatrics and Child Health have suggested that the term 'sufficiently informed', as opposed to 'fully informed' would be more applicable to many RCTs in neonatal care. The Euricon Study Group (over 40 neonatologists, ethicists and lawyers from nine EU countries), of which the author is a member, recently produced a consensus statement based on the Euricon research and colloquia discussions. The following list, taken from some of these discussions and my own personal views provides a practical insight into how the whole consent process for neonatal research may be improved:

- At the present time it should be standard practice for researchers to obtain informed consent from parents prior to research being conducted. In general, the consent must be written.
- A record must be kept of all signed consent forms. Copies should be stored in the case notes and given to the parent(s).
- All researchers should examine their study to identify potential areas where consent would be problematic against the criteria of fully valid consent. Where possible, an attempt to overcome these problems should be sought.
- RECs should be made aware of any anticipated problems with fully valid consent for a particular project.
- All those involved in research must recognize that for some RCTs the informed consent may not be fully valid, but simply represent 'best possible' (or sufficiently informed) consent.
- The ability to communicate appropriately with parents, preferably separately from providing information on the infant's condition, is a key component to obtaining best-possible informed consent. It would be hoped that by improved communication the recruitment rates for neonatal trials would be improved.
- If identification of subjects likely to be eligible for an RCT is possible antenatally, information and discussion on the trial should take place before delivery. The signing of the consent form will, in the majority of studies, be necessary after birth. This approach simply provides the prospective parent(s) with more time to evaluate the trial.
- Particularly for urgent and/or high-risk research where valid consent is often problematic, repeated approaches should be made to parents to discuss the study (staged approach). This could take place over a number of days or weeks after entry. Re-providing the option to withdraw from further aspects of the study should be clearly stated.
- Obtaining consent from parents must not be seen as safeguarding the well-being of their baby. All trials must be subjected to critical appraisal and approval by all the appropriate research bodies and/or RECs before proceeding.

- Regular audits of the validity of the consent process should form part of all research and development programmes in units undertaking neonatal research.

It is hoped that neonatal research will continue to the present generally high standards. We must not allow the problems around informed consent to prevent appropriate neonatal trials being performed. Failure to do so is likely to see major sequelae to newborn infants from new treatments that would have been avoided had these been subjected to formal RCTs. The example of acetazolamide and furosemide for the management of posthaemorrhagic ventricular dilatation is a pertinent example of a treatment that was used for many years before being subjected to an RCT. This trial demonstrated a negative effect on neurological outcome in the treated group.[16] The present worldwide debate regarding postnatal dexamethasone and adverse neurological outcome will continue until an appropriate RCT has been performed.[17]

CONCLUSIONS

Properly conducted research is vital for the progression of medicine, and it could be argued that it is even more so for progression of neonatal care, given the longevity of the effects of some treatments on future quality of life. Fully valid informed consent for all RCTs is probably an unrealistic goal, but the validity of consent can be improved with understanding and changes to the approach of RECs and researchers towards parents.

The following quote obtained from one of the parent interviews for the Euricon project highlights the majority view of parents regarding consent for neonatal research.:

I am sure there are times when you would want to say 'You decide' but you can't. They're your children, your responsibility right from the moment they're born. You should be involved in the decision but you should have a lot of help making it. The more information you have the easier it will be for you to make that decision.

It is hoped that, through greater awareness of the issues around informed consent in neonatal research, clinical trials will be undertaken with improved validity of the consent than would presently appear to be the case. Improvements in the validity of consent will, hopefully, increase public confidence in neonatal research.

Chapter Thirty Eight

Consent for the examination or treatment of teenagers

Bryan Vernon • Jan Welbury

SUMMARY

Examination and treatment of any patient requires their consent. This may be verbal or written and involves giving adequate information and ensuring that this is understood. The patient must consent freely, may withdraw consent at any time and should be competent. At 16 years of age young people are competent to consent, but their refusal of treatment may be overridden by their parents, those with parental responsibility or the courts until they are 18 years old. Below age 16 years, young people may be competent, and this is a judgement for the clinician to make using recognized criteria. Any treatment should be in the best interests of a young person. Teenagers value honesty and appreciate involvement in decisions about their care. There is a balance between empowering young people to make adult decisions and protecting them. It is good practice to offer to see young people and their parents separately. There is scope for honest disagreement in applying these principles.

INTRODUCTION

The care of teenagers can challenge clinicians, who may feel that they face at least two sets of interests that are not always in harmony. This challenge is most acute in consent to an examination or treatment. The aim of this chapter is to clarify who can give or withhold consent, and how far it is possible or appropriate to impose decisions, and the implications for unwilling parties. Professionals need to be familiar with the legal position, the moral debate and perceived good practice to support them in their quest to serve the best interests of young people.

IS CONSENT FOR TEENAGERS DIFFERENT?

The answer to this question is 'Yes' and 'No'.

'No' in that the underlying principles should be the same whatever the age of the patient.

'Yes' as to whose consent is required. With a competent, conscious adult, a small child or indeed an unconscious patient needing emergency treatment the decision is straightforward. However, clinicians are less confident about gaining consent from a young person with a reasonable understanding of the issues when they disagree with their parents' decision or are adamant that they do not wish their parents to know. Uncertainty increases where the decision involves sexual health or potential mental health issues, particularly in suspected child abuse.

The Department of Health guidance *Seeking Consent: Working with Children* helpfully sets out a list of those who have parental responsibility under the Children Act, 1989,[1] pointing out that a mother who is under 16 years old may give consent for treatment of her child if she is herself Gillick competent. Those with parental responsibility can arrange for others to exercise that responsibility, for instance a childminder or teacher on a school trip. Those who do not have parental responsibility but who have care of a child are allowed to 'do what is reasonable in all the circumstances of the case for the purpose of safeguarding or promoting the child's welfare'.[2] Throughout this chapter we use the term 'parents' to mean anyone with parental responsibility.

WHAT DOES CONSENT MEAN?

Seeking consent for consultation, examination and treatment shows respect for the autonomy of an individual, and rests on a claim to the right of non-interference and the right to participate in decision-making. This is stronger than a claim to the right to select a particular treatment, which is a positive rather than a negative right. Clinicians cannot be compelled to provide treatment they regard as inappropriate. Such treatment may be worse than no treatment, futile, as it is ineffective, or not cost-effective. Sometimes agreement to such treatment may be appropriate, say where it can cause no harm and where it has assumed a high level of importance to the patient.

Informal or implied consent

Informal or implied consent is part of everyday working practice. It arose from the assumptions that patients and clinicians make that doctors can ask for and receive information and perform examinations – no matter how intimate – without prior discussion or explanation. A more respectful form of informal consent involves a brief agreement or clarification of the needs of the consultation and an explanation of the process, emphasizing the patient's right to question, seek clarification or refuse any part of the process.

Formal consent

Formal consent for an operation or a procedure requiring anaesthetic or sedation is a concept that is much more familiar to clinicians. A signature is evidence of consent and appropriate explanation, and not the act of consent itself. Written and verbal consent are equally valid.

WHAT ARE OUR LEGAL OBLIGATIONS?

Seeking consent is important because intentionally touching another person without consent is a criminal act, technically called a battery. This has always been part of English law and healthcare professionals who ignore this may have to defend their actions. Practices such as intimate examination under anaesthesia by medical students, without consent, and treatments forced on unwilling, competent patients have never been lawful. That consent was 'implied' in these cases is unlikely to be a successful defence. Such practice is indefensible, with those acting in this way relying on their patient's confidence in their integrity, their ignorance and the general reluctance of patients to complain.

In most cases gaining consent is not a problem. Consent comprises four elements:

- 'Sufficient' information is given to the patient. What is 'sufficient'? The General Medical Council (GMC) in their booklet *Seeking Patients' Consent: The Ethical Considerations*[3] list 12 points under the heading: 'The information which patients want or ought to know, before deciding whether to consent to treatment or an investigation, *may* include ...' (our italics). For clinicians following guidelines for a particular treatment such uncertainty can be unsettling, but it is not possible to provide a list that applies to every case. Those who seek a checklist for what they must disclose may give the impression that they are trying to provide the minimum information possible. More constructively, clinicians could ask themselves why they wish to withhold a piece of information. If the information is relevant to the patient's decision, withholding it needs justification. The GMC would allow withholding information where disclosure would seriously harm the patient, but note that the fact that the patient would become upset or refuse further treatment is not what they mean by serious harm. Where information is withheld, this should be recorded in the notes along with the reason.
- The information is understood. Clinicians do not generally mean to give incomprehensible explanations to patients, although they may unwittingly use phrases unfamiliar to lay people. It can be difficult for patients to admit that they have not understood something. Asking a person whether they have understood invites the answer 'Yes'. No one wants to look stupid. A device clinicians can use is to say, 'I don't always explain these things very well. Can you tell me what you think I have said, just to make sure I have made things clear?' This puts the emphasis on the clinician's skills, rather than the patient's intelligence.
- Consent is given freely, without pressure from the clinician or others, and may be withdrawn at any time. Recommending a treatment option is not necessarily putting pressure on a patient, and may be helpful.[4] On the other hand, what is seen by a clinician as an appropriate, clinically soundly based recommendation may be received as overbearing pressure. Aware-ness of this possibility is essential. The patient should be asked about their understanding of the recommendation and their feelings and/or fears of consenting to that course of action.
- The person giving consent is competent. Doubts about the competence of people under 18 years old have led to decisions being made on their behalf. Competence does not appear suddenly at a particular age. It develops and fluctuates. For this reason it is good practice to involve children in decisions about their treatment and care from an early age, where they may be able to assent to treatment and even decide on details about its timing. This practice of involvement is part of a process of empowerment that enables young people to take more responsibility for their own care as they develop. The desire to empower young people can, on occasions, prove to be in conflict with the desire to protect them. As McCabe points out,[5] there are some decisions that adults with responsibility to care find very difficult. In such cases it would be easy to ask young people to make the decision under the pretext of empowerment whilst actually abdicating responsibility for making a difficult decision.

The British Medical Association (BMA) summarizes the points that need to be considered when assessing competence.[6] Individuals should be able to:

- understand in simple language what the medical treatment is, its purpose, nature and the reason that it is proposed
- understand its principal benefits, risks and alternatives
- understand in broad terms what will be the consequences of not receiving the proposed treatment
- retain the information long enough to make an effective decision
- make a free choice (i.e. free from pressure).

In all cases a decision as to competence is specific to the treatment in question.

WHAT ARE OUR LEGAL OBLIGATIONS TOWARDS TEENAGERS?

The legal position of teenagers in England and Wales regarding consent is not difficult to describe, but its interpretation can lead to value conflicts. *At 16 years of age*, every person is presumed able to give their consent to treatment.[7] However, *before age 18 years*, parents, the courts or others with parental responsibility can override the *refusal* of a minor,[8] even a competent minor. The BMA explains why this apparent inconsistency is defensible:

> *When giving consent to proposed treatment, the patient is accepting the advice of a qualified professional. Refusal, on the other hand, is a rejection of expert advice from a necessarily less well-informed position and may have grave consequences.*[9]

At 18 years of age teenagers may consent and refuse in the same way as an adult. Such refusal may be irrational, but cannot be challenged unless competence is in question. Refusal to follow medical advice is not in itself a sign of incompetence. We do not propose to discuss the position of those over 18 years old any further.

It is not yet clear whether the Human Rights Act will affect the ability of others to override a competent minor's wishes. Article 5 of the Act provides for the right of security of the person, while Article 8 relates to respect for privacy, Article 9 to freedom of conscience and Article 14 to non-discrimination in respect of the enjoyment of these rights. Such conflicts will come to court eventually, but this will require a decision by someone prepared to mount a test case. It would be hard to predict the timing or the outcome of such a case, which would depend on its precise circumstances.

In 1985 the House of Lords established that a person under the age of 16 years may be competent to give consent to treatment by a clinician. In *Gillick v West Norfolk and Wisbech Area Health Authority*,[10] Mrs Victoria Gillick had sought a declaration that it would be unlawful for any of her daughters under the age of 16 years to be given contraceptive advice or treatment without her agreement. The case went to the House of Lords, where Mrs Gillick was unsuccessful. In his judgement in this case, Lord Fraser set out the following criteria:

- The young person understands the advice being given.
- The young person cannot be convinced to involve parents/carers or allow the medical practitioner to do so on their behalf.
- It is likely that the young person will begin or continue having intercourse with or without treatment/contraception.
- Unless he or she receives treatment/contraception their physical or mental health (or both) is likely to suffer.
- The young person's best interests require contraceptive advice, treatment or supplies to be given without parental consent.

Although parents should normally be involved in decisions about the treatment of children under 16 years old, there are exceptions. In such cases assessment of competence should be carried out. (See the BMA criteria outlined in the previous section.[6]) The decision about whether a young person is 'Gillick competent' is a clinical one, and is therefore unlikely to be challenged successfully unless it is clearly unreasonable. The clinician should document discussion about involving parents and the young person's wishes.

There is a high risk of unwelcome and hostile media attention for clinicians in some cases.[11, 12] The ruling has significant implications for dealing with young people's health issues, including consultation, confidentiality, consent and treatment. For example, the Health Advisory Service has applied the principles of this case to needle-exchange programmes,[13] and there is widespread agreement that the 'Fraser guidelines' are generally applicable and not restricted to giving contraceptive advice. It is now clear from a case in 2006 that Gillick competence applies to abortion, and no doubt to any other procedure involving a young person under 16 years old.[14]

If a person under 16 years old is not competent, parents may give consent for treatment or refuse. Such a decision must be in the best interests of the minor, and a doctor who believes that parental refusal is not in the minor's best interests may seek the consent of a court to treat. In an emergency, it is lawful to treat under the Common Law doctrine of necessity, but clinicians should appreciate that it is possible to get a judgement within hours and define an emergency accordingly. The clinician may believe that there is enough room for disagreement about best interests that going to court is not warranted, even though he or she would prefer, on balance, to treat.[15]

WHAT IS GOOD PRACTICE?

It is good practice to work in the best interests of the young person. The legal provisions relating to consent allow clinicians consid-

erable freedom of interpretation, and it is here that value judgements are made, implicitly or explicitly, involving ethical choices. 'Best interests' can be interpreted in a variety of ways.

The BMA suggest 13 factors to consider, in a list which is not exhaustive:[16]

- the patient's own ascertainable wishes, feelings and values
- the patient's ability to understand what is proposed and weigh up the alternatives
- the patient's potential to participate more in the decision, if provided with additional support and explanations
- the patient's physical and emotional needs
- the risk of harm or suffering for the patient
- the views of parents and family
- the implications for the family of treatment or non-treatment
- relevant information about the patient's religious or cultural background
- evidence of the effectiveness of the proposed treatment, particularly in relation to other options
- the prioritizing of options that maximize the patient's future opportunities and choices
- evidence concerning the likelihood of improvement with treatment
- evidence about the anticipated extent of improvement
- risks arising from delayed treatment or non-treatment.

Such a list helps to identify the difficulties in assessing best interests when some factors point towards treatment and some to non-treatment, but it cannot resolve them.

Like adults, young people value honesty. A survey published in 1995 showed that the personal quality ranked as most important in adolescents' healthcare providers was honesty.[17] It is important that young people know the extent of their power to decide. There is evidence that young people are less likely to return to healthcare providers who offer only conditional confidentiality.[18] On the other hand, a breach of confidentiality, which had been understood to be unconditional, would seriously jeopardize a young person's future trust in healthcare providers. Many young people do not believe that they have the power to withhold consent to breach of confidentiality, and an assurance of confidentiality makes them more likely to discuss sexually transmitted infections, pregnancy prevention and substance abuse.[19]

The American Academy of Pediatrics gives the following advice:

Although confidentiality is important in adolescent health care, for adolescents at risk to themselves or others, confidentiality must be breached. Pediatricians need to inform the appropriate persons when they believe an adolescent is at risk of suicide.[20]

Understandably, many doctors would prefer to be in court defending their decision to save the life of a teenager than defending their decision to give a young person the power to refuse life-saving treatment.

When teenagers attend a consultation without a parent the clinician needs to assess their competence. Where consent to treatment is required it is essential in the under 16 year old to advise sharing the information and decision-making with the parent(s) and to document clearly that this has been addressed.

The majority of young people will be happy and reassured to have a parent with them throughout most consultations and examinations, but the opportunity to choose is an appropriate demonstration of respect of their increasing autonomy. When they attend with a parent it can be helpful to offer to see the young person and the parent individually at some stage as part of routine practice. This allows:

- clarification of the aims of the consultation, particularly where there is a discrepancy between the parties
- negotiation with the parent regarding any potential examination – particularly an intimate examination – to ensure that they will be in agreement with a possible decision by the young person not to have them present; it is good practice to provide a chaperone, and suggesting this may reassure the parent
- elucidation of any parental fears or anxieties, for example where their own previous experience of examination or treatment has been distressing
- questioning the young person about matters they wish to keep confidential or find embarrassing to discuss with their parent present, such as sexual activity, or alcohol or drug use.

HOW IS IT DIFFERENT FOR TEENAGERS?

Although others may consent on behalf of someone under the age of 18 years, the practical consequences of trying to treat a resistant teenager can be challenging. There will be occasions when young people will accept treatment once someone else has given consent, particularly when they feel that their views have been taken into account, even if not followed. Even when consent has been obtained from another, it is appropriate to keep a young patient as informed as possible about the process of treatment. There may be occasions when withholding consent enables a young person to test clinicians' respect for their autonomy, although this could be a game with fatal consequences. Refusing consent may also be a protest against other aspects of care, rather than a strong desire to avoid proposed treatment.

It is important to be realistic about the consequences of not examining or treating a teenager. Respecting a young Jehovah's Witness's wishes may not in fact lead to their death from exsanguination, but a longer recovery period. In this case the consequences of refusing blood are not life-threatening. A key communication skill is negotiation. Clinicians may see this as a way of winning a teenager over to their point of view, but true negotiation involves both sides being prepared to change positions.

An intimate examination of a young person where there are suspicions of sexual abuse may yield clinical information to support this possibility. However, such an examination conducted without appropriate explanation and negotiation may be perceived by the young person as a further act of abuse. This can further disempower the young person and lead to distrust of the medical profession. In such circumstances a pragmatic strategy of winning their confidence by promising not to examine without their con-

sent would be more constructive, although the promise must then be kept despite any external pressures.

Sometimes a realistic assessment of the effect of refusing treatment is that it will lead to death. No doctor is unmoved by a patient who makes such a decision. UK judges have given consent for life-saving treatment in cases where minors have refused, but have been careful to stress that each case has been decided on its particular facts. In 1999, a 15 year old who was refusing a heart transplant had her refusal overruled by the High Court.[21] She now appears reconciled to this decision. Courts accept the principle of a young person competently refusing life-saving treatment. This lends support to the advice of the Royal College of Paediatrics and Child Health, which allows young people to request withdrawal or withholding of treatment in a situation they regard as 'unbearable'.[22]

Traugott and Alpers[23] discuss three cases where 15 and 16 year olds had refused treatment. One refused chemotherapy for Hodgkin's disease, one refused immunosuppression after a liver transplant and a further transplant, and one refused chemotherapy for ovarian cancer. In each case the proposed interventions had serious adverse effects for the young person concerned, had to be given for an extended period and, in the latter two cases, did not necessarily offer a high prospect of success. In both cases the young people concerned were adamant in their refusal of treatment, to the extent that two of them ran away from home. The authors are sympathetic to each refusal, but believe that:

> ... even adolescents who can understand alternative treatments and their consequences may have flawed decision-making capacity. For example, teenagers' concerns about physical appearance, peer acceptance, and social life may cause them to reject a long-term prospect of improved health in favor of a short-term benefit from the adverse effects of medication.[23]

The examples of 'flawed decision-making capacity' are interesting. Such a value system pursued by an adult could not be challenged.

CONCLUSION

The law affords clinicians considerable freedom in the decisions they make regarding young people and consent. This is a freedom that is exercised responsibly when clinicians are honest and can demonstrate and record a coherent, well-considered process of decision-making within accepted legal guidelines and a reasoned ethical framework that respects the wishes of the young person whilst acting in their best interests. Where there are divergent beliefs about the best interests of a young person, such decisions will be open to question and may provoke controversy. Respectful debate regarding practice should continue in the light of experience and case law. The General Medical Council are consulting about the guidance it should issue as this goes to press.[24]

Chapter Thirty Nine

Treating children: whose consent counts?

Sir Mark Hedley

SUMMARY

Consent lies at the heart of the relationship between patient and clinician. It is the right of any adult who has capacity to refuse any treatment they choose, irrespective of need or catastrophic outcome. For the paediatrician, however, the issue is not so simple, as the question of what, if any, consent is required quite often arises not least in an emergency. This chapter is written from the perspective of a lawyer with many years of experience in child-care cases and some past experience as a member of a Children's Rights Advisory Forum (CRAF) at a large hospital, as well as dealing with these medical cases in the High Court since 2002.

Doctors are guided not only by the restraints of the law but by good practice, dictated both by formal medical policy and personal experience. The legal framework is governed in the criminal law by the law of Assault, and in the civil field by the duties to take reasonable care of a patient by the exercise of proper professional competence and to act in the best interests of the patient. This, however, provides only a floor of professional obligation. Two cases illustrate the point.

- a 14-year-old girl is admitted alleging that she has overdosed but, after initial treatment, she refuses advised blood tests despite the consent of the parent
- a 10-year-old boy is brought in by his mother who asserts that he has been the recent victim of anal abuse, but then he vigorously resists intimate examination.

In either of these cases a doctor who in good faith treated or examined using minimum reasonable force would probably not contravene the criminal law, but I doubt that many would support such an approach. Most would rely on negotiation and, in the second case, if unsuccessful, would desist. The first would require a clinical judgment that balanced risk to the young person against respect for their autonomy.

There has in recent years been a heightened awareness of children's rights through such instruments as the United Nations (UN) Convention on the Rights of the Child. On 20 October 2000 the Human Rights Act 1998 came into force. With its Right to Life (Article 2) and Right to Personal Autonomy (Article 8) it becomes the guideline legislation. However, since the sort of case under consideration almost invariably involves a potential conflict between various rights, the Act produces no clear answer. It follows that the decision-makers must strike a balance between rights, having considered each right individually before so doing. Nevertheless, the European Court of Human Rights has made it clear that, in the case of minors, their welfare may be the determining factor in the balance. My own view is that the Act (in this specific area of children and consent) will affect the language but probably not (at least significantly) the substance of this debate, which was in any event governed by just such considerations. Time alone will tell.

The basic legal propositions are relatively simple to state:

- by Section 8 of the Family Law Reform Act 1969 a young person over 16 years old may consent to any treatment without the need for any other person's consent
- a young person under 16 years old may nevertheless give a valid consent if 'Gillick competent'
- as a general rule no minor has the binding right to refuse treatment if a valid adult consent has been given
- however, there are some specific limited provisions under the Children Act 1989 which give a child a right to refuse, usually in connection with assessments.

The concept of Gillick competence is not an easy one. The name is that of the unsuccessful litigant, Mrs Gillick, in the House of Lords when she sought to prevent confidential contraceptive advice being given to her 16-year-old daughter who had requested it. It is basically defined as a child who has reached 'a sufficient understanding and intelligence to be capable of making up his own mind on the matter requiring decision'. It follows that the same child may be competent to decide some matters but not others in relation to his own treatment, depending on the complexity of the questions and the consequences of the particular course under consideration. A child who is competent in this sense does not necessarily oust the right of a parent to give or withhold consent; they run in parallel. Inevitably this rather loose framework leaves many areas of uncertainty.

Occasions will inevitably arise when clinicians are confronted either with disputes over consent or purported refusals of consent that (in their view) are contrary to the best interests of the patient. At all times doctors will principally be guided by his or her duty to act in the best interests of their patient. Most disputes can and should be resolved by negotiation and compromise, and the case that cannot is very much the exception. Some hospitals have informal procedures, such as a Children's Rights Advisory Forum (CRAF), available to patient, parent or clinician. However, there will be cases, hopefully rare, where questions of strict legal entitlement need to be resolved.

The courts have always been reluctant to become involved in these matters but have had to do so and, it seems, increasingly so. Where parents disagree with each other, it is possible to obtain a Specific Issue Order from the court on the application of a parent under the Children Act 1989. The court's duty under that Act is to treat the welfare of the child as its 'paramount' consideration, and in so doing to take into account the wishes and feelings of the child in the light of their age and understanding. If parent and child disagree with one another, a similar course may also be available. Where, in the case of a young or mentally disordered child, parents refuse consent to necessary treatment, it may become necessary to take advice from the legal advisor or from social services, who may then suggest involving the court, perhaps through its wardship (or parental) jurisdiction. Interestingly, the duty on the court under our domestic law is higher than that required by the UN Convention, which merely requires the best interests of the child to be a 'primary' consideration. In any dispute, however, the court has, so far as I know, never required a clinician to treat contrary to his or her clinical judgement, although the possibility has been mooted.

The real difficulties lie in those areas where consent is being refused by a child whom the clinician believes to have the capacity to consent. It is a grave step to override that refusal, and the problem is at its most acute where permanent or even fatal consequences may ensue from a failure to treat. It is in these circumstances that the court is most likely to be involved. There have been three groups of cases that have highlighted these difficulties: first, the refusal of blood products by those with a conscientious objection to such forms of treatment; secondly, the refusal of nutrition by those with eating disorders; and, thirdly, the refusal of major surgery or significant invasive treatment on the basis that death is to be preferred to the medical consequences, recent vivid examples being a 15-year-old girl refusing a heart transplant and a 15-year-old boy refusing cancer treatments. As a matter of fact the court has overridden each such refusal by finding that the child concerned did not have the capacity fully to understand the implications of their choices, and so were not in respect of that particular decision Gillick competent. It should be stressed, however, that the court order authorized but did not require treatment to be given.

A compelling example of the first category can be seen in the case of an intelligent, articulate 16-year-old Jehovah's Witness. He had a chronic condition that required a blood transfusion on an emergency basis. Supported by his parents, he steadfastly refused his consent, making clear both his reasons for so doing and his understanding of the consequences of his refusal. It required some judicial ingenuity (exercised at 2 a.m. as the medical team waited) to find that he was not Gillick competent, but the judge simply could not bring himself to do otherwise. In fact, 2 years later the circumstances repeated themselves and the young man, now 18 years old, took the same stance and died. The second category can be equally distressing, but in a different way. There have been

several cases of anorexic girls refusing nutrition. In some ways a finding that they are not Gillick competent is easier to make, given their mental and physical condition; however, the overriding of their consent often involves the repeated use of force to treat, a most unhappy prospect for any paediatrician. The third category is the least common, and once again these children were found not to be competent to refuse as they did not fully grasp the implications of their refusal. I have to recognize that the decisions both in these cases and the Jehovah's Witness case do present logical problems, as there is clearly a cogent argument that a young person can appreciate the implications of death as well as an 18 year old can. It merely illustrates, if such be needed, that in this area none of us can be purely cerebral, and the natural human instinct to preserve life asserts itself.

The other area in which consent can be a real problem is where there is no one to give a valid consent. Perhaps the patient is deeply unconscious and likely to remain so, or is mentally impaired to the extent of not being able to do so, or perhaps there is no guardian or no one prepared to take the responsibility of consenting. The clinician's duty remains to act in the best interests of the patient, and if he acts in an emergency without consent he would not be liable. If, however, there is time, reference to the court, perhaps via social services, may be necessary. In a case where a baby with chronic brain damage was on a ventilator and her position was considered to be medically hopeless, a court overrode the parents' wish for ventilation to be continued and granted leave to discontinue the treatment, although the consequences would be fatal. The Human Rights Act 1998 has not apparently altered this approach, since implicit in the Right to Life in such a case must surely be a right to a dignified death unencumbered by futile treatment. Every doctor would be most anxious to elicit a consent in these circumstances, but the court is there for the extreme case.

Any such application to the court is usually referred to the Family Division of the High Court, which provides 24 hour a day, 7 day a week cover in such circumstances, and every hospital legal advisor should know how to access this procedure. I would want to stress again that this approach should be seen as wholly exceptional.

I have tried to offer an overview of some of the difficulties arising out of the treatment of young people and the need to balance their welfare, their autonomy and the clinician's legal, professional and moral responsibilities. The first responsibility for dealing with this lies with the family and the treating doctor, and almost every case can and should be resolved in discussion and negotiation between them. The courts are anxious to intervene as little as possible between doctor and patient. However, the consequences of proceeding without a valid consent could be serious, both criminally and in terms of incurring liability to pay damages as well as risking adverse publicity. If confronted with a troubling issue of consent, or lack of it, in a specific case, it may be wise to obtain specialist advice.

Chapter Forty

The ethics of population screening

Alexandra Murray • Angus Clarke

SUMMARY

The ethical issues raised by population screening programmes are complex, with implications for individuals, healthcare professionals and society as a whole. While personal autonomy has to be respected in these programmes, especially the need for informed consent, population screening will often be justified on the basis of benevolence. The public health criteria and the ethical considerations applicable to any screening programme are outlined, especially in the context of genetic conditions. The issues raised by some current screening programmes are discussed, and the problems that may arise with genetic screening programmes in the future are considered.

PRACTICE POINTS

- Newborn screening tests are not just laboratory tests.
- Adding new disorders to newborn screening programmes can raise issues of consent.
- New protocols may need to be developed to handle positive cases.

THE ETHICS OF POPULATION SCREENING

Population screening is the practice of offering a test or investigation to apparently healthy individuals in order to detect unrecognized disease or its precursors, with the intention of improving the outcome for individuals identified in this way. Screening tests will often modify the risk that an individual has the disorder in question, shifting the group with positive screening results from low (standard or population) risk to a high (increased) risk, without this amounting to a firm, positive diagnosis. In such screening programmes, further investigations may be required to confirm or exclude the suspected diagnosis. Population screening programmes are made available to the whole population or to large subgroups (e.g. all newborn infants, all pregnant women) where there is no specific reason to think that the individuals screened are likely to be affected. Where there is reason to single out an individual as already being at risk of the condition, then diagnostic testing may be appropriate without the screening procedure.

Given that many individuals will be recruited into a screening programme for each identified case of disease recognized in the end, serious consideration must be given to the possibility that screening is too costly, that the small burden it imposes on many is cumulatively too great to justify its benefits, or that too many individuals have to be subjected to further, possibly hazardous, diagnostic testing for the programme to be justified. Concerns of this nature led Wilson and Jungner,[1] on behalf of the World Health Organization, to draw up criteria to be met before screening would be regarded as worthwhile. These criteria have been used as the basis of public health decision-making ever since, and have been reworked into a number of more contemporary formulations.[2, 3] The crux of such criteria is the concern that screening is offered to individuals who are healthy and asymptomatic; screening is not a response to pre-existing concerns from those who think they might be ill, or those who do have symptoms of disease or a relevant family history; these groups should instead be assessed through conventional healthcare channels.

In many screening programmes, the disease being targeted is a genetic condition. There are several differences between screening programmes for genetic conditions and other population screening programmes. One important difference is that a positive result in a screening programme for a genetic condition may have implications for other family members as well as the health of the individual being screened. In newborn screening for the X-linked disorder Duchenne muscular dystrophy, the immediate and extended family may benefit from the early diagnosis, perhaps through genetic counselling and better-informed reproductive decisions, although the affected child is as yet unlikely to benefit directly himself. In prenatal screening, a positive result may lead to a decision to terminate a pregnancy, and those opposed to pregnancy termination may accuse the screening programme of having eugenic intentions or consequences. In both these cases, it may be argued that the programme fails to meet the Wilson and Jungner criteria for screening.

SUMMARY OF CRITERIA FOR A SCREENING PROGRAMME

Before the introduction of any population screening programme it should be clear that (based on Wilson and Jungner[1] and National Screening Committee[3]):

- The condition being screened for is an important health problem resulting in significant mortality or morbidity. The natural history of the disease should be adequately understood, and it should be possible to improve outcomes through intervening in the natural history before affected individuals would otherwise be recognized.

- The test is simple, safe, precise and validated. There should be a defined cut-off level and an agreed policy on further diagnostic investigations appropriate to identified individuals (with a positive screening test result) and on the choices available to them.

- The treatment or intervention available to these individuals leads to better outcomes than late treatment, and there should be agreement, based on evidence, as to what intervention should be made available to early diagnosed cases. This optimal, clinical management should be available to all affected individuals before screening is introduced.

- The complete screening programme (test, diagnostic procedures, treatment) is acceptable to the population and health professionals, and it should have been shown in randomized, controlled trials (RCTs) that it leads to a reduction in mortality or morbidity when compared to conventional diagnostic routes. These benefits should outweigh any physical or psychological harm caused by the test or the subsequent diagnostic procedures or treatments. Furthermore, the opportunity costs of the programme should be balanced in relation to healthcare expenditure as a whole, and there should be adequate staffing facilities to manage the programme, deliver the benefits and ensure a high quality of operation.

The ethical principle that must be protected with most particular care in the context of population screening programmes is individual autonomy. Where a healthcare system decides that a screening test is justified, it would be all too easy for the offer of screening to be presented to the public in such a way that it could hardly be declined – either through being made routine or, perhaps, through the application of coercive pressure. Any decision to offer screening is likely to be justified on the grounds of benevolence, which could easily slide into an inappropriate paternalism if the staff offering the test assumed that everyone should accept it. This situation contrasts with specialist genetic counselling, in which the possibility of genetic testing may be discussed but any decision about testing will be made by the client. In the different context of screening programmes, the fact that the test is being offered proactively by healthcare professionals conveys the powerful message that screening is recommended by the professionals and by society. This recommendation may be entirely appropriate where early diagnosis is known to improve the prognosis for affected individuals (e.g. as with Guthrie screening for phenylketonuria), but this is not true for reproductive genetic screening or for newborn screening for currently incurable conditions such as Duchenne muscular dystrophy. In such contexts, it is important that clients do not enter into screening passively, by default, but that they only participate through making an active decision.

The non-directive ethos appropriate in much genetic counselling practice[4, 5] cannot easily be transferred across to those population screening programmes where it would also be valuable. This ethos seeks to ensure that an individual's decisions are her own rather than those determined in advance by medical professionals or the healthcare system. Population screening programmes carry an implicit recommendation in the very offer of the test, and must strive to leave space for individual autonomy where that is required.

A related issue is that of informed consent. Individuals should be aware that they have a choice about whether or not to take part.

Screening may be such a part of routine care that both the professionals and the participants accept it as standard practice without giving much thought to the issues involved, as in newborn screening for treatable disorders (phenylketonuria, hypothyroidism); indeed, such screening is mandatory in some jurisdictions. Difficult situations arise when screening tests for different categories of disease are made available at the same time, perhaps on the same blood sample and with the same consent process. It may then be helpful to emphasize the differences between the diseases for which screening is available by using different consent procedures for the various tests. Another context in which informed consent is a serious problem is that of antenatal screening for Down syndrome and congenital malformation. Several studies have expressed concern that women undergoing serum screening for Down syndrome have poor understanding of what the test involves, that the 'offer' of screening is made routine, and that it discourages discussion and reflection as to the implications of a positive test result.[6-8] Just as worrying is the evidence of poor factual knowledge about maternal serum screening on the part of some health professionals.[9]

It is also necessary to consider the rate of uptake of a screening test. Traditionally, it has been considered desirable to maximize the uptake of screening programmes, after the fashion of immunization programmes, and in many cases it is only when the uptake rates are high that a screening programme is deemed to be successful. Unfortunately, a high uptake rate may be more a reflection of it being made routine – of a lack of informed consent – than of a successful or worthwhile screening programme. Especially where screening touches on personal reproductive issues, so that a non-directive ethos would be desirable, the outcome and worth of screening must be assessed in other ways than by measures of uptake.

Other commonly used means to assess the worth of a screening programme are monetary, such as cost–benefit and cost–effectiveness analyses. While most clinicians would agree that cost should never be a priority, resources are not infinite, so that any money or effort expended in one area of healthcare is necessarily not available for use elsewhere. All screening programmes, therefore, need to be able to demonstrate their efficient and effective use of resources, but it is highly contentious and may cause great moral offence to use the cost–benefit approach as the measure of the worth of reproductive genetic screening programmes. Despite these concerns, it has often been argued that it is cheaper to prevent the births of individuals with certain genetic disorders than to care for them, so that screening 'for' these disorders is justified. This reasoning is particularly applied to the 'prevention' of Down syndrome – on the assumption that terminating a pregnancy in which the fetus has Down syndrome amounts to its 'prevention'. Such arguments, that the financial costs of prenatal screening for Down syndrome amount to less than the likely costs of care for affected individuals, typically omit many of the true costs of screening – such as the training of staff to offer screening in an appropriate manner; the loss of wanted, healthy pregnancies after invasive diagnostic procedures; the offence and distress caused to individuals with Down syndrome and their families by these screening programmes; and the anxiety and distress caused to individuals and families confronted by unsought, difficult decisions (whatever the outcome of these pregnancies). Even when such crude cost–benefit arguments are not used in the justification of a screening programme, assumptions about the value of human lives and the social implications of screening may be present but implicit; such silent, value-loaded assumptions can be corrosive unless made explicit.[10]

Finally, the process through which decisions are made about population screening programmes should be considered. In the UK, the National Health Service now makes these decisions at a national level through the National Screening Committee (NSC), although decisions about most paediatric and genetic screening programmes were introduced before the existence of the NSC. Ideally, the process should include examination of the relevant medical evidence together with representation of the views of patient and professional organizations, public interest groups, industry and government agencies. The enthusiasm for a new screening test expressed by doctors, scientists and businessmen may not be reflected in the general population. Just because a test is technologically possible, it does not necessarily follow that it should be introduced for general population screening. The essentially political nature of the processes leading to the introduction of screening tests, including commercial pressures and professional enthusiasm, is demonstrated in studies of the introduction of cystic fibrosis carrier screening in Denmark[11] and of widespread testing for the fragile X syndrome.[12]

NEWBORN SCREENING

Newborn screening has been well established in the UK for over 30 years and it has generally been the least contentious of the various screening programmes currently in operation. Testing is carried out on dried blood spots obtained by heel prick from newborn babies at 6–7 days. Currently, all babies in the UK are screened for phenylketonuria and congenital hypothyroidism, and screening for additional disorders is being introduced (e.g. cystic fibrosis and sickle cell disease). Screening for Duchenne muscular dystrophy is made available for boys born in Wales. While screening for phenylketonuria and hypothyroidism has transformed the prognosis for babies born with these conditions, there have been many debates about the rights and wrongs of screening for conditions such as cystic fibrosis or Duchenne muscular dystrophy. The purpose of newborn screening for cystic fibrosis is to give affected infants the benefit of early intervention with prophylactic antibiotics and nutritional supplements. Experience suggests that this results in reduced morbidity in the first 2 years and improved nutritional and respiratory status up to the age of 10 years.[13] Although there is no certainty that these early benefits will persist in the long term, and there are some potential disadvantages, such as the recognition of some healthy carrier infants, the arguments in favour of screening are strong. It would take a long time for cast-iron evidence of the eventual outcomes to emerge – by which time the treatments available for newborn infants would have changed, so that the gold standard of RCT 'proof' may simply never be available. Decisions, therefore, must be made on the balance of probabilities.

The evidence of benefit from the early diagnosis of sickle cell disease, permitting early antibiotic prophylaxis, is not in doubt. In the past, debate has centred on whether universal newborn screening for the disease is appropriate in areas where the ethnic composition of the population is such that few infants are at risk. Some have suggested that it might be better to test only those infants thought by healthcare professionals to come from the relevant population groups, but this raises questions about the equity of access to healthcare and the priority given to minority ethnic groups. The NSC has now recommended that sickle cell disease screening should be offered to all newborns, and this is being implemented across England, with similar programmes being considered in Wales, Scotland and Northern Ireland.

Different arguments are used to justify newborn screening for Duchenne muscular dystrophy, because there is no evidence that the early recognition of boys affected by Duchenne muscular dystrophy leads to any improvement in their health. If it is justified, it will be on other grounds.[14] Firstly, parents are spared the distress and bitterness so often found in families where the diagnosis has been delayed; and, secondly, early detection allows parents to make informed reproductive choices in future pregnancies. The potential disadvantages are the possible damage an early diagnosis may cause to the parent–child relationship and the child's early development, as well as the extra worry and distress the family will suffer. Newborn screening for Duchenne muscular dystrophy has been available in Wales for over 10 years and has been subject to a social evaluation. Reports of this programme show no evidence of such harms, no evidence of parents withdrawing their infants from all newborn screening so as to avoid tests for Duchenne muscular dystrophy, a high level of parental satisfaction with the early diagnosis and a high uptake of this opt-in test (over 90%).[15] As discussed above, this level of uptake could represent a problem with informed consent or the test being made routine. Since all the newborn screening tests are carried out on the same dried bloodspots, it is essential that parents are made aware, at the time of consent, of the difference between the tests for phenylketonuria and congenital hypothyroidism, where therapeutic intervention is possible, and the tests for conditions such as Duchenne muscular dystrophy, where it is not. Modification of the consent process for Duchenne muscular dystrophy testing, to enhance the distinction between the tests done for the benefit of the child and the Duchenne muscular dystrophy test, leads to only a modest reduction in uptake.[16] The most important lesson from this screening programme has been the absolute need for careful coordination, ensuring that a protocol for handling positive results is developed and monitored.[17] Newborn screening for Duchenne muscular dystrophy and similar disorders must not be regarded as just a laboratory test, but must entail a process of midwife education, communication with the primary care team and coordination with the relevant paediatric teams. Otherwise, the potentially adverse consequences of screening could emerge all too easily.

The next group of conditions being considered for inclusion in the newborn screening programme are some of the inherited metabolic disorders. The introduction of tandem mass spectrometry (TMS) has made it feasible to detect a number of these conditions, although useful interventions will not be available for all of them. In 2004, the NSC decided to commission a study to examine the effectiveness of screening for the fatty acid oxidation disorder medium-chain acyl-CoA dehydrogenase (MCAD) deficiency using TMS. The pilot study[18] will report in 2008, but on the basis of the interim results the NSC has decided that all newborns will be screened for MCAD deficiency by March 2009. The NSC intends to use the data gathered from the MCAD study to explore the most effective and efficient way of making decisions about other rare inherited disorders, such as amino acid metabolism disorders. Procedures for handling infants with abnormal biochemistry but atypical or mild (low penetrance) mutations will need to be worked out, and the responses of families to minor illnesses in their affected infant, when they have no experience of the disease, will need to be monitored. It will be essential to ensure that the consent procedure is appropriate for each additional disorder included in the screening programme, and to evaluate the consequences of screening for such new conditions.

There is the distinct possibility that, in the future, it could become too simple to add in new conditions to the screening programme, without first determining whether there is likely to be any advantage in making an early diagnosis. The use of TMS is likely to increase and, as costs decrease, DNA microarray technology may also be applied to newborn and other population screening programmes. It is hard to predict all the possible uses of these technologies in the future, but there would be major ethical concerns if they were to be employed in the detection of adult-onset disorders or other genetic susceptibilities. These issues need to be debated sooner rather than later.[19]

SCREENING IN CHILDHOOD

Children in many countries are screened for a variety of non-genetic conditions. These may include screening for congenital dislocation of the hip, impairments of vision and hearing, dental problems, head lice and scoliosis.[20] Such programmes are unlikely to present specific ethical challenges beyond the usual ones that apply to any screening programme – is there evidence that the programme is worthwhile, given the resources required to operate it? Nevertheless, before any new screening programme is implemented, it is essential to ensure there are sufficient resources available to provide the necessary follow-up and optimal intervention for those infants identified by the screening programme. There should also be a method of evaluation in place, which should include measures of acceptability and distress caused by screening.

REPRODUCTIVE SCREENING

Fetal anomaly screening

The purpose of antenatal screening by ultrasound scanning and/or maternal serum screening is to detect those fetuses with Down syndrome or structural malformations. Those who are found to be at high risk of having a baby with Down syndrome are offered an amniocentesis to confirm or exclude the diagnosis. When a chromosome anomaly is identified or a major structural malformation (e.g. a neural tube defect) is detected, the woman and her partner are offered a termination of the pregnancy. These screening programmes are now so much a part of routine antenatal care that couples can all too easily enter a screening programme and then find themselves faced with a most difficult decision – whether or not to have amniocentesis, whether or not to terminate the pregnancy – without having ever understood the purpose of the initial screening test. Indeed, ultrasound fetal anomaly scans may be performed 'to make sure that baby is alright' (a deeply ambiguous phrase) and can become social events 'to promote bonding' or to provide a photo opportunity. Staff and parents may collude to avoid confronting sensitive subjects that are difficult to discuss, such as the possibility that screening may place the woman on a conveyor belt leading to the termination of a wanted pregnancy. It is important to ensure that pregnant women understand the voluntary nature of screening, the fact that a normal test result is not a guarantee of a normal baby, that sometimes test results are misleading or equivocal (perhaps requiring further investigations for their interpretation), and that staff are likely to offer a termination of pregnancy if a problem is suspected. There is evidence that staff find it difficult to tackle these issues without training and support – and to promote prenatal screening without such training and support would clearly be wrong.

Since the main conditions targeted by prenatal screening programmes are Down syndrome and neural tube defects, the discussion should also include information on these conditions and on the help and support that is available to families who have an affected child.

The offer of prenatal screening should enable mothers/couples to make informed decisions about continuing or terminating a pregnancy if a fetal anomaly is found; it is important that they should feel supported whatever their decision. Some will choose to terminate an affected pregnancy, perhaps then experiencing regret or guilt, while others will continue with the pregnancy while fearing stigmatization, isolation and a lack of support. We should recognize that 'choice' in this context can be a burden, leading to great anxiety and distress. We should also recognize that prenatal screening programmes have implications for individuals with these and other disabilities, and may cause deep offence to them and their families. While this should not necessarily restrict the freedom of pregnant women to make reproductive decisions, we should recognize the tension between their reproductive autonomy and the respect due our fellow human beings, whatever their physical or intellectual capacities. Society needs to work hard to develop an accommodation between these perspectives.

Carrier screening

Population screening for healthy carriers of the haemoglobinopathies and Tay–Sachs disease has been possible for decades with the use of haemoglobin electrophoresis and enzyme assays, and the advent of molecular genetic technologies has led to the development of carrier screening for other autosomal-recessive conditions, such as cystic fibrosis, where a majority of heterozygotes carry one of a small set of common mutations. Even this restriction is disappearing as gene chip technologies are introduced into diagnostic laboratories. The goal of carrier screening programmes is to identify couples whose children would be at 25% risk of developing the particular disease.

There are three basic strategies that can be employed for carrier screening:

- cascade screening of the relatives of affected individuals
- screening of couples before conception, before marriage or during pregnancy
- comprehensive population screening of all individuals of reproductive age.

Cascade screening is standard practice wherever clinical genetics services exist, although it is generally agreed that 'at-risk' individuals have the right not to participate, i.e. the 'right not to know'. At present, comprehensive population screening programmes for this type of condition remain a matter for debate. Several countries offer screening to couples or individuals if they are from high-risk communities, e.g. screening for Tay–Sachs disease for the Ashkenazi Jewish community and haemoglobinopathy screening for the African, Afro-Caribbean, South Asian and Mediterranean communities in Britain. Some countries are now also introducing screening programmes for cystic fibrosis in antenatal clinics.

Detection of a healthy heterozygote has virtually no implications for an individual's own health, so the benefits of such a screening programme come from giving couples an awareness of their risk of having an affected child. As with antenatal screening, this enables them to make informed reproductive choices. It is important that these choices are respected. Problems can arise, especially when screening is made available to an ethnic minority group; the stigmatization of carriers can reinforce or provoke racial discrimination, as with mandatory screening for sickle cell anaemia in the USA in the 1970s. There remain concerns that the tension between individual autonomy and the desire of the healthcare system to prevent disease cannot be easily resolved.[21]

One of the reasons for caution in relation to the introduction of carrier screening is the possible stigma experienced by carriers. A positive result may cause anxiety or low self-esteem or lead to social discrimination, with carriers regarded as undesirable marriage partners. In order to avoid stigmatization and discrimination, every effort must be made to ensure that results remain confidential. As with other forms of reproductive screening, a desire on the part of public health experts to maximize the 'cost savings' from genetic screening could lead to the routinization of testing or coercion to ensure a high uptake. The cost pressures to promote reproductive screening and the termination of affected pregnancies will increase, paradoxically, as the treatment of cystic fibrosis and other such disorders improves, because the associated cost of care will be greater. As a family's reasons for choosing to have a termination of pregnancy weaken with progress in healthcare, society's reasons for promoting reproductive screening will strengthen. Our society's resolution of that tension will give some insight into our collective mores.

Susceptibility screening for individual health

The era of genetic susceptibility screening – generating each individual's profile of disease risks – has not yet arrived. The prospect of such a scenario has been somewhat inflated, and there are very real limitations as to what biotechnology will be able to deliver over the next few decades. Testing to predict an individual's responses to specific drugs, however, including their toxicity and efficacy, may gradually enter routine clinical practice in a limited range of contexts. Such tests are likely to generate information about an individual's prognosis as well as their response to therapy, and careful thought will be required as to the use made of this information. Experience of screening for hypertension and for high blood cholesterol levels has demonstrated mankind's capacity to respond unhelpfully to risk information, showing that a low risk of disease can be interpreted as invulnerability and a high risk of disease as an inevitability, with either result leading (in some individuals) to damaging health-related behaviours.[22] The knowledge that parents can damage a child's health through forcing 'excessive compliance' to a suggested diet warns us that information about a child's disease susceptibility profile, in so far as such information becomes available, may also prove unhelpful. Fortunately, population genetic screening for disease susceptibility is unlikely to be applied on a wide scale in childhood in the absence of good research evidence of substantial health benefits to the screened population. In the near future, it is more likely that research studies will wish to recruit children to track their health and accumulate evidence about the influence of genotype on the development of the common, complex (multifactorial) disorders. Participation in such research also raises ethical issues, but they cannot be tackled here.

41 Chapter Forty One

The ethics of genetic testing of families

Annie M. Procter

SUMMARY

The ethics of genetic testing relate in particular to the need to obtain a balance between the possible benefits conferred on and the potential harm done to an individual and their family as a consequence of both the process and the results obtained from genetic investigations. It is not always possible to predict the effect of the receipt of genetic information upon the individual or the family, and therefore the investigation of families for genetic disorders should not be undertaken without careful consideration of the implications of such testing. The implications of genetic testing depend on several factors, including the type of genetic investigation proposed, the reasons for the test request and the age of the individual concerned. The purpose of this chapter is to highlight the key issues involved in the genetic testing of families.

PRACTICE POINTS

- Every request for a genetic investigation in a child and family should be carefully considered in its individual context.
- Care should be taken to adequately explore and discuss each request and its implications with the family, and with the child if appropriate. This will help to ensure that the most appropriate joint decision is made with regard to genetic testing.
- Predictive testing of children for adult-onset disorders for which there is as yet no beneficial therapeutic intervention is generally considered to be inappropriate.
- Predictive testing of children for adult-onset disorders for which beneficial interventions exist may be considered appropriate.
- The implications of carrier testing of healthy children are complex. Where possible, the decision to undergo carrier testing is best taken by the children themselves when mature enough to make such a decision.
- Where a decision not to perform a test is made, provision must be agreed with the family to enable the children to gain adequate information in the future to allow them to make a decision regarding genetic testing for themselves.

INTRODUCTION

It is now possible to use an increasing number of investigations both to diagnose the presence and predict the onset of genetic disorders. However, the receipt of genetic information can have an enormous and unpredictable impact on the individual tested, an impact that may visit its effects throughout the extended family and across the generations. Genetic information also has a wider impact on society and its politics.[1,2] Therefore the desirability or otherwise of performing genetic investigations is governed by many issues, not the least of which is the ethics of making such a decision.

The definition of what constitutes a genetic investigation has broadened enormously over recent years and is not limited to the analysis of chromosomes or DNA. Important inclusions in a broad definition of genetic tests are such things as renal ultrasound scanning and echocardiography that can be used to identify conditions such as polycystic kidney disease and cardiomyopathy, respectively, in otherwise apparently healthy individuals.

There are several important factors to take into account when considering the implementation of investigations for genetic disorders. The first important issue is the type of test involved. In some situations the use of a genetic investigation serves to diagnose a disorder in a sick individual and allows the subsequent development of a medical management plan. However, in other situations genetic investigations are performed in apparently healthy individuals, either to predict the likelihood of developing a particular disorder in the future (predictive testing) or to ascertain whether that individual will pass a genetic disorder on to his or her offspring (carrier testing).

Another factor that poses problems, both for those requesting tests and those to whom the request is made, is the definition of the reasons for and the benefits of a particular genetic investigation. It is frequently difficult to balance the perceived need for a genetic test against the perceived benefits of such an investigation. This issue can cause particular problems when the relative merits of a genetic investigation are viewed differently by an individual or family, and the professional to whom the request for a genetic test has been made.

The key factor in the consideration of whether to perform or withhold a genetic investigation is perhaps the age of the individual concerned. The implications of testing an adult for a genetic disorder can be very different to those that relate to performing the same genetic investigation in a child.

Much of this chapter concentrates on the ethical problems surrounding the genetic testing of children. Adults who are considering genetic testing generally do so either to aid in the diagnosis of a medical disorder or to remove uncertainty about their risk of either passing a disorder on to their children or developing a particular disorder themselves in the future. It is usual, particularly in the situation in which an adult is considering predictive testing, for such an individual to take part in an extensive counselling process prior to making the final decision about whether to undergo genetic testing or to decline it. One aim of the counselling process, particularly with regard to predictive testing, is to ensure that the individual recognizes the possible effects of receiving a positive or a negative result, either of which could have enormous and unexpected consequences for the individual.[3]

There are complex psychological and social implications associated with genetic disease and the receipt of genetic test results. Major life decisions can be hugely influenced, both by the fear of harbouring a genetic disorder and by the results of genetic investigations; for example, some individuals have avoided close relationships and parenthood because of 'unfavourable' genetic test results. Individuals who undergo genetic investigations need also to consider the effect that the results of such tests will have on their ability to obtain insurance, buy a house and choose a career.

The results of genetic tests may remove one uncertainty, 'Will I get the disease?', only to replace it with another, 'When will I get the disease?'. Genetic counselling offers individuals who are considering genetic testing the opportunity to confront all these possibilities and use the experience to aid their decision-making. A child who is subjected to genetic testing during childhood may be denied the opportunity to benefit from this vital process. It is thus the testing of children, particularly predictive and carrier testing, which is the area of genetic investigation that demands the most intense ethical scrutiny.

PREDICTIVE TESTING

In 1986, in the context of the neurodegenerative disorder Huntington's disease,[4] it was recognized that predictive testing might be performed inappropriately on children. As the range of disorders for which genetic testing is available has increased, so the concern and debate relating to childhood testing has expanded to encompass other disorders[5] and more general issues such as population screening.[6]

The predictive testing of apparently healthy children may be justified if the results of such testing achieve a positive balance between the 'enabling' aspects of testing and the potential harm caused by carrying out such investigations. The introduction of some beneficial medical intervention or life-style change might be considered an 'enabling' consequence of genetic testing. Hence, in some of the familial cancer disorders such as familial adenomatous polyposis coli (FAP), screening for tumours in early or mid-childhood may be warranted for those children known to carry disease-associated gene mutations. However, for those genetic disorders for which there are as yet no useful interventions, for example Huntington's disease and prion-associated dementia, the benefits to the child of genetic testing during childhood are much less clear.

Performing a genetic investigation on a young child in particular deprives that child of the right to make the decision when they are older. It is entirely possible that a child when of an age to make such a decision, might wish not to know their genetic status with regard to a particular condition. A genetic test performed earlier in their childhood will have robbed them of the right to say 'no' and of the right to say 'yes' with confidentiality assured.[7, 8] In a family in which

a disorder such as Huntington's disease is a part of 'normal life', predictive testing may appear to be a very rational and obvious course of action. It is vital, therefore, to consider who is the real beneficiary of a genetic test result, and to ensure that it is the individual undergoing the investigation rather than another person or simply the expansion of medical and scientific knowledge.

Individuals for whom predictive testing is an option, whether they be a child or an adult, will often have first-hand experience of the 'family disease'. This may have a considerable influence on the views these individuals hold with regard to the disease, the desirability of predictive testing and the way they react to the test results.[9] Some families may hold the view that genetic testing in a 'family environment' in which a disorder is known is the most supportive situation in which such testing could occur. Indeed, not to test might be considered by some individuals to be 'abnormal'. However, grave concerns have been expressed about the desirability of predictive testing during childhood. These concerns relate particularly to the potential harm of labelling a healthy child as sick[10] and causing them to live their lives under the shadow of the uncertain timing of the onset and development of the disorder.[11] There are a number of reports concerning the psychological effects of predictive testing on adults.[12] However, partly because the opportunity to perform childhood testing is a relatively recent phenomenon, the possible effects on children are not fully understood[9, 13, 14] and the most beneficial approach to the management of such testing in childhood continues to be explored.[15–17]

CARRIER TESTING

Carrier testing generally, by definition, will have no implications for the health of the individual being tested, but the results may have an enormous effect on the reproductive decisions that such an individual feels able to make. As with predictive testing, adults who make a decision about the desirability of having their carrier status assessed generally do so as a result of a counselling process or some type of informative discussion process with healthcare professionals. Such opportunities for appropriate, informed decision-making may not be possible for a young child. Thus performing a carrier test on a child can deprive them of such autonomy and the right to make that choice for themselves when they are older. In addition, as is the case for predictive testing, that child has to live for many years with genetic information they may not, as an adult, wish to have or wish other people to know about.

The question of whether to perform carrier testing during early childhood is an issue about which families and professionals may hold very different views. A family in which a child has suffered, and perhaps died, of a debilitating genetic disorder may see carrier testing of that child's siblings as hugely advantageous. Such a family will often approach the paediatrician who helped them care for the sick child with the request that the paediatrician perform carrier testing on the other children in the family. The paediatrician can feel that to be seen to refuse such testing could undermine the relationship with the family to such a degree that, despite any misgivings they might have on behalf of the child to be tested, they feel impelled to perform the carrier testing as requested. Other paediatricians and healthcare professionals might feel that to test any child for their carrier status is a mistake, whatever the reasons for the request.[19]

CONSENT TO TESTING

Whether a child or an adult can maintain their autonomy and give consent to a genetic investigation depends on the degree to which they can become informed about the details and the implications of such testing. The degree to which a child can contribute to the decision-making process depends very much on the child's age and maturity at the time. This contribution will also be greatly influenced by the child's experience of the disease in their family, as well as their unique personality and their experience of personal and interpersonal conflict.[19] The Gillick standard is an accepted legal test of competence to consent. That said, there is a need to recognize the abilities of younger or less mature children to be involved in the decision-making process and to give or to withhold their consent to a test.[20]

The views of children with regard to assessing their own genetic status should be explored whenever feasible. It has been demonstrated that even young children have the capacity to contribute to important decisions about their healthcare.[21, 22] There is also strong evidence that requests from adolescents for genetic testing should be thoroughly and sympathetically followed up.[23, 24] The adolescent may benefit from both the opportunity to explore the possibilities confronting them and the respect afforded them by the professional who is prepared to consider their views.

GENERAL ISSUES

In 1994, the Clinical Genetics Society formed a Working Party that carried out a survey of professional attitudes to childhood genetic testing.[18] The results of this survey demonstrated very substantial differences of opinion, both within and between different professional groups in Britain. Despite these differences, the Working Party was able to establish a consensus approach to some areas of genetic testing during childhood. With regard to childhood predictive testing for adult-onset disorders, the consensus view was that in the absence of a useful medical intervention such testing would generally be regarded as inappropriate. The consensus view with regard to carrier testing during childhood was very similar but it was put forward with a greater degree of caution than was the case for childhood predictive testing. The Working Party felt that children should not undergo investigations for which the results were of reproductive significance only, and therefore unlikely to be of benefit to the child until they achieved adulthood.

This survey was repeated in 1998 on behalf of the Advisory Committee on Genetic Testing[25] and a very similar consensus view emerged. However, it is evident that with regard to predictive testing, the consensus between professional groups is increasing. The 1994 survey revealed considerable division between paediatricians and geneticists with regard to the desirability of childhood genetic testing. There is now strong evidence from the 1998 survey that professionals consider that it is frequently 'more important to have the discussions than to do the tests'.

It is important that 'availability' of genetic testing does not translate directly into 'advisability' of genetic testing without due consideration. This distinction is important whether the testing is being considered in a child or in an adult. For many professionals one particular area of difficulty is experienced in the attempt to reconcile an enthusiastic approach to antenatal testing with a much more conservative approach to genetic testing once a child is born.

In the practice of medicine, situations will arise in which an individual is identified as having a condition that is recognized as an inherited disorder for which there exists a genetic test. In such situations it may be possible to offer testing to other family members, including both adults and children. To avoid the potential for considerable distress and confusion, the decision to have such testing is best made in an informed and supportive manner at a time that is right for each and every individual concerned.

The consideration of when and how best to approach family members with regard to genetic testing must also apply to the application of 'new' or 'research' tests. Some families find that being re-approached about tests in situations where they have come to accept that there may never be a diagnostic test, much less a cure, is extremely distressing. This distress can be exacerbated by the fact that the offer of an investigation may add very little to the understanding or management of the disorder for the individuals concerned. These issues will become increasingly important as the availability of genetic testing continues to outstrip our abilities to treat or cure many genetic disorders.

An individual or family may be so determined to have an investigation performed that they will find the means to achieve their wishes. It is therefore vital that the issues surrounding genetic testing, particularly genetic testing during childhood, are discussed in a fulsome and non-confrontational manner. This will allow families the freedom to consider and discover the optimal way to do what they believe will benefit their child most.[25]

It is important to give careful thought to the management of those families in which a decision to perform genetic testing has been delayed. This generally applies to children who are considered too young to have genetic testing but for whom an investigation may be an option at some time in the future when they are able to make such a decision for themselves. It is vital that provision is made for the required information to be relayed to the family or individual at the appropriate time and in the appropriate manner to allow such decisions to be made.

When considering the genetic testing of children, families and professionals need to work together with the interests of the child jointly held as their highest priority. In such circumstances there is a need for all the participants to understand and accept that the professional has the responsibility for aiding the family in a thorough and well-informed consideration of all the implications of performing genetic testing during childhood. Recent research has underlined the need for support and training in the ethical complexities of genetic testing within families for all professionals who may have a role in such investigations.[27, 28]

Anyone considering predictive and carrier testing within a family, and most particularly during childhood, should approach such investigations with caution. It is important that a dialogue is established between all the parties concerned to allow discussion and consideration of the benefits gained and the opportunities presented against the possible disadvantages of the receipt of genetic information. A vital part of such interactions is the recognition that individuals within the family have the right to have their own discussions and make their own, independent decisions with regard to the desirability of a genetic investigation.

Chapter Forty Two

Ethics in undergraduate medical education: sowing the seeds

42

David P. Davies

SUMMARY

This chapter discusses an approach to the teaching of ethics and associated legal issues in a new integrated medical curriculum. The importance of having a clear definition of learning outcomes and the integration of principles of core values of ethics with their practical application throughout the course is emphasized. The need to develop assessment tools to signal to students the importance of ethics study is also paramount. Important limitations to improving and enhancing ethics awareness is a lack of human resources appropriately trained in ethics, the law and moral philosophy. Staff development, 'teaching the teacher', is critical.

PRACTICE POINTS

- Ethics in clinical medicine is, in its simplest form, about some sort of moral choice about right and wrong conduct in medical care.
- Understanding basic ethical principles and associated issues of law along with their practical application in medical practice and research need to be part of core teaching in the medical curriculum. But how best this instruction should be given remains to be determined.
- Experience shows that many students do have difficulty in ethical analysis, perhaps not surprisingly, since few teachers in medical schools have much experience of how to teach ethics, the law and moral philosophy.
- Formal examination is paramount to signify to students the importance of medical ethics.
- Staff development, 'teaching the teachers', and how to involve other professionals and non-professionals in teaching and learning roles is critical.

INTRODUCTION

This chapter will not enter the 'moral maze' of how ethics in medicine should be defined: few words are tossed around with such impunity. So ingrained in the practice of medicine is its ethical dimension that familiarity almost breeds a contempt of definition. Not a day passes without the media dwelling on presumed moral and ethical dilemmas raised in the course of medical practice and in complex issues raised by research and its application to medicine. Ask a prospective medical student at interview to give an example of an ethical matter they have recently read about: cloning, the human genome, euthanasia, rationing of health services, all trip off the tongue.

My starting point, a naive and simplistic one I admit, but one that I hope will strike a sympathetic cord of consensus, is that ethics in clinical medicine is, in its simplest form, about some sort of moral choice, about right and wrong conduct in medical care. Of course, in even this barest of definitions there will be controversy, since a relativism of moral viewpoint is inevitable, especially when theological, ethnic and cultural perspectives are embraced – as they must always be. Thus, for example, with a steady decrease in organized religion in many western countries, some of the basic tenets that have underpinned ethics values for so long, such as, for example, the notion of the absolute sanctity of human life, become untenable. The law allows, under certain conditions, the termination of pregnancy (an act that some would hold to be unethical). Yet the law will not usually uphold the right of a terminally ill person to take his or her own life – an act that some attending physicians might be sympathetic towards and, indeed, not question the ethical desirability of. A minefield indeed.

What I would like to do in this chapter is to raise a debate on how best we can sow the seeds of ethics and moral reasoning in the minds of undergraduate medical students in their training in order to help prepare them for the time when in their later professional practice they will be confronted with such problems. The fact that medicine has always to be practised within a legal framework is why issues of law are usually combined with ethics, as is the case in this chapter (although with much more emphasis given to ethics).

Rather than adopt a general overview, what I thought might be of more practical interest to readers would be to use as a basis for discussion how in our medical school we have approached and implemented in a new medical curriculum the improved appreciation of the ethical dimension of medical practice. Issues that emerge, difficulties, failures as well as successes, will, I am sure, resonate with others who, in a world of limited educational resources in medical ethics, are also grappling with this educational challenge.

HISTORICAL FOCUS

Recent decades have seen a steady increase in the time given to instruction in medical ethics in the standard medical curriculum in British medical schools. As long ago as 1950, the General Medical

Council recommended that medical ethics should be taught to all medical students.[1] In 1986, the British Medical Association called for all medical schools to provide curriculum teaching time for ethical and legal aspects of medical practice.[2] The Pond Report gave detailed information in 1987 on the current state of medical ethics teaching in British medical schools and gave advice how this instruction might best be given: not as a subject with a set syllabus added to an already overburdened curriculum, but by integration with all aspects of medical practice.[3] Local initiatives were especially to be encouraged, building on existing arrangements in individual medical schools.

June 1998 saw a seminal publication, a consensus statement for a core curriculum in medical ethics and law by teachers in British medical schools.[4] The main impetus leading to this publication were recommendations by the General Medical Council (especially those contained in *Tomorrow's Doctors*[5] that offered, in 1995, a blueprint for the radical revision of the undergraduate medical syllabus), which was continuing to emphasize the importance of ethics and key legal issues in medical education as core components in the medical curriculum. This is because the practice of good medicine, the quality of patient care, has invariably to embrace ethical and legal dimensions, and to help begin to resolve these an understanding of basic ethical principles is essential. Also, the recognition that to be a good doctor promoting the health and medical welfare of the people they serve, and societies in which they live, there must be fair and just respect of patient autonomy, beneficence, non-maleficence and justice – the four cardinal principles that underpin good medical practice. The good doctor must also embrace the virtues of honesty, humility and compassion and the core day-to-day working values of confidentiality, informed consent and non-prejudice. From the earliest stages of their medical training students need to appreciate these pillars on which the structure of the practice of good medicine is based.

SOWING SEEDS

A new integrated medical curriculum in Cardiff was introduced in 1995.[6] This anticipated, and was already implementing, many of these important recommendations. In the early planning stages, the curriculum planning committee decided to include medical ethics and key aspects of law in medical practice as an important core theme to extend through the 5 years of the medical course, starting in the first term. The coordination of ethics teaching is by one of 13 subject panels, the Health in Society Panel. Some of these topics were covered in the previous traditional curriculum, but mostly by serendipity in the course of clinical practice along with lectures in forensic medicine. But there was no coordinated plan.

We decided to introduce a theoretical basis of ethics in the first year, moving, in later years, into more patient-based clinical learning situations to illustrate and to make relevant these theoretical principles. This teaching of basic principles is given as a series of seminars, lectures and clinical demonstrations, spread over the first year, from a large number of teachers in the major clinical disciplines, supported by an honorary member of our teaching staff with special understanding of healthcare ethics and moral philosophy. In the latter half of the first year, each student spends a day (eight in total) in the major medical specialties, where they are also encouraged to reflect on both good and bad practices they see and ethical issues that might emerge from contact with patients.

Detailed learning outcomes are provided:

- understanding the various forms of consent to medical intervention, examination, investigation and treatment
- confidentiality and truth-telling and respect for the individual
- an early awareness of clinical ethical issues facing clinicians
- an introduction to some of the major principles that underlie ethical analysis – especially, patient autonomy, beneficence, non-maleficence and justice against a background understanding of human rights
- an introduction to the law relating to death, especially that relating to death certification, handling of cadavers for dissection, disposal of the dead and the coroner system
- religious issues in a multidenominational population (including transplant ethics, organ harvesting, importance of religious belief and organ-donation legislation); the important recognition that clinicians will often continue to be involved with families of the dead, indicating the continuity of care and compassion
- research issues, including clinical trials on patients and the role of research ethics committees; how advances in information technology are dramatically changing medical practice, especially the rapid advances being made in stem cell research; and to appreciate the issues of confidentiality, electronic medical records and the relation of clinical records to both research and healthcare systems
- to recognize that allocation of limited resources to a population, including dilemmas facing medical priorities in rich versus poor countries, requires prioritization; understanding the doctor has a duty of the just allocation of resources, personnel, equipment and medication, balancing professional care with the best possible clinical care.

We were mindful from the outset of the Pond Report recommendations[3] that some type of formal assessment was necessary to signal to students the importance of the study of medical ethics, and with special emphasis on powers of reasoning. From the beginning this was difficult because (a point discussed later) of limited human resources in our medical school to help design such assessment. Health ethicists hardly grow on trees in medical faculties. Most clinicians are not sufficiently well informed about the science of moral reasoning.

In the first couple of years of the new curriculum, students were required to select from one of their 8 days of clinical attachments an item of ethical interest, including examples of good or bad medical practice, analysing issues of ethical concern and how they were resolved, and to write a short commentary on this (which contributed to the summative assessment in the first professional examination in year 1). However, increasing concerns from both within and without (external examiners) that this written work was difficult to mark with no 'penalties' for students having worrying, negative perceptions of ethics, led us to discontinue this mode of assessment after 5 years. Instead, students are now given a few carefully prepared problems and must dissect out the ethical issues as short note written answers. How useful this new method of assessment is remains to be seen.

The next 2 years of our medical course sees an increase in clinical contact and lays down the foundations of the clinical method in medicine and surgery. Teaching and learning in ethics now moves away from more theoretical considerations to its application in day-to-day medical practice, including especially the core values that underpin good clinical practice: this helps students better conceptualize ethical problems in relation to specific patients. The family case study (where each student is allocated to, and follows for a year, a mother and her newborn baby) and a cancer project (which provides students with opportunities to look at the quality of end-of-life care) are two important additional clinical catalysts in these years to enhance ethics awareness. At the end of this 2-year period of study, students should be starting to develop a better practical understanding of ethics, to incorporate ethical and legal aspects in their interactions with all patients and to begin to appreciate issues of resource allocation. Additional opportunities are provided in 5-day special study components offered to pairs of medical students by the Department of Forensic Medicine, which involve up to 10–12 visits to the post-mortem room, the coroner's court, criminal court and/or scenes of suspicious death (if they occur during the attachment) and, most importantly, a day in the Medical Centre at the prison in Cardiff. At the end of the third year, our students have their second professional examination: included in this is an objective-structured examination (OSE) station examining ethics and legal understanding.

In clinical years 4 and 5, attachments of a more specialist nature in reproductive medicine, child health, mental disorders, palliative care, and medical and surgical specialities further broaden understanding and awareness of ethics and legal issues in special situations. In the final years, there is an 8-week 'Medicine in the Community' integrated attachment between general practice, community specialities and hospital medicine, which offers increasing contact with palliative care, ageing, special needs, community and institutional care. Students are expected to include in a learning portfolio reflections on ethical issues that have been observed during the attachment. During all their clinical attachments, students should have discussions of their experiences with ethics and law aspects with their clinical teachers. In years 1, 3 and 5, all students attend a series of professional awareness days, which give a particular emphasis on medico-legal aspects of the practice and duties of a doctor.[7] Towards the end of the final year, they consolidate core knowledge of legal documentation and its completion as part of their 6-week preparation for pre-registration.

DISCUSSION

In appraising our core teaching of ethics and law, we are, so far, reasonably reassured that the virtues of confidentiality, honesty and dealing kindly with patients seem to have been adopted and accepted widely, and acted on, by medical students. Palliative care, especially ethics surrounding disclosure of bad news and issues regarding death and end-of-life care, seems to have been particularly well assimilated. However, in their written work, students continue to show difficulty in grasping the basic building blocks of ethics understanding, which leads to weak analysis of ethical matters. We do need to provide more opportunities to discuss ethics and legal issues in the clinical years, but not as an isolated exercise. It is better to integrate this into the general curriculum, consistently forging links between rigorous moral and legal analysis and good medical and surgical practice, at the same time recognizing that a theoretical basis of understanding still has to be given. I would personally like a portfolio of ethics experiences to be collected over the whole 5 years of the curriculum and presented as a requirement for completion of medical studies. We need to

encourage, more than we do, all clinical disciplines to address relevant ethical and legal issues.

We conducted a student appraisal of the core course in ethics and law in the year 1999–2000 when the first students enrolled in the new curriculum were completing their final year. Overall, the 5-year course was well received, but there emerged some significant problem areas that we continue to address. An important issue relates to the bulk of theoretical ethics instruction taking place in the first year, at a time when students themselves perceive their own personal appreciation of ethics in medicine to be limited. Without much clinical exposure they recognize a difficulty to grasp practical application of theoretical principles. This leads to the possibility that the order is perhaps wrong. Perhaps ethics theory should lead on from, and not anticipate, clinical experience. But with our course structure, this is difficult.

Throughout the course, students are recognizing that ethics awareness is an integral part of patient management – the cement that binds together the skill of treating patients with the art of caring for them. There is, after all, an ethical element in almost every act of medical care. But this is not perceived by students as being sufficiently emphasized by clinicians during clinical attachments, although, when this does occur, it is not always recognized as such by the students. One problem could be that because in their day-to-day practice doctors themselves see ethics merging imperceptibly with clinical practice, separate consideration is seen not to be appropriate. I wonder also whether we have sometimes overestimated students' ability to grasp issues. On a warning note as well, patients do not like to think of themselves as 'ethics problems', so teaching in these areas needs careful and very sensitive consideration.

Compared with our 'old' curriculum, there is no comparison in the time allowed for students to reflect on ethical and relevant legal topics, their theoretical basis and their relevance to qualities of medical practice. But it is difficult to easure how effective this teaching is. The fact that in our professional examinations there are questions relating to medical ethics sends a signal to students of its importance – it was a strong recommendation of the 1987 Pond Report[3] that formal examination or assessment be made in order to signal to students the importance of medical ethics. But we do recognize that a particular challenge is to develop valid reliable measures for evaluating ethical awareness during education and training. In this assessment, powers of ethical reasoning are to be emphasized. Several tools have been described that enable aspects of students' moral reasoning powers to be given an objective score, such as the ethical sensitive rating used at the University of Toronto[8] and Kholberg's moral judgement interview.[9] These devices do, however, seem rather contrived and clumsy to the average clinician. Also, and a very important point, who in the curriculum will lead this formal assessment? Academic appreciation of ethics by the average clinical teacher is, at best, sketchy. Health ethicists who might be able to assess quality are few and far between. Our students quickly recognized that many of their teachers themselves have had little or no educational experience of how to teach ethics in a medical curriculum, and many teachers were therefore seen to be insecure in teaching in this area. Cardiff, I am sure, is not unique in this, and we are addressing the matter. Staff development, 'teaching the teachers', is critical.

Along with teachers drawn from clinical and social sciences, should other professionals also be involved? For example, theologians and lawyers? I am sure they should. Parents, and even children and young people themselves, could be involved if we could organize this. Clinicians who doubt their ability to justify their ethical judgements often benefit from this approach by learning in multidisciplinary settings. In turn, I am sure non-medical people may also gain greater insight into medical practice to help them better understand clinical, ethical dilemmas as they really are. There does, however, seem to be general agreement that the optimum format for learning is one that encourages student participation in small-group, case discussions led by a knowledgeable facilitator and based on actual cases. An example is given as Case Illustration 42.1.

Medical Declaration of newly qualified doctors of their intention to apply the highest possible standard of ethical behaviour in medical practice.[11] These have evolved from earlier declarations of the Hippocratic Oath.

But, in the final analysis, the best time to develop awareness and understanding of ethics and relevant matters of law in medicine is when the student has become a doctor and is actually faced with real dilemmas in day-to-day clinical practice. It is important to deal effectively and sensitively with these, the seeds that are being sown in the undergraduate years, which must be allowed to germinate in postgraduate professional training. But this is another story.

CONCLUSION

The importance the current generation of students in Britain attribute to ethics and the law in medicine, and their commitment to responsibilities and obligations in their future medical practice is encouragingly being reflected in an increased popularity of the

ACKNOWLEDGEMENTS

In preparing this manuscript I am most grateful for the help and wise counsel given to me by Professor Helen Houston and Dr Lorna Tapper-Jones from the Department of General Practice, Cardiff University.

Case illustration 42.1

A social dilemma in clinical paediatric practice: highlighting an ethical issue of parental responsibility versus responsibility of social services

The case

EC is an 18-month-old boy. The consultant had been asked by social services to evaluate EC as a suspected victim of child abuse. He was brought in by a social worker. On entering the consulting room, the immediate impression was that he was a happy, alert, well-nourished, clean, normal little boy. The social worker proceeded to tell the following story.

EC had been born to an unmarried, cohabiting couple who were both long-standing intravenous drug abusers. As a result, he had been put on the 'At Risk' Register and a social worker had visited him at home regularly throughout his short life. During this period the social worker had observed that EC had developed a very strong bond with his mother. He had always been adequately cared for, although the house was noticeably dirty and there were few toys for him to play with. His father had a known criminal record and seemed to spend very little time at home. His relationship with EC seemed to be virtually non-existent. A month before EC was brought in to see the consultant, social services had begun receiving distressing phone calls from the neighbours. They reported that EC's parents had started arguing a lot; this was taking place in the middle of the night and things were being thrown around in the house. EC had been crying a lot during these arguments, and witnesses said that some of this verbal abuse was being hurled at EC. The neighbours were also very worried that the parents may also have begun abusing EC.

As a result, EC was immediately removed from the parents' care by social services, with only supervised visits allowed. So it came about that EC ended up in hospital for an evaluation; on examination, the consultant found no evidence of physical or emotional abuse or any signs of neglect. Despite this, the social worker said it was unlikely that EC would be returned to his parents.

The ethical issue

Was it the right thing to do to take EC away from his parents?

Resolution and comment

In favour of this, we have the argument that the parents were living a life that is unacceptable to society, and the fact that the violent arguments which were taking place between the parents would not be good for EC's emotional development. Also EC would be brought up in a household where intravenous drug abuse was an everyday reality. Against this decision we have the following arguments: no evidence had been found that EC was being abused in any way by his parents. EC had bonded very strongly with his mother, so was it right to break that bond? Finally, does anybody have the right to break up a family at a time when the results of a breakdown in family values are all too evident?

In my view, I believe it was probably the right thing to do but, at the back of my mind, I wonder if he will think the same when he has grown up without his true family. Possibly EC will be left with emotional scars, whichever path was chosen.

Chapter Forty Three

The ethical principles for research with children

43

Neil McIntosh

SUMMARY

Good research with children is critical for the advancement of their care. Research must be properly performed, whether it is therapeutic or non-therapeutic. The sanction of a properly constituted ethics advisory committee should be in place before any research project is started. Consent in research with children is given by the parents, but in non-therapeutic research the child's assent is also mandatory, although this is not absolute in therapeutic research.

PRACTICE POINTS

- Before starting a research project, the answers to the following questions should be in the affirmative:
  - the question to be answered is important
  - there are enough patients available to answer the question
  - I have enough money to enable the answer to be found
  - my methodology will be rigorous
  - my analysis will be secure
  - I have local research ethics committee approval.
- During the research:
  - do not deviate from the protocol
  - give feedback to the patients/parents as to how the project is going
  - watch for side-effects if you are testing a new management strategy.

INTRODUCTION

Without research, medicine will stagnate. This is true as much for the management of the defenceless preterm newborn infant, as it is for the treatment of the child and adult. For this reason, it is my belief that in all medical practice it is unethical not to do research. To omit research in a particular group prejudices that group. This said, there are obvious qualifications to this approach, of which the most essential is that the research is carried out in the most

effective way possible on any individual or group of individuals. In infants and children there are some extra principles that are important, and these are outlined in Box 43.1. The key to all research is that it must be carried out in a proper fashion. A bad study will, at best, tell you nothing, and at worst, it may tell you things that are incorrect.

The four index Hippocratic ethical principles of autonomy, beneficience, non-maleficience and justice, should apply equally to children as to adults. They should also apply as much to research as to clinical management, although inevitably the emphasis may differ.

Autonomy

In our society, autonomy is the key principle relating to the individual. It recognizes that a person (of any age) is an individual first (*cogito ergo sum* – I think, therefore I am) and a member of society second (*sumus ergo sum* – we are, therefore I am). The autonomy of the individual is reflected in medicine by the need for consent to treatment and research. Consent in relation to research in children is considered below.

Beneficience

The Hippocratic tradition of medicine enshrines the sanctity of human life with a medical duty of care and a duty to act in the patient's best interests. In clinical medicine, the doctor is called on

---

BOX 43.1

Principles of paediatric research[1]

- Research involving children is important for the benefit of all children and should be supported, encouraged and conducted in an ethical manner.
- Children are not small adults; they have an additional unique set of interests.
- Research should only be done on children if comparable research on adults could not answer the same question.
- A research procedure, which is not intended directly to benefit the child subject, is not necessarily either unethical or illegal.
- All proposals involving medical research on children should be submitted to a research ethics committee.
- Legally valid consent should be obtained from the child, parent or guardian, as appropriate. When parental consent is obtained, the agreement of school-age children who take part in research should also be requested by researchers.

to evaluate treatment options for his patient. To do this, the physician needs to know (on the basis of probability) what is in the best interests of his patients, whether newborn infant, child or adult, balancing the benefits of the proposed treatment with the known risks. A neuroblastoma is a nasty malignancy. Following the diagnosis the chosen cytotoxic agent may well cause nausea and vomiting, mouth ulcers and alopecia but, the balance of benefit, may get rid of the tumour.

The dilemma in research is that we do not know whether it is in the best interests of the patient to be given the new treatment, or to carry on with the old until the research has been completed. If we did know, it would be unethical to give the second-rate treatment or diagnostic manipulation to 50% of the patients as this would not be in their best interests. To make researchers feel better, however, there are now two studies in the literature, one in oncology,[2] and one in neonatology,[3] which suggest that whatever arm of treatment you are in for a clinical trial, you will probably fare better as a patient within the trial than if you were receiving the treatment outside the trial.

Non-maleficence

Balancing the bad effects of a proven therapy with the benefits is relatively easy. The child's best interests can be served.

In research we may know the side-effects or we may not. We may not know their extent. It may be that the new cytotoxic agent has a far better cure rate than the old, but we do not know this until the research is done, neither do we know whether the side-effects may be much worse than with the conventional drug. Non-maleficence in research is critically important and is reflected in the outcome internationally of the Nuremberg Trials (for a good historical reference, see Shuster[4]) and the original recommendations of the Helsinki Declarations[5] (with the most recent update[6]). In addition, and most specifically, in most countries non-maleficence is reflected by local regulations, which in the UK and pertaining to children are set out in the Royal College of Paediatrics and Child Health Guidelines.[1]

In research, the possible downsides of the new treatment, should, in general, be no greater than those of the known treatment, unless the chances of successful treatment are significantly greater.

Justice

When a recognized therapy is available, it should be equally available to all children in need of it, not based on their race, social class or the social class of their doctor. The best available therapies must be on offer to children, but such therapy must have been evaluated by research. For the individual child, entering a trial of treatment is likely to give a child a better outcome.[2, 3] For children, in general, entry into a trial or study allows medical progress.

Overall, the ethics of treatment relate to a presumption that medical opinion has the answer to what is in the best interests of the child in a particular situation, whereas in research, because of equipoise, there is a presumption that medical opinion does not know what is in the best interests of the child, and therefore to do the research on the child (as part of a group) may well be ethical. If you give an unlicensed therapy outside a trial, all the patients get the benefit, but all take the risks and, as the therapy is not yet proven, all may get an inferior treatment. In a research trial, 50% of the patients get the benefit, and 50% only take the risks. But at the end of the trial, there is likely to be a clear answer as to whether the new treatment is beneficial or not.

TYPES OF TREATMENT AND DEGREES OF HARM

Research is often divided into therapeutic and non-therapeutic. In therapeutic research, the individual patient involved may get the benefit of a therapy within the trial. Alternatively, in non-therapeutic research there is no therapeutic benefit to the individual patient, but the body of knowledge may be increased from the work, possibly leading to more logical future management of children in general. With therapeutic research it may be appropriate to accept a significant downside of harm because of the morbidity of the condition or the side-effects of previous management strategies. With non-therapeutic research, however, it would be wrong to subject the child to any significant harm.

Risks are often estimated as being of high, low or minimal degree. High-risk procedures, such as liver or lung biopsy, or cardiac catheterization, would not be warranted for non-therapeutic research purposes alone. They might, however, be appropriate when the research is testing treatment that is intended to benefit the child. Low-risk procedures may cause brief pain and may leave bruises or scars. Such procedures would also not be appropriate, unless there was some direct benefit to the child in the research. Minimal-risk procedures, including observing and questioning children, can usually be carried out in a sensitive and non-stressful way. Similarly, collecting a urine sample (except by suprapubic aspiration) or a blood sample, when done at the same time as other samples are taken as part of treatment, is also not stressful in excess of the basic sampling, and we would view these as of minimal risk. The Royal College of Paediatrics and Child Health also clearly states its belief, that a single well-performed venesection, using local anaesthetic cream may be only minimally invasive and thus ethical.[1] But, if the child in anticipation of this procedure is distressed, or if he or she becomes distressed during the procedure, the procedure becomes low risk rather than minimal risk. For non-therapeutic research, only minimally invasive risk procedures are appropriate, and thus it behoves the researcher in performing such research to be honest with the child and the parents, and to promptly desist in the blood taking if the child does become distressed.

ETHICS COMMITTEES

Children are a vulnerable group as, in general, they are not allowed to make decisions on their own behalf. For research they are best protected (as are the researchers) by having the research protocols reviewed critically before starting a project by peers, funding bodies, scientific bodies and hospital ethics advisory committees (in North America these are called institutional review boards).

In the UK, local research ethics committees (LRECs) assess all projects before their commencement. Projects involving children should be assessed by committees that have within their membership people experienced in children's medicine, either/or both nursing or medical. The duties of the local committee are to satisfy themselves that the project sets out to answer a useful question or questions, that the project is designed in the best possible way to answer the question, and that the research will work in practice.

Quite often good studies involve more than one centre, and if more than five are involved a multi-centre research ethics committee (MREC) has the task of reviewing this research prior to the involvement of the LREC. Although this potentially works to the advantage of the research worker, who may not have to traverse so much red tape, the MRECs often do not have an experienced child-orientated member. Protocols approved by a MREC cannot be amended by the LREC, although the latter should ensure that there are no local objections to the study based on research facilities, known problems with investigators, or ethnic factors involved in the research. Research ethics committees safeguard both the patients and the researcher, and it is negligent for any research to be carried out without their sanction.

CONSENT AND CHILDREN'S INTERESTS

Children are the only people in British Law on whose behalf other individuals may consent to medical procedures. With many decades ahead of them, they are likely to experience the most lasting benefits from good research or, alternatively, harms from poor research. Research should not be performed on children, but with children, the researcher learning from the responses and attending to their interests as perceived by both the child and the child's parents as the research project progresses. This partnership should be such that the interests of the subject always prevail over those of society and science – i.e. they should be in accord with the Declaration of Helsinki.[5]

The law relating to research on children has never been clearly established, but children with sufficient understanding and intelligence to understand what is proposed should certainly be involved in the consenting process for any research, even though it is their parents who are required to consent by law. If a child can give a reasoned refusal to be involved in research, then it is clear that they have understanding, and it would be unwise in this situation to rely on parental consent. A younger child may be insufficiently mature to have any understanding, and in this situation valid parental consent must be obtained. Thus, research with children may normally be carried out only with the consent of the parents, but should also be with the assent of the child.

An exception to formal consent may be necessary where a research project is exploring the best treatment in an emergency. In this situation there may be nobody to give consent, or if there is the concept of informed consent may be impracticable or meaningless.[7] This does not sanction research without consent if there is a parent present. When research is carried out in emergency situations, consent is an ongoing phenomenon. Similarly, informed consent for an early entry into a randomized, controlled trial following the birth of a newborn baby cannot be as informed as consent obtained later, but it is still important at this point: later clarifications and information come from the 'continuing consent' process. Early consent is not likely to be educated, or with complete understanding, but continued dialogue with the parents about the trial protocol, and thus the concept of continuing permission, is important and makes the consent more valid.

Only someone with detailed knowledge of the research study should be obtaining the consent of the patient or parents, in the same way that it is the duty of the surgeon who will perform an operation to obtain the consent for that operation. When the researcher has obtained a signature on a form, this is not the end of it, and it does not mean that research can go on and on. Part of good practice on a consent form is a statement to the effect that the patient can withdraw from a study at any time without prejudice to their treatment. Parents should be supported throughout the research on their children by regular visits and discussions with the research team. Such discussions should proceed for as long as their child is involved in a research project and, similarly, beyond it with progress reports and time to ask further questions. In many cases it is important to inform the parents of the results of the trial when these are complete.

THE DOCTOR AS ADVISOR AND COUNSELLOR, OR PATERNALISM

Part of good clinical medicine is the doctor counselling as to what is in the best interests of the patient – this is not necessarily paternalism, but it may be. With an established doctor–patient relationship, trust is an essential element of good care, and in many cases the patients value this advice.

In the context of research, the research doctors are not free to offer counselling about involvement in a research project. This might logically be because in research (comparing two treatments), one does not know what is in 'the best interests of the patient'. In fact, it is because counselling is regarded as coercion and it would be suspected that the patient would not be consenting voluntarily to the research. This double standard might seem inappropriate. After all, when a patient is outside a research study a doctor can recommend an unproven medication to 100% of their cases. Surely, it is more ethical to recommend it to 50% of their cases in the context of a randomized, controlled trial?[8] How do we get round this problem? The short answer and the legal answer is, at the moment, we do not.

Some have postulated[9, 10] that a sensible way around the dilemma would be to have the research ethics committee taking responsibility for the decision, by positively recommending the treatment to the parents, but offering them the opportunity to reject the recommendation. Thus, Modi[9] suggests that an honest approach would be for the doctor to say.

We do not know which medicine is best, but we want to give your baby and every other baby in the same situation, a fair chance of getting the better treatment, whichever it is. For this reason we are recommending that all babies like yours are offered one or other treatment in a properly conducted way. My colleagues and I, and our Research Ethics Committee all believe this is the correct approach.

Zupancic et al.[11] explored the determinants of parental consent, and found that a significant proportion of parents agreed with the statement 'I would prefer to have doctors advise me whether my baby should be in the study, rather than asking me to decide'. An Australian study showed that 15% of parents had faith in their physician's advice, and thought that consent was unnecessary.[12] In a study at Edinburgh,[13] the parents of 150 babies entered into a randomized, controlled trial of surfactant, were followed-up at 18 months. Although 12% of parents could not remember having their infants involved in the trial (even though they had signed consent forms), most said that they wanted to be part of the decision on the enrolment.

The Zelan post-randomization consent process may be a way of allowing doctors to avoid explaining abstract concepts, such as randomization, to parents.[14] It also spares the doctor from the need to confess to medical uncertainty, which characterizes randomized controlled trials – 'I don't know which medicine is best'. Mason[15] suggested it might be appropriate to waive consent when comparing treatments, both of which can be considered as part of standard treatment. Others have suggested an opting out procedure, where parents sign only when they refuse, rather than grant, consent to the research.[16] All this is, at present, only a debate.

Doyle[17] viewed only three circumstances where patients (or a parental 'proxy') consent could be waived. Firstly, research carried out on patients incompetent to give consent (this would include children, but someone with parental authority is in a position to give consent); secondly, research without patient involvement, such as retrospective epidemiological research from medical records; and, lastly, the use of human tissues derived from surgical interventions or other stored clinical materials. The US Food and Drug Administration proposed four criteria where informed consent is unnecessary:[7]

- where the human subject is confronted by a life-threatening situation necessitating the use of the test article
- where informed consent cannot be obtained because of an inability to communicate with or obtain legally effective consent from the subject
- where time is not sufficient to obtain consent from the subject's legal representative
- where there is no available alternative method of approved or generally recognized therapy that provides an equal or greater likelihood of saving the subject.

CONCLUSIONS

Valid consent from parents is required before research is performed on any children. Where children have understanding, they should also assent to the research. The consenting procedure is not a single response, as it involves willing commitment that may falter during a long and difficult project. The families therefore need to be supported and informed frequently of how the research is going. No research should be carried out without ethical sanction from the LREC, MREC or, in the USA, the institutional review board.

Despite these constraints, to carry out research and to perform it well is critical for the improvement of practice. Only good research is ethical, and for the reasons detailed above it is negligent not to do research.

References, further reading and useful information

CHAPTER 1

References

1. Hart C, Chesson R. Children as consumers. *BMJ* 1998; **316**: 1600–1603.
2. Department of Health. *Choosing Health: Making Healthy Choices Easier*. London: Stationery Office, 2004. Available at: http://www.dh.gov.uk/PublicationsAndStatistics/Publications/PublicationsPolicyAndGuidance/PublicationsPAmpGBrowsableDocument/fs/en?CONTENT_ID=4097491&chk=KPBy7H (accessed January 2007), p. 67.
3. Scally G, Donaldson LJ. The NHS's 50th anniversary: clinical governance and the drive for quality improvement in the new NHS in England. *BMJ* 1998; **317**: 61–65.
4. National Health Service Executive. *A First Class Service: Quality in the New NHS*. Consultation document. London: Department of Health, 1998.
5. The Health Act. Chapter c8, London: The Stationery Office, 1999.
6. Kennedy I. *Learning from Bristol: The Report of the Public Inquiry into Children's Heart Surgery at the Bristol Royal Infirmary 1984–1995*. Command Paper 5207-1. London: The Stationery Office, 2001. Available at: http://www.bristol-inquiry.org.uk (accessed January 2007).
7. Dyer C. Government orders inquiry into removal of children's organs. *BMJ* 1999; **319**: 1518.
8. *The Royal Liverpool Children's Inquiry (Redfern Report). Summary and Recommendations ordered by The House of Commons*. 30 January 2001. Available at: http://www.rlcinquiry.org.uk/download/sum.pdf (accessed January 2007).
9. Laming WH (Chair). *The Victoria Climbié Inquiry Report*. Cm 5730 London: The Stationery Office, 2003. Available at: http://www.victoria-climbie-inquiry.org.uk (accessed January 2007).
10. Department of Health. *Getting the Right Start. National Service Framework for Children. Standard for Hospital Services*. London: DoH, April 2003, para 4.11:23. Available at: http://www.dh.gov.uk/PolicyAndGuidance/HealthAndSocialCareTopics/ChildrenServices/ChildrenServicesInformation/fs/en (accessed January 2007).
11. Department of Health. *Learning from Bristol: The Department of Health's Response to the Report of the Public Inquiry into Children's Heart Surgery at the Bristol Royal Infirmary 1984–1995*. London: DoH, 2002, Chap. 3. Available at: http://www.dh.gov.uk/PublicationsAndStatistics/Publications/PublicationsPolicyAndGuidance/PublicationsPolicyAndGuidanceArticle/fs/en?CONTENT_ID=4002857&chk=k6BnqM (accessed January 2007).
12. *Keeping Children Safe: The Government's Response to the Victoria Climbié Inquiry Report and Joint Chief Inspectors' Report Safeguarding Children*. London: The Stationery Office, 2003.
13. Bichard M. *The Bichard Inquiry Report*. London: The Stationery Office, 2004; Healthcare Commission NHS National Staff Survey, 2004; Commission for Healthcare Audit and Inspection, 2005.
14. Children Act 2004, Chapter 31. London: The Stationery Office, 2004. Available at: http://www.hmso.gov.uk/acts.htm (accessed January 2007).
15. Department for Education and Skills. *Every Child Matters: Change for Children*. London: The Stationery Office, 2003.
16. Department of Education and Skills. *Every Child Matters: Change for Children – An Overview of Cross Government Guidance, 2005*. Available at: http://www.everychildmatters.gov.uk (accessed January 2007).
17. Borrill CS, Carletta J, Carter AJ, et al. *The Effectiveness of Health Care Teams in the National Health Service*. Report. Universities of Aston, Glasgow, Edinburgh, Leeds and Sheffield.
18. National Confidential Enquiry into Patient Outcome and Death. *Functioning as a Team? The 2002 Report of the National Confidential Enquiry into Perioperative Deaths*. London: NCEPOD, 2002. Available at: http://www.ncepod.org.uk (accessed January 2007).
19. Healthcare Commission. *NHS National Staff Survey 2004*. Commission for Healthcare Audit and Inspection, 2005.
20. *Hidden Harm: Responding to the Needs of Children of Problem Drug Users*. Executive Summary of the Report of an Inquiry by the Advisory Council on the Misuse of Drugs. London: Home Office, 2003.
21. Commission for Social Care Inspection. *Safeguarding Children*. The second Joint Chief Inspectors' Report on Arrangements to Safeguard Children. Commission for Social Care Inspection, July 2005. Available at: http://www.safeguardingchildren.org.uk (accessed January 2007).
22. Department of Health. *Getting the Right Start: National Service Framework for Children. Standard for Hospital Services*. London: DoH, April 2003, para 4.11:23. Available at: http://www.dh.gov.uk/PolicyAndGuidance/HealthAndSocialCareTopics/ChildrenServices/ChildrenServicesInformation/fs/en (accessed January 2007).
23. Department of Health. *Shifting the Balance of Power: The Next Steps*. London: DoH, 2002.
24. Department of Health. *Standards for Better Health*. London: DoH, 2004.
25. Department of Health. *National Standards, Local Action: Health and Social Care Standards and Planning Framework 2005/06–2007/08*. London: DoH, 2004.
26. National Institute for Health and Clinical Exellence (NICE): http://www.nice.org.uk (accessed January 2007).
27. Aynsley-Green A. *Children's Charter for Health and Social Care Unveiled Today*. Press release 2004/0336. London: DoH, 15 September 2004.
28. Acting Chief Executive, CHI, Her Majesty's Chief Inspector of Constabulary, Acting Chief Inspector of Social Services. *The Victoria Climbié Inquiry Report. Key Findings from the Self Audits of NHS Organisations, Social Services Departments and Police Forces*. London: Commission for Health Improvement, 2003.
29. National Patient Safety Agency: http://www.npsa.nhs.uk (accessed January 2007).
30. Commission for Healthcare Audit and Inspection. *Healthcare Commission. Strategic Plan 2005/2008*. Available at: http://www.healthcarecommission.org.uk (accessed January 2007).
31. Healthcare Commission. *Improvement Review. Services for Children in Hospital. Management Summary*. May 2005. Available at: http://www.healthcarecommission.org.uk (accessed January 2007).

Further information

Clinical governance resources: http://www.ouls.ox.ac.uk/hcl/services/clinical_updates/clin_gov_pubs (accessed January 2007).

Institute for Healthcare Improvement (USA): http://www.ihi.org (accessed January 2007).

King's Fund, clinical governance reading lists: http://www.kingsfund.org.uk/resources/information_and_library_service/reading_lists/index.html (accessed January 2007).

National Audit Office, reports on clinical governance: http://www.nao.gov.uk (accessed January 2007).

NHS Clinical Governance Support Team: http://www.cgsupport.nhs.uk (accessed January 2007).

Royal Society Of Medicine, Clinical Governance Bulletin: http://www.clinical-governance.com (accessed January 2007).

CHAPTER 2

References

1. Children Act 1989. Available at: http://www.opsi.gov.uk/acts/acts1989/Ukpga_19890041_en_1.htm (accessed January 2007).
2. Children (Jersey) Law 2002. Available at: http://www.jerseylegalinfo.je/Law/display.aspx?URL=lawsinforce%5cconsolidated%5c12%5c12.200_ChildrenLaw2002_RevisedEdition_1January2006.htm (accessed January 2007).
3. Every Child Matters website – glossary – significant harm. Available at: http://www.everychildmatters.gov.uk/deliveringservices/multiagencyworking/glossary/?asset=glossary&id=22657 (accessed January 2007).
4. Information about parental responsibility, guidance from the BMA ethics department, 2006. Available at: http://www.bma.org.uk/ap.nsf/Content/Parental#Basicprinciples (accessed January 2007).
5. The Children (Northern Ireland) Order 1995. Available at: http://www.opsi.gov.uk/si/si1995/Uksi_19950755_en_1.htm (accessed January 2007).
6. Children (Scotland) Act 1995 s1(1). Available at: http://www.opsi.gov.uk/acts/acts1995/Ukpga 19950036_en_1.htm (accessed January 2007).
7. Gillick v West Norfolk and Wisbech Area Health Authority [1986] AC112.
8. Re W [1992] 3 WLR 758.
9. Shield JPH, Baum JD. Children's consent to treatment. *BMJ* 1994; **308**: 1182–1183.
10. Fraser Guidelines. Available at: http://www.confidentiality.scot.nhs.uk/publications/fraser%20guidelines.doc (accessed January 2007).
11. Wheeler R Gillick or Fraser? A plea for consistency over competence in children. *BMJ* 2006; **332**: 807.
12. Sterrick MJ. Competence in children has a Scottish twist. *BMJ* 2006; **332**: 975.
13. Cawson. *Child Maltreatment in the UK: A Study of the Prevalence of Child Abuse and Neglect*, NSPCC, 2000.
14. Department of Health, Home Office, Department for Education and Employment. *Working Together to Safeguard Children: A Guide to Inter-agency Working to Safeguard and Promote the Welfare of Children*. London: The Stationery Office, 1999. Available at: http://www.dh.gov.uk/PublicationsAndStatistics/Publications/PublicationsPolicyAndGuidance/PublicationsPolicyAndGuidanceArticle/fs/en?CONTENT_ID=4007781&chk=BUYMa8 (accessed January 2007).
15. Emergency Protection Order. Available at: http://www.opsi.gov.uk/si/si1991/Uksi_19911414_en_1.htm (accessed January 2007).
16. Every Child Matters website, Emergency Protection Order: http://www.everychildmatters.gov.uk/deliveringservices/multiagencyworking/glossary/?asset=glossary&id=22642 (accessed January 2007).
17. Section 8 orders. Available at: http://www.opsi.gov.uk/ACTS/acts1989/Ukpga_19890041_en_3.htm (accessed January 2007).
18. Children Act 1989, Section 17, Support for the child in need. Available at: http://www.opsi.gov.uk/acts/acts1989/Ukpga_19890041_en_4.htm (accessed January 2007).
19. Allen N. *Making Sense of the Children Act 1989*, 4th edn. London: Wiley, 2006.
20. Directgov, Government information website, information on Care Orders. Available at: http://www.direct.gov.uk/Parents/AdoptionAndFostering/AdoptionAndFosteringArticles/fs/en?CONTENT_ID=10027535&chk=sUcw31 (accessed January 2007).
21. Department of Health. *Promoting the Health of Looked after Children*. London: DoH, 2002. Available at: http://www.dh.gov.uk/PublicationsAndStatistics/Publications/PublicationsPolicyAndGuidance/PublicationsPAmpGBrowsableDocument/fs/en?CONTENT_ID=4098019&chk=hn54wN (accessed January 2007).
22. Adoption and Children Act 2002. Summary of legislation. Available at: http://www.compactlaw.co.uk/free_legal_information/adoption_law/adoptf16.html (accessed January 2007).
23. Mather M, Batty D, Payne H. *Doctors for Children in the Public Care*. London: BAAF, 2000.
24. British Association for Adoption & Fostering (BAAF): http://www.baaf.org.uk (accessed January 2007).
25. Every Child Matters: http://www.everychildmatters.gov.uk/strategy/guidance (accessed January 2007).
26. Every Child Matters. Local Safeguarding Children Boards. Available at: http://www.everychildmatters.gov.uk/socialcare/safeguarding/lscb (accessed January 2007).
27. Protection of Children Act 1999. Available at: http://www.opsi.gov.uk/acts/acts1999/19990014.htm (accessed January 2007).
28. Department of Health. *The Protection of Children Act 1999: A Practical Guide to the Act for all Organisations Working with Children*. Available at: http://publications.teachernet.gov.uk/default.aspx?PageFunction=searchresults&ft=protection+children+act&pn=1&rpp=1&ShowHide=4&Area=1 (accessed January 2007).
29. Criminal Justice and Court Services Act 2000. Available at: http://www.opsi.gov.uk/acts/acts2000/20000043.htm (accessed January 2007).

CHAPTER 3

References

1. Graham P. Mental health must be 'centre stage' in child welfare. *Arch Dis Child* 2000; **83**: 4–6.
2. Davis H, Day C, Cox A, et al. Child and adolescent mental health needs: assessment and service implications in an inner city area. *Clin Child Psychol Psychiatry* 2000; **5**: 169–188.
3. Meltzer H, Gatward R, Goodman R, et al. *The Mental Health of Children and Adolescents in Great Britain*. London: The Stationery Office, 2000.
4. Ross DP, Scott K, Kelly M. *Child Poverty: What are the Consequences?* Ottawa: Centre for International Statistics, Canadian Council on Social Development, 1996.
5. Lewis G, Sloggett A. Suicide, deprivation and unemployment: record linkage study. *BMJ* 1998; **317**: 1283–1286.
6. Scahill L, Schwab-Stone M, Merikangas KR, et al. Psychosocial and clinical correlates of ADHD in a community sample of school-age children. *J Am Acad Child Adolesc Psychiatry* 1999; **38**: 976–984.
7. Korenman S, Miller JE, Sjaastad JE. Long-term poverty and child development in the United States: results from the NLSY. *Child Youth Service Rev* 1995; **17**: 127–155.
8. Sure Start: http://www.surestart.gov.uk (accessed January 2007).
9. Taylor J, Spencer NJ, Baldwin N. The social, economic and political context of parenting. *Arch Dis Child* 2000; **82**: 113–120.
10. Babb P, Martin J, Haezewindt P. *Focus on Social Inequalities*. Office of National Statistics. London: The Stationery Office, 2004.
11. Bynner J, Joshi H, Tsatsas M. *Obstacles and Opportunities on the Route to Adulthood: Evidence from Rural and Urban Britain*. London: The Smith Institute, 2000.
12. Rose G. *The Strategy of Preventive Medicine*. Oxford: Oxford Medical Publications, 1992.
13. UNICEF. *Child Poverty in Rich Nations*. Florence: UNICEF Innocenti Research Centre, 2005.

CHAPTER 4

References

1. Stone B. Child neglect: practitioners' perspectives. *Child Abuse Rev* 1998; **7**: 87–96.
2. Rosenberg D, Cantwell H. The consequences of neglect – individual and societal. In: *Baillière's Clinical Paediatrics International Practice and Research: Child Abuse* (eds Hobbs CJ, Wynne JM). London: Ballière Tindall, 1993, Chap. 10.
3. *Childhood Matters – Report of the National Commission of Inquiry into the Prevention of Child Abuse*, Vol. 1. London: The Stationery Office, 1996.
4. *Working Together 1991. Working Together under the Children Act 1989. A Guide to Inter-agency Co-operation for the Protection of Children from Abuse*. London: HMSO, 1991.
5. Strauss MA, Kantor GK. Definition and measurement of neglectful behaviour: some principles and guidelines. *Child Abuse Neglect* 2005; **29**: 19–29.

6. *Child Protection: Messages from Research. Studies in Child Protection.* London: HMSO, 1995.
7. Cawson P, Wattam C, Brooker S, et al. *Child Maltreatment in the United Kingdom. A Study of the Prevalence of Child Abuse and Neglect.* London: NSPCC, 2000.
8. Oliver JE. Successive generations of child maltreatment: the children. *Br J Psychiatry* 1988; **153**: 543–553.
9. Department of Health. *Children and Young People on the Child Protection Registers Year Ended 31st March 2003.* London: DoH, 2003.
10. Spencer N. Poverty and child health in developed countries. In: *Poverty and Child Health* (ed. Spencer N). Oxford: Radcliffe Medical, 1996.
11. Frank DA, Zeisel SH. Failure to thrive. *Pediatr Clin North Am* 1988; **35**: 1–14.
12. Hobbs CJ, Hanks HGI, Wynne JM. Failure to thrive. In: *Child Abuse and Neglect: A Clinician's Handbook* (eds Hobbs CJ, Hanks HGI, Wynne JM). London: Churchill Livingstone, 1999, pp. 23–61.
13. Iwaniec D. An overview of emotional maltreatment and failure to thrive. *Child Abuse Rev* 1997; **6**: 370–388.
14. Pollit E, Eichler AW, Chan CK. Psychosocial development and behaviour of mothers of failure to thrive children. *Am J Orthopsychiatry* 1975; **45**: 525–537.
15. Benoit D, Zeanah CH, Barton W. Maternal attachment disturbances in failure to thrive. *Infant Mental Health J* 1989; **10**:185–202.
16. Hobbs CJ, Hanks HGI. A multidisciplinary approach to children who fail to thrive. *Child Care Health Dev* 1996; **22**: 273–284.
17. Dowdney L, Skuse D, Heptinstall E, et al. Growth retardation and developmental delay amongst inner-city children. *J Child Psychol Psychiatry* 1987; **28**: 529–541.
18. Taylor J, Daniel B. Interagency practice in children with non organic failure to thrive: is there a gap between health and social care? *Child Abuse Rev* 1999; **8**: 325–338.
19. Sure Start: http://www.surestart.gov.uk (accessed January 2007).

Further reading

Brown KD, Lynch M (eds). Editorial and review articles on child neglect. *Child Abuse Rev* 1998; **7**: 73–115.
Iwaniec D. *The Emotionally Abused and Neglected Child.* Wiley Series in Child Care and Protection. Chichester: Wiley ,1995.
Iwaniec D. *Children Who Fail to Thrive – A Practice Guide.* Chichester: Wiley, 2004.

CHAPTER 5

References

1. Caffey J. Multiple fractures of long bones of children suffering from subdural haematoma. *AJR* 1946; **56**: 163–167.
2. Caffey J. On the theory and practice of shaking infants. *Am J Dis Child* 1972; **124**: 161–169.
3. Jayawant S, Rawlinson A, Gibbon F, et al. Subdural haemorrhages in infants: population based study. *BMJ* 1998; **317**: 1558–1561.
4. Barlow KM, Minns RA. Annual incidence of shaken impact syndrome. *Lancet* 2000; **56**: 1571–1572.
5. Haviland J, Russell RIR. Outcome after severe non accidental head injury. *Arch Dis Child* 1997; **77**: 504–507.
6. Bonnier C, Nassogne M, Evrard P. Outcome and prognosis of whiplash shaken infant syndrome: late consequences after a symptom-free intervals. *Dev Med Child Neurol* 1995; **37**: 943–956.
7. The Ophthalmology Working Party. Child abuse and the eye. *Eye* 1999; **13**: 3–10.
8. Billmire ME, Myers PA. Serious head injury in infants: accident or abuse? *Pediatrics* 1985; **75**: 340–342.
9. Kivlin JD. A 12 year ophthalmological experience with shaken baby syndrome at a regional children's hospital. *Trans Am Ophthalmol Soc* 1999; **97**: 545–581.
10. Kleinman PK. Diagnostic imaging in infant abuse. *AJR* 1990; **155**: 703–712.
11. Fenton S, Murray D, Thornton P, et al. Bilateral massive retinal hemorrhages in a 6-month-old infant: a diagnostic dilemma. *Arch Ophthalmol* 1999; **117**: 1432–1434.
12. Morris AAM, Hoffmann GF, Naughten ER, et al. Glutaric aciduria and child abuse. *Arch Dis Child* 1999; **80**: 404–405.
13. Ommaya AK, Faas F, Yarnel P. Whiplash injury and brain damage: an experimental study. *JAMA* 1968; **204**: 285–289.
14. Duhaime AC, Alanio AJ, Lewander WJ, et al. Very young children: mechanism, injury types and ophthalmologic findings in 100 hospitalised patients younger than 2 years of age. *Pediatrics* 1992; **20**: 179–185.
15. Guthkelch AN. Infantile subdural haematoma and its relationship to whiplash injuries. *BMJ* 1971; **ii**: 430–431.
16. Brown JK, Minns RA. Non accidental head injury, with particular reference to whiplash shaking injury and medico-legal aspects. *Dev Med Child Neurol* 1993; **35**: 849–869.
17. Showers J. Shaken baby syndrome: the problem and a model for prevention. *Children Today* 1992; **21**: 34–37.

CHAPTER 6

References

1. *Childhood Matters. Report of the National Commission of Inquiry into the Prevention of Child Abuse.* London: The Stationary Office, 1996.
2. Working Together 2000. Children Act 1989. Available at: http://www.opsi.gov.uk/acts/acts1989/Ukpga_19890041_en_1.htm (accessed January 2007).
3. Royal College of Physicians. *Physical Signs of Sexual Abuse in Children,* 2nd edn. London: Royal College of Physicians, pp. 5, 21.
4. Paradise JE. Winter MR, Finkel MA, et al.. Influence of the history on physicians' interpretations of girls' genital findings. *Pediatrics* 1999; **103**: 980–986.
5. Frothingham TE, Hobbs CJ, Wynne JM, et al. Follow up study eight years after diagnosis of sexual abuse. *Arch Dis Childhood* 2000; **83**: 132–134.
6. Christian CW, Lavelle JM, De Jong AR, et al. Forensic evidence findings in prepubertal victims of sexual assault. *Pediatrics* 2000; **106**: 100–104.
7. Girardin BW, Faugno DK, Seneski PC, et al. *Colour Atlas of Sexual Assault.* Edinburgh: Mosby, 1997.
8. Pugno PA. Genital findings in prepubertal girls evaluated for sexual abuse. *Arch Fam Med* 1999; **8**: 403–406.
9. McCann J, Voris J, Simon M, et al. Perianal findings in prepubertal children selected for nonabuse. *Child Abuse Neglect* 1989; **13**: 179–193.
10. Berenson AB. Normal anogenital anatomy. *Child Abuse Neglect* 1998; **22**: 589–596.
11. Muram D. Child sexual abuse: relationship between sexual acts and genital findings. *Child Abuse Neglect* 1989; **13**: 211–216.
12. Centres for Disease Control and Prevention. 1998 Guidelines for the Treatment of Sexually Transmitted Diseases. *MMWR* 1997; **47**(RR1): 116.
13. Hammerschlag MR. Sexually transmitted diseases in sexually abused children: medical and legal implications. *Sex Transm Infect* 1998; **74**: 167–174.

CHAPTER 7

References

1. Department for Education and Skills. *Incredibly Caring.* A Training Pack in FII. Oxford: Radcliffe, 2006.
2. Wilson RG. Fabricated or induced illness in children. *BMJ* 2003; **323**: 296–297.
3. Royal College of Paediatrics and Child Health. *Fabricated or Induced Illness by Carers.* 2002. Available at: http://www.rcpch.ac.uk/publications/recent_publications/fii.pdf (accessed January 2007).
4. Department for Education and Skills. *Safeguarding Children in Whom Illness is Induced or Fabricated by Carers with Parenting Responsibilities.* London: Department of Health, 2001.
5. Department of Education and Skills. *Working Together to Safeguard Children.* London: Department of Health, 2006.
6. Coulthard M, Haycock G. Evaluation of hypernatraemia. *BMJ* 2003; **326**: 157–160.
7. McClure RJ, Davis PM, Meadow SR, et al. Epidemiology of Munchausen syndrome by proxy. *Arch Dis Child* 1996; **75**: 57–61.
8. Carpenter R, Waite A, et al. Repeat sudden unexpected and unexplained infant deaths; natural or unnatural. *Lancet* 2005; **365**: 29–35.

9. Foundation for the Study of Infant Deaths. *Responding When A Baby Dies*. Available at: http://www.fsid.org.uk/responding-baby-dies.html (accessed January 2007).

10. Royal College of Pathologists and Royal College of Paediatrics and Child Health. *Sudden Unexpected Death in Infancy. A Multiagency Protocol for Care and Investigation*. Report chaired by Baroness Helena Kennedy. London: RCP and RCPCH, 2004. Available at: http://www.rcpath.org/resources/pdf/sudi%20report%20for%20web.pdf (accessed January 2007).

11. British Paediatric Association. *Evaluation of Suspected Imposed Upper Airway Obstruction*. London: BPA, 1994.

12. Department of Health. *Framework for the Assessment of Children in Need and their Families*. London: The Stationery Office, 2000.

13. Eminson DM, Postlethwaite RJ. Munchausen Syndrome by Proxy Abuse. London: Arnold, 2000.

14. Southall DP, Plunkett MCB, Banks MW, et al. Covert video recordings of life-threatening child abuse: lessons for child protection. *Pediatrics* 1997; **100**: 735–760.

15. Eminson DM, Jureidini J. Concerns about research and prevention strategies in Munchausen syndrome by proxy. *Child Abuse Neglect* 2003; **27**: 413–420.

16. Confidential Enquiry into Stillbirths and Deaths in Infancy. *Sudden Unexpected Deaths In Infancy*. The CESDI. SUDI Studies 1994–96 London: HMSO, 2000.

17. Horwath J, Lawson B (eds). *Trust Betrayed*. London: National Children's Bureau, 1995.

CHAPTER 8

References

1. Butler I, Williamson H. *Children Speak: Children, Trauma and Social Work*. Harlow: Longman/NSPCC, 1994.

2. *Childhood Matters: Report of the National Commission of Inquiry into the Prevention of Child Abuse*. London: HMSO, 1996.

3. Welsh Child Protection Systematic Review Group. Core Info: http://www.core-info.cf.ac.uk (accessed January 2007).

4. Maguire S, Mann MK, Sibert J, et al. Are there patterns of bruising in childhood which are diagnostic or suggestive of abuse? A systematic review. *Arch Dis Child* 2005; **90**: 182–186.

5. Maguire S, Mann MK, Sibert J, et al. Can you age bruises accurately in children? A systematic review. *Arch Dis Child* 2005; **90**: 187–189.

6. Smith SM, Hanson R. 134 battered children: a medical and psychological study. *BMJ* 1974; **3**: 366–370.

7. Lynch A. Child abuse in the school age population. *J School Health* 1975; **45**: 141–148.

8. Carpenter RF. The prevalence and distribution of bruising in babies. *Arch Dis Child* 1999; **80**: 363–366.

9. Sugar NF, Taylor JA, Feldman KW. Bruises in infants and toddlers: those who don't cruise rarely bruise. Puget Sound Paediatric Network. *Arch Pediatr Adolesc Med* 1999; **153**: 399–403.

10. Dunstan FD, Guildea ZE, Kontos K. A scoring system for bruise patterns: a tool for identifying abuse. *Arch Dis Child* 2002; **86**: 330–333.

11. Atwal GS, Rutty GN, Carter N. Bruising in non-accidental head injured children: a retrospective study of the prevalence, distribution and pathological associations in 24 cases. *Forensic Sci Int* 1998; **96**: 215–230.

12. de Silva S, Oates K. Child homicide – the extreme of child abuse. *Med J Aust* 1993; **158**: 300–301.

13. Sussman SJ. Skin manifestations in the battered child syndrome. *J Pediatr* 1968; **72**: 99–100.

14. Johnson CF, Showers J. Injury variables in child abuse. *Child Abuse Neglect* 1985; **9**: 207–215.

15. Ellerstein NS. The cutaneous manifestations of child abuse. *Am J Dis Child* 1979; **133**: 906–909.

16. Kogutt MS, Swischuk LE, Fagan CJ. Patterns of injury and significance of uncommon fractures in the battered child syndrome. *AJR Radium Ther Nucl Med* 1974; **121**: 143–149.

17. Loder RT, Bookout C. Fracture patterns in battered children. *J Orthop Trauma* 1991; **5**: 428–433.

18. Prosser I, Maguire S, Harrison SK, et al. How old is this fracture? Radiologic dating of fractures in children: a systematic review *AJR* 2005; **184**: 1282–1286.

19. Ingram JD, Connell J, Hay TC, et al. Oblique radiographs of the chest in non-accidental trauma. *Emerg Radiol* 2000; **7**: 42–46.

20. Kemp AM, Butler A, Morris A, et al. Which radiological investigations should be performed to identify fractures in suspected child abuse? *Clin Radiol* 2006; **61**: 723–736.

21. British Society of Paediatric Radiology. NAI Standard for Skeletal Surveys. Available at: http://www.bspr.org.uk (accessed January 2007).

22. Worlock P, Stower M, Barbor P. Patterns of fractures in accidental and non-accidental injury in children: a comparative study. BMJ 1986; **293**: 100–102.

23. Eastwood D. Breaks without bruises are common and can't be said to rule out non-accidental injury. *BMJ* 1998; **317**: 1095–1096.

24. Matthew MO, Ramamohan N, Bennet GC. Importance of bruising associated with paediatric fractures: prospective observational study. *BMJ* 1998; **317**: 1117–1118.

25. Cadzow SP, Armstrong KL. Rib fractures in infants: red alert! The clinical features, investigations and child protection outcomes. *J Paediatr Child Health* 2000; **36**: 322–326.

26. Barsness KA, Cha ES, Bensard DD, et al. The positive predictive value of rib fractures as an indicator of non-accidental trauma in children. *J Trauma Injury Infect Critical Care* 2003; **54**: 1107–1110.

27. Reece R, Sega R. Childhood head injuries. *Arch Pediatr Adolesc Med* 2000; **200**: 11–15.

28. Hobbs CJ. Skull fracture and the diagnosis of abuse. *Arch Dis Child* 1984; **59**: 246–252.

29. Helfer RA, Slovis TL, Black M. Injuries resulting when small children fall out of bed. *Paediatrics* 1977; **60**: 533–535.

30. Tenenbein M, Reed MH, Black GB. The toddler's fracture revisited. *Am J Emerg Med* 1990, 8: 208–212.

31. Gabos PG, Tuten HR, Leet A, et al. Fracture–dislocation of the lumbar spine in an abused child. *Pediatrics* 1998; **101**: 473–477.

32. Levin TL, Berdon WE, Cassell I, et al. Thoracolumbar fracture with listhesis – an uncommon manifestation of child abuse. *Pediatr Radiol* 2003; **33**: 305–310.

33. Diamond P, Hansen CM, Christofersen MR. Child abuse presenting as a thoracolumbar spinal fracture dislocation: a case report. *Pediatr Emergency Care* 1994; **10**: 83–86.

34. Maguire S, Mann M, John N, et al. Does cardiopulmonary resuscitation cause rib fractures in children? A systematic review. *Child Abuse Neglect* 2006; **30**: 739–751.

35. Jayawant S, Rawlinson A, Gibbon F, et al. Subdural haemorrhages in infants: population based study. *BMJ* 1998; **317**: 1558–1561.

36. Geddes JF, Hackshaw AK, Vowles GH, et al. Neuropathology of inflicted head injury in children. I. Patterns of brain damage. *Brain* 2001; **124**: 1290–1298.

37. Geddes JF, Vowles GH, Hackshaw AK, et al. Neuropathology of inflicted head injury in children. II. Microscopic brain injury in infants. *Brain* 2001; **124**: 1299–306.

38. Kemp AM, Stoodley N, Cobley C, et al. Apnoea and brain swelling in non accidental head injury. *Arch Dis Child* 2003; **88**: 472–476.

39. Punt J, Bonshek RE, Jaspan T, et al. The 'unified hypothesis' of Geddes et al. is not supported by the data. *Pediatr Rehabil* 2004; **7**: 173–184.

40. Kemp AM. Investigating subdural haemorrhage in infants. *Arch Dis Child* 2002; **86**: 98–102.

41. Datta S, Stoodley N, Jayawant S, et al. Neuroradiological aspects of subdural haemorrhages. *Arch Dis Child* 2005; **90**: 947–951.

42. Morris AAM, Hoffman GF, Naughten ER, et al. Glutaric aciduria and suspected child abuse. *Arch Dis Child* 1999; **80**: 404–405.

43. Hight SW, Bakalar HR, Lloyd JR. Inflicted burns in children. *JAMA* 1979; **242**: 517–520.

44. Keen JH, Lendrum J, Wolman B. Inflicted burns and scalds in children. *BMJ* 1975; **4**: 268–269.

45. Yeoh C, Nixon JW, Dickson W, et al. Patterns of scald injuries. *Arch Dis Child* 1994; **71**: 156–158.

46. Barnes PM, Norton CM, Dunstan FD, et al. Abdominal injury due to child abuse. *Lancet* 2005; **366**: 234–235.

47. Whittaker DK, Aitken M, Burfitt E, et al. Assessing bite marks in children: working with a forensic dentist. *Ambulatory Child Health* 1997; **3**: 225–230.

CHAPTER 9

References

1. Wilson MH, Baker SP, Tenet SP, et al. *Saving Children. A Guide to Injury Prevention*. Oxford: Oxford University Press, 1991.

2. Foot H, Tolmie A, Thomson J, et al. Recognising the hazards. *Psychologist* 1999; **12**: 400–402.

3. Sinnott W. Safety aspects of domestic architecture. In: *Children, the Environment and Accidents* (ed. Jackson RH). London: Pittman Medical, 1977, pp. 76–90.

4. Towner E, Dowswell T, Errington G, et al. *Injuries in Children Aged 0–14 Years and Inequalities*. London: Health Development Agency, 2005.

5. Dowswell T, Towner E, Cryer C, et al. *Accidental Falls: Fatalities and Injuries An Examination of the Data Sources and Review of the Literature on Preventive Strategies*. Report No.: URN 00/805. London: Department of Trade and Industry, 1999.

6. Office for National Statistics. *Mortality Statistics*. Cause Series DH2 No. 29 Table 2.19. London: Office for National Statistics, 2004.

7. Office for National Statistics. *Mortality Statistics*. Cause Series DH2 No. 30 Table 2.19. London: Office for National Statistics, 2005.

8. Office for National Statistics. *Mortality Statistics: Injury and Poisoning 1997 and 1998*. London: HMSO, 1999 and 2000.

9. Roberts I, DiGuiseppi C, Ward H. Childhood injuries: extent of the problem, epidemiological trends and costs. *Injury Prevent* 1998; **4**: S10–S16.

10. Office of Population Censuses and Surveys. *Occupational Mortality: Childhood Supplement. Registrar General's Decennial Supplement for England and Wales, 1970–72*. London: HMSO, 1988.

11. UNICEF. *A League Table of Child Deaths by Injury in Rich Nations*. Innocenti Report Card. Report No. 2. Florence: UNICEF Innocenti Research Centre, 2001.

12. Malbut K, Falaschetti E. Non-fatal accidents. In: *The Health Survey for England 2002. Vol. 1: The Health of Children and Young People* (eds Sproston K, Primatesta P). London: The Stationery Office, 2003, Chap. 6.

13. Towner E. The role of health education in childhood injury prevention. *Injury Prevention* 1995; **1**: 53–58.

14. Towner E, Dowswell T, Simpson G, et al. *Health Promotion in Childhood and Young Adolescence for the Prevention of Unintentional Injuries*. London: Health Education Authority, 1996.

15. Millward LM, Morgan A, Kelly MP. *Prevention and Reduction of Accidental Injury in Children and Older People*. Evidence Briefing. London: Health Development Agency, 2003.

16. Brownscombe J, Simpson N, Lenton S, et al. The potential of emergency department injury surveillance data: an illustration using descriptive analysis of data in 0–4 year olds from the Bath injury surveillance system. *Child Care Health Dev* 2004; **30**: 161–166.

17. Bass JL, Christoffel KK, Widome M, et al. Childhood injury prevention counseling in primary care settings: a critical review of the literature. *Pediatrics* 1993; **92**: 544–550.

18. Schelp L. Community intervention and changes in accident pattern in a rural Swedish municipality. *Health Promotion* 1987; **4**: 109–125.

19. Child Safety Week: http://www.capt.org.uk/csweek/default.htm (accessed January 2007).

20. Spencer N. The role of the paediatrician in reducing the effects of social disadvantage on children. *Curr Paediatr* 1999; **9**: 62–67.

21. Sibert J, Craft A, Jackson R. Child-resistant packaging and accidental child poisoning. *Lancet* 1977; **ii**: 289–290.

22. Child Accident Prevention Trust: http://www.capt.org.uk (accessed January 2007).

23. Machonachie I. Accident prevention. *Arch Dis Child* 2003; **88**: 275–277.

24. Lee A, Mann N, Takriti R. A hospital led promotion campaign aimed to increase bicycle helmet wearing among children aged 11–15 living in West Berkshire 1992–98. *Injury Prevention* 2000; **6**: 151–153.

25. Frederick K, Bixby E, Orzel M, et al. An evaluation of the effectiveness of the Injury Minimization Programme for Schools (IMPS). *Injury Prevention* 2000; **6**: 92–95.

26. Colver A, Hutchinson P, Judson E. Promoting children's home safety. *BMJ* 1982; **285**: 1177–1180.

CHAPTER 10

References

1. The Right Honorable Lord Justice Wall. *Enforcement of Contact Orders*. Family Law. January 2005.

2. Cockett M, Tripp JH. *The Exeter Family Study*. Exeter: University of Exeter Press, 1994.

3. Emery RE, Fincham FD, Cummings EM. Parenting in context: thinking about parental conflict and its influence on children. *J Consult Clin Psychol* 1992; **60**: 909–912.

4. Jenkins JM, Smith MA, Graham PJ. Coping with parental quarrels. *Am J Adolesc Psychiatry* 1989; **28**:182–189.

5. Grych JH, Fincham FD. Marital dissolution and family adjustment: an attributional analysis. In: *Close Relationship Loss. Theoretical Perspectives* (ed Orbuch T). New York: Springer Verlag, 1993.

6. Rutter M. Resilience in the face of adversity: protective factors and resistance to psychiatric disorders. *Br J Psychiatry* 1989; **147**: 598–611.

7. Wallerstein JS, Lewis JM, Blakeslee S. *The Unexpected Legacy of Divorce: A 25 Year Landmark Study*. New York: Hyperion, 2000.

8. Hester M, Pearson C, Harwin N. *Making an Impact: Children and Domestic Violence – A Reader*. Philadelphia, PA: Jessica Kingsley, 1999.

9. Department for Education and Skills. *Every Child Matters – Next Steps*. London: The Stationery Office, 2004.

10. Amato P, Keith B. Parental divorce and the well being of children: a meta analysis. *Psychol Bull* 1991; **10**: 26–46.

11. Rogers B, Pryor J. *Divorce and Separation: The Outcomes for Children*. York: Joseph Rowntree Foundation, 1998.

12. Harold G, Pryor J, Reynolds J. *Not in Front of the Children? How Conflict between Parents Affects Children*. London: One Plus One Marriage and Partnership Research, 2001.

13. Pryor J, Rogers B. *Children in Changing Families: Life after Parental Separation*. Oxford: Blackwell, 2001.

14. Mansfield P, Collard J. *The Beginning of the Rest of Your Life*. Basingstoke: Macmillan, 1988.

15. Office for National Statistics. *Population Trends 117*, Autumn 2004, London: HMSO.

16. Smart C, Stevens P. *Cohabitation Breakdown*. London: Family Policy Studies Centre, 2000.

17. Amato P, Sobolewski JM. The effects of divorce and marital discord on adult children's psychological well-being. *Am Sociol Rev* 2001; **66**: 900–921.

18. Fincham D, Osborne L. Marital conflict and children: retrospect and prospect. *Clin Psychol Rev* 1993; **13**: 75–88.

19. Wallerstein JS, Kelly JB. *Surviving the Break Up: How Children and Parents Cope with Divorce*. London: Grant Mcintyre, 1980.

20. Emery R. *Marriage, Divorce and Children's Adjustment*. Thousand Oaks, CA: Sage, 1988.

21. Amato R. Children's adjustment to divorce: theories, hypotheses, and empirical support. *J Marriage Faro* 1993; **55**: 23–38.

22. Wadsworth MEJ, Maclean M, Kuh D, et al. Children of divorced and separated parents: summary of review findings from a long term follow up in the UK. *Fam Pract* 1990; **7**: 104–109.

23. Block JH, Block J, Gjerde PF. The personality of children prior to divorce: a prospective study. *Child Dev* 1986; **57**: 827–840.

24. Amato PR. Reconciling divergent perspectives: Judith Wallerstein, quantitative family research, and children of divorce *Fam Relations* 2003; **52**: 332–339.

25. Kelly JB, Emery RE. Children's adjustment following divorce: risk and resilience perspectives. *Fam Relations* 2003; **52**: 352–362.

26. Zill N, Morrison DR, Coiro MJ. Long-term effects of parental divorce on parent child relationships, adjustment, and achievement in young adulthood. *J Fam Psychol* 1993; **7**: 91–103.

27. The Home Office. *Supporting Families*. London: HMSO, 1998.

28. Dunn J, Deater-Deckard K. *Children's Views of their Changing Families*. Findings No. 931. York: Joseph Rowntree Foundation, 2001.

29. Campbell A. World Mediation Forum, University of South Australia, Adelaide, 2003.

30. Bridge J. Domestic Violence and Contact, 2005. Avaiable at: http://www.divorce.co.uk (accessed January 2007).

31. Maclean M. *Together and Apart: Child and Parents Experiencing Separation and Divorce*. Findings No. 314. York: Joseph Rowntree Foundation, 2004.

32. Walker J, McCarthy P. Marriage support services and divorce: a contradiction in terms? *Sex Relation Ther* 2001;**16**: 329–348.

33. Cockett M, Kuh D, Tripp JH. *Bridge over Troubled Waters*. London: HMSO, 1986.

34. Goodyer IM (ed). *The Depressed Child and Adolescent*, 2nd edn. Series in Child and Adolescent Psychiatry. Cambridge: Cambridge University Press, 2002.

35. *Family Law Bill*. London: HMSO, 1996.
36. Davis GC. Love in a cold climate – disputes about children in the aftermath of parental separation. In: *Family Law – Essays for the New Millennium* (ed. Cretney SM). Bristol: Family Law, 2000, pp. 127–142.
37. Davis GC, Bevan G, Dingwall R, et al. *Monitoring Publicly Funded Family Mediation*. London: Legal Services Commission, 2000.
38. Davis G. Reflections in the aftermath of the family mediation pilot. *Child Fam Law Q* 2001; **13**: 371–381.
39. Walker J. *Reflections on Research on Mediation*. Back to the Future. Newcastle: Centre for Family Studies, 2004.
40. Douglas A. *Walking the Tightrope of Family Disputes*. Family Law Week, July 2005. Available at: http://www.familylawweek.co.uk/library.asp (accessed January 2007).
41. Mellanby A, Phelps F, Crichton N, et al. School sex education: an experimental programme with educational and medical benefit. *BMJ* 1995; **311**: 414–417.
42. Trinder L, Beek M, Connolly J. *Making Contact: How Parents and Children Negotiate and Experience Contact after Divorce*. York: York Publishing Services, 2003.

CHAPTER 11

References

1. Royal College of Paediatrics and Child Health. *Strengthening the Care of Children in the Community: A Review of Community Child Health*. London: RCPCH, 2001.
2. Children's Rights Development Unit. UK Agenda for Children. London, 1994.
3. Guildea ZES, Fone DL, Dunstan FD, et al. Social deprivation and the causes of infant mortality. *Arch Dis Child* 2001; **84**: 307–310.
4. Spencer N. *Poverty and Child Health*, 2nd edn. Abingdon: Radcliffe Medical, 2001.
5. l'Hoir MP, Engelberts AC, van Well GT, et al. Case–control study of current validity of previously described risk factors for SIDS in the Netherlands. *Arch Dis Child* 1998; **79**: 386–393.
6. Murphy J, Newcombe R, Sibert JR. The epidemiology of sudden infant death syndrome. *J Epidemiol Commun Health* 1982; **36**: 17–21.
7. Kendrick D, Marsh P. How useful are socio-demographic characteristics in identifying children at risk of unintentional injury? *Public Health* 2001; **115**: 103–107.
8. Avery G, Vaudin JN, Fletcher JL, et al. Geographical and social variations in mortality due to childhood accidents in England and Wales 1975–1984. *Public Health* 1990; **104**: 171–182.
9. Smith GD, Hart C, Blane D, et al. Adverse socio-economic conditions in childhood and cause specific adult mortality: prospective observational study. *BMJ* 1998; **316**: 1631–1635.
10. Sherriff A, Emond A, Bell JC, et al. Should infants be screened for anaemia? A prospective study investigating the relation between haemoglobin at 8, 12, and 18 months and development at 18 months. *Arch Dis Child* 2001; **84**: 480–485.
11. Leach CE, Blair PS, Fleming PJ, et al. Epidemiology of SIDS and explained sudden infant deaths. CESDI SUDI Research Group. *Pediatrics* 1999; **104**: e43.
12. Heath PT, McVernon J. The UK Hib vaccine experience. *Arch Dis Child* 2002; **86**: 396–399.
13. Sibert JR, Craft AW, Jackson RH. Child resistant packaging and accidental child poisoning. *Lancet* 1977; **2**: 289–290.
14. Sibert JR, Payne EH, Kemp AM, et al. The incidence of severe physical abuse in Wales. *Child Abuse Neglect* 2002; **26**: 267–276.
15. Tudor Hart J. Commentary: three decades of the inverse care law. *BMJ* 2000; **320**: 18–19.
16. Webb E, Shankleman J, Evans MR, et al. The health of children in refuges for women victims of domestic violence: cross sectional descriptive survey. *BMJ* 2001; **323**: 210–213.
17. Polnay L, Ward H. Promoting the health of looked after children. Government proposals demand leadership and a culture change. *BMJ* 2000; **320**: 661–662.
18. Hodes M. Refugee children. *BMJ* 1998; **316**: 793–794.
19. Sibert JR, Mott A, Rolfe K, et al. Preventing injuries in public playgrounds through partnership between health services and local authority: community intervention study. *BMJ* 1999; **318**: 1595.

CHAPTER 12

References

1. Thomas M, Pierson J. *Collins' Educational Dictionary of Social Work*. New York: Harper Collins.
2. HM Government. *Working Together to Safeguard Children: A Guide for Inter-agency Working to Safeguard and Promote the Welfare of Children*. Available at: http://www.everychildmatters.gov.uk/resources-and-practice/IG00060 (accessed January 2007).

Further reading

Baldwin N (ed.). *Protecting Children. Promoting their Rights*. London: Whiting and Birch, 2000.
Barker J, Hodes D. *The Child in Mind. A Child Protection Handbook*. New York: Routledge, 2003.
Crompton S (ed.). Compass 2000: Career Opportunities for the Personal Social Services. Supported by BASW and TOPSS. Hucksters, 2000.
Fowler J. *A Practitioner's Tool for Child Protection and the Assessment of Parents*. Philadelphia, PA: Jessica Kingsley.
Hester M, Pearson C, Harwin N. *Making an Impact: Children and Domestic Violence – A Reader*. Philadelphia, PA: Jessica Kingsley, 1999.
Stanley N, Penhale B, Riordan D, et al. *Mental Health Services and Child Protection: Responding Effectively to the Needs of Mothers*. Bristol: Policy Press, 2003.

CHAPTER 13

References

1. Payne H, Butler I. Literature Reviews of Services for Children with Special Health Needs in Wales. Lot 7: Children who are Looked After in Placements, March 2002. Health and Social Services Committee, National Assembly for Wales. Available at: http://www.wales.gov.uk/servlet/HealthAndSocialServicesCommittee?area_code=37D6A89F00087B550000121400000000&document_code=3CBECEB40005FD7D0000372E00000000&p_arch=pre&module=dynamicpages&month_year=4|2002 (accessed January 2007).
2. Mather M. Adoption – a forgotten paediatric specialty *Arch Dis Child* 1999; **81**: 492–495.
3. Mather M, Batty D, Payne H. *Doctors For Children In Public Care – A Resource Guide Advocating, Protecting and Promoting Health*. London: BAAF, 2000.
4. Triseliotis J, Feast J, Kyle F. *The Adoption Triangle Revisited – A Study of Adoption, Search and Reunion Experiences*. London: BAAF, 2005.
5. *Holy Bible*, Exodus, Chaps 1–14. Available at: http://www.holybible.com (accessed January 2007).
6. Sophocles. Oedipus Tyrannos. Available at: http://www.users.global.net.co.uk/~loxias/myth.htm (accessed January 2007).
7. William Shakespeare. *As You Like It*. Available at: http://www.shakespeare.org.uk (accessed January 2007).
8. Charles Dickens. *Oliver Twist*. Available at: http://www.online-literature.com/dickens/olivertwist (accessed January 2007).
9. Reich D, Batty D. *The Adoption Triangle. A Training Pack on Adoption. Services – One Day Module*. London: BAAF, 1980.
10. Batty D. The interface between medicine and social work in working with looked after children. *Adopt Foster* 2002; **26**: 26–34.
11. British Association for Adoption and Fostering. *The Placement of Children with Disabilities*. BAAF Practice Note 34. London: BAAF, undated.
12. British Association for Adoption and Fostering. *The Children Act 1989. Implications for Medical Practitioners*. BAAF Practice Note 28. London: BAAF, undated.
13. Payne H. The health of children in public care. *Curr Opin Psychiatry* 2000; **13**: 381–388.
14. Monck E, Reynolds J, Wigfall V. *The Role of Concurrent Planning – Making Permanent Placements for Young Children*. London: BAAF, 2003.
15. Children Act 1989. Available at: http://www.opsi.gov.uk/acts/acts1989/Ukpga_19890041_en_1.htm (accessed January 2007).
16. Masson J. The Impact of the Adoption and Children Act 2002. Part 1: parental responsibility. *Fam Law* 2003; **8**: 580–584.
17. Selwyn J, Quinton D. Stability, permanence, outcomes and support: foster care and adoption compared *Adopt Foster* 2004; 28: 6–15.

18. Bailey-Harris R, Barron J, Pearce J. From utility to rights? The presumption of contact in practice. *Int J Law Policy Fam* 1999; **13**: 111–131.
19. Ball C. The Adoption and Children Act 2002 – a critical examination. *Adopt Foster* 2005; **29**: 6–17.
20. Neil E. Contact after adoption: the role of agencies in making and supporting plans. *Adopt Foster* 2002; **26**: 25–38.
21. Payne H, Butler I. *Mental Health of Children in Need*. Quality Protects Briefing No. 9. London: Department for Education and Skills, 2004.
22. Richardson J. *The Mental Health of Looked After Children. Bright Futures: Working with Vulnerable Young People*. London: Mental Health Foundation, 2002.
23. Department for Education and Skills. *Quality Protects*. Available at: http://www.dfes.gov.uk/qualityprotects (accessed January 2007).
24. Welsh Assembly Government. *Children First*. Available at: http://www.childrenfirst.wales.gov.uk (accessed January 2007).
25. Ruggles A, Po M. *Quality Protects. Health of Looked After Children. Work programme*. Available at: http://www.dfes.gov.uk/quality protects/work_pro/project_7.shtml (accessed January 2007).
26. Melzer H, Corbin, T, Gatwood R, et al. *The Mental Health of Young People Looked After by Local Authorities in England. Summary Report*. Norwich: The Stationery Office, 2003. Available at: http://www.statistics.gov.uk/downloads/theme_health/Mental_health_children_in_LAs.pdf (accessed January 2007).
27. Children (Leaving Care) Act 2000. London: The Stationery Office, 2000. Available at: http://www.opsi.gov.uk/acts/acts2000/20000035.htm (accessed January 2007).
28. Department of Health. Children (Leaving Care) Act 2000. Regulations and Guidance. Available at: http://www.dfes.gov.uk/qualityprotects/pdfs/regs2000.pdf (accessed January 2007).
29. Department of Health. *Promoting the Health of Looked After Children*. London: The Stationery Office, 2002. Available at: http://www.dh.gov.uk/assetRoot/04/08/92/61/04089261.pdf (accessed January 2007).
30. British Association for Adoption and Fostering. *Using the BAAF Health Assessment Forms – Setting Standards of Health Practice Across all Agencies*. BAAF Practice Note 47. London: BAAF, 2004.
31. Department of Health. National Standards for the Provision of Children's Advocacy Services (2002). Available at: http://www.dh.gov.uk/assetRoot/04/01/88/93/04018893.pdf (accessed January 2007).
32. The Adoption Agencies Regulations (2005). Available at: http://www.opsi.gov.uk/si/si2005/20050389.htm (accessed January 2007).
33. The Adoption Agencies (Wales) Regulations (2005). Available at: http://www.uk-legislation.hmso.gov.uk/legislation/wales/wsi2005/20051313e.htm#9 (accessed January 2007).
34. Butler I, Payne H. The health of children looked after by local authorities. *Adopt Foster* 1997; **21**: 28–35.
35. Piaget J. Child psychodevelopmental stages. Available at: http://www.uca.ac.uk/edu/learn/morphett/piaget.htm (accessed January 2007).
36. Phillips R, McWilliam E (eds). *After Adoption: Working with Adoptive Families*. London: BAAF, 1996.
37. Phillips R (ed.). *Children Exposed to Parental Substance Misuse – Implications for Family Placement*. London: BAAF, 2004.
38. Harper PS. *Practical Genetic Counselling*, 6th edn. London: Arnold, 2004.
39. Clarke A, Payne H. Predictive genetic testing in adoption. In: *Secrets in the Genes – Adoption, Inheritance and Genetic Disease* (ed. Turnpenny P). London: BAAF, 1995.
40. British Association for Adoption and Fostering. *Undertaking Competence Assessments*. BAAF Practice Note 40 London: BAAF, 2000.
41. British Association for Adoption and Fostering. *Health Screening of Children Adopted from Abroad*. BAAF Practice Note 46. London: BAAF, undated.
42. Tragedy of the babies bought for a pittance, sold for a fortune. *The Times* 17 July 2005. Available at: http://www.timesonline.co.uk (accessed January 2007).

Further information

British Agencies for Adoption and Fostering (BAAF). Membership of BAAF is available from: BAAF, Skyline House, 200 Union Street, London SE1 0LX. Subscription includes *Adoption and Fostering*, the quarterly house journal, which is multidisciplinary and peer reviewed. http://www.baaf.co.uk (accessed January 2007).

CHAPTER 14

References

1. Department for Education and Skills. *Sex and Relationship Guidance*. London: HMSO, 2000.
2. Ofsted. *Sex and Relationships. A Report*. London: HM Chief Inspector of Schools, 2002.
3. Kirby D. *Emerging Answers: Research Findings on Programs to Reduce Teen Pregnancy*. Washington DC: National Campaign to Prevent Teen Pregnancy, 2001.
4. Stephenson J, Strange V, Forrest S, et al. Pupil-led sex education in England (RIPPLE study): cluster-randomised intervention trial. *Lancet* 2004; **364**: 338–346.
5. Rees JB, Mellanby AR, White J, et al. Added Power And Understanding in Sex Education (APAUSE): a sex education intervention staffed predominantly by school nurses. In: *Evidence-based Child Health Care* (eds Glasper A, Ireland L). Basingstoke: Macmillan, 2000, pp. 203–223.
6. Blenkinsop S, Wade P, Benton T, et al. *Evaluation of the APAUSE Sex and Relationships Education Programme*. Slough: National Foundation for Educational Research, 2004.

Further reading

Ajzen I. Theory of planned behaviour. *Organisation Behav Human Decision Process* 1991; **50**: 179–211.
Bandura A. Health promotion by social cognitive means. *Health Educ Behav* 2004; **31**: 143–164.
Mellanby AR, Phelps FA, Crichton NJ, et al. School sex education: an experimental programme with educational and medical benefit. *BMJ* 1995; **311**: 414–417.
Mellanby AR, Newcombe RG, Rees JB, et al. A comparative study of peer-led and adult-led school sex education. *Health Educ Res* 2001; **16**: 481–492.
Phelps FA, Mellanby AR, Crichton NJ, et al. Sex education: the effect of a peer led programme on pupils (aged 13–14 years) and their peer leaders. *Health Educ* 1994; **53**: 127–139.
Rees JB, Mellanby AR, Tripp JH. Peer led sex education in the classroom. In: *Teenage Sexuality, Health, Risk and Education* (eds Coleman JC, Roker D). London: Harwood, 1998, pp. 137–162.
Wellings K, Wadsworth J, Johnson AM, et al. Provision of sex education and early sexual experience: the relation examined. *BMJ* 1995; **311**: 417–420.
Whitehead BD. The failure of sex education. *Atlantic Monthly* 1994; **274**: 55–80.
Wight D, Raab GM, Henderson M, et al. Limits of teacher delivered sex education: interim behavioural outcomes from randomised trial. *BMJ* 2002; **324**: 1430.

Further information

APAUSE programme. http://www.pms.ac.uk/apause (accessed January 2007).

CHAPTER 15

References

1. Scott S. Aggressive behaviour in childhood. *BMJ* 1998; **316**: 202–206.
2. Moffit TE. Adolescence-limited and life-course-persistent antisocial behavior: a developmental taxonomy. *Psychol Rev* 1993; **100**: 674–701.
3. Moffit TE, Caspi A. Childhood predictors differentiate life-course persistent and adolescence-limited antisocial pathways among males and females. *Dev Psychopathol* 2001; **13**: 355–375.
4. Moffit TE, Harrington HL. Delinquency across development: the natural history of antisocial behaviour in the Dunedin multidisciplinary health and development study. In: *The Dunedin Study: From Birth to Adulthood* (eds Stanton W, Silva PA). Oxford: Oxford University Press, 1994.
5. Farrington DP. The development of offending and anti-social behaviour from childhood: key findings from the Cambridge Study in Delinquent Development. *J Child Psychol Psychiatry* 1995; **36**: 929–964.
6. Stallard P, Thomason J, Churchyard S. The mental health of young people attending a Youth Offending Team: a descriptive study. *J Adolesc* 2003; **26**: 33–43.

7. Hill P. Attention deficit hyperactivity disorder. *Arch Dis Child* 1998; **79**: 381–384.

8. Woolfenden SR, Williams K, Peat JK. Family and parenting interventions for conduct disorder and delinquency: a meta-analysis of randomised controlled trials. *Arch Dis Paediatr* 2002; **86**: 251–256.

9. Farrinton DP. The challenge of teenage anti-social behaviour. In: *Psychosocial Disturbances in Young People: Challenges for Prevention* (ed. Rutter M). Cambridge: Cambridge University Press, 1995.

10. Taylor J, Spencer N, Baldwin N. Social, economic and political context of parenting. *Arch Dis Paediatr* 2000; **82**: 113–120.

11. Hoghughi M, Speight ANP. Good enough parenting for all children – a strategy for a healthier society. *Arch Dis Child* 1998; **78**: 293–296.

12. Labour Party Press Briefing. Labour party calls for national debate on parenting: discussion paper on parenting by Jack Straw and Janet Anderson. 1996. Available at: http://pages.britishlibrary.net/altcamden/2002/labparent.htm (accessed January 2007).

13. Hall DMB, Roberts H. What is Sure Start? *Arch Dis Child* 2000; **82**: 435–437.

14. Sure Start. Available at: at http://www.surestart.gov.uk (accessed January 2007).

15. UNICEF. *Child Poverty in Rich Countries 2005*. Innocenti Report Card, No.6. Geneva. UNICEF, 2005.

16. Spencer N. The role of the paediatrician in reducing the effects of social disadvantage on children. *Curr Paediatr* 1999; **9**: 62–67.

17. Toward Equity in Health: A Joint Meeting of the Royal College of Paediatrics and Child Health and the American Academy of Pediatrics September 2000. *Pediatrics* 2003; **112**(Suppl): 701–772.

18. Hill P, Taylor E. An auditable protocol for treating attention deficit/hyperactivity disorder *Arch Dis Child* 2001; **84**: 404–409.

19. *Paediatric Clinics of North America*, October 1999 (themed issue on ADHD).

20. Simonoff, E. Children with psychiatric disorders and learning disabilities. *BMJ* 2005; **330**: 742–743.

21. Hall DMB, Elliman D. *Health for All Children*, 4th edn. Oxford: Oxford University Press, 2004.

22. Webb E, Shankleman J, Evans MR, et al. The health of children in refuges for women victims of domestic violence: cross sectional descriptive survey. *BMJ* 2001; **323**: 210–213.

23. Hayes S. *Hayes' Ability Screening Index (HASI) Manual*. Sydney: Department of Behavioural Sciences in Medicine, University of Sydney, 2000.

24. Goodman R. The Strengths and Difficulties Questionnaire: a research note. *J Child Psychol Psychiatry Allied Disciplines* 1997; **38**; 581–586.

25. Gould J, Payne H. Health needs of children in prison. *Arch Dis Child* 2004; **89**: 549–550.

26. Goldsen B. *Vulnerable Inside: Children in Secure and Penal Settings*. London. The Children's Society, 2002.

27. Stuart M, Baines C. *Safeguards for Vulnerable Children: Three Studies on Abusers, Disabled Children and Children in Prison*. York. Joseph Rowntree Foundation, 2004.

28. Webb E. Health services: who are the best advocates for children? *Arch Dis Child* 2002; **87**: 175–177.

29. Webb EVJ. Discrimination against children: developing a conceptual framework *Arch Dis Child* 2004; **89**: 804–808.

30. Howard League for Penal Reform: http://www.howardleague.org (accessed January 2007).

CHAPTER 16

References

1. Behnke M, Eyler FD, Garvan CW, et al. The search for congenital malformations in newborns with fetal cocaine exposure. *Pediatrics* 2001; **107**: e74.

2. Chasnoff IJ, Bussey ME, Savich R, et al. Perinatal cerebral infarction and maternal cocaine use. *J Pediatr* 1986; **108**: 456–459.

3. Stone ML, Salerno LJ, Green M, et al. Narcotic addiction in pregnancy. *Am J Obstet Gynecol* 1971; **109**: 716–723.

4. Olsen GD, Sommer KM, Wheeler PL, et al. Accumulation and clearance of morphine 3-β-D-glucuronide in fetal lambs. *J Pharmacol Exp Ther* 1988; **247**: 576–584.

5. Claman AD, Strang RI. Obstetric and gynecologic aspects of heroin addiction. *Am J Obstet Gynecol* 1962; **83**: 2520150257.

6. Van Baar AL, Fleury P, Soepatmi S, et al. Neonatal behaviour after drug dependent pregnancy. *Arch Dis Child* 1989; **64**: 235–240.

7. Hammer RP, Ricalde AA, Seatriz JV. Effects of opiates on brain development. *Neurotoxicology* 1989; **10**: 475–484.

8. Ornoy A, Michaelevskaya V, Lukashov I, et al. The developmental outcome of children born to heroin dependant mothers, raised at home or adopted. *Child Abuse Neglect* 1996; **20**: 385–396.

9. Frank DA, Augustyn MG, Wanda GK, et al. Growth, development, and behavior in early childhood following prenatal cocaine exposure. *JAMA* 2001; **285**: 1613–1625.

10. Jones HE, Johnson RE, Jasinski DR, et al. Buprenorphine versus methadone in the treatment of pregnant opioid-dependent patients: effects on the neonatal abstinence syndrome. *Drug Alcohol Depend* 2005; **79**: 1–10.

11. Finnegan LP. Neonatal abstinence. In: *Current Therapy in Neonatal–Perinatal Medicine* (ed. Nelson NM). Toronto: BC Decker, 1985, pp. 262–270.

12. Ostrea EM. Infants of drug-dependent mothers. In: *Current Paediatric Therapy*, Vol. 14 (eds Burg FD, Ingelfinger JR). Philadelphia, PA: WB Saunders, 1993, pp. 800–801.

13. Lipsitz PJ. A proposed narcotic withdrawal score for use with newborn infants: a pragmatic evaluation of its efficacy. *Clin Pediatr* 1975; **14**: 592–594.

14. Rivers R. Infants of drug addicted mothers. In: *Textbook of Neonatology* (eds Rennie JM, Roberton NRC). London: Churchill Livingstone, 1999, pp. 443–451.

CHAPTER 17

References

1. Spencer NJ. *Poverty and Child Health*, 2nd edn. Oxford: Radcliffe Medical, 2000.

2. Smith T. Influence of socioeconomic factors on attaining targets for reducing teenage pregnancies. *BMJ* 1993; **306**: 1232–1235.

3. Department of Health. *Health Survey for England: The Health of Young People '95–'97*. London: TSO, 1998

4. Berg I. School refusal and truancy. *Arch Dis Child* 1997; **76**: 90–91.

5. Kolvin I, Miller FJW, Fleeting M, et al. Risk/protective factors for offending with particular reference to deprivation. In: *Studies of Psychosocial Risk* (ed. Rutter M). Cambridge: Cambridge University Press, 1988.

6. UNICEF. *Child Poverty in Rich Nations, 2005*. Innocenti Report Card No. 6. Florence: UNICEF Innocenti Research Centre, 2005.

7. Flaherty J, Viet-Wilson J, Dornan P. *Poverty: The Facts*, 5th edn. London: Child Poverty Action Group, 2004.

8. Kuh D, Ben-Shlomo Y. *A Life Course Approach to Chronic Disease Epidemiology*. Oxford: Oxford University Press, 1997.

9. Garrett P, Ng'andu N, Ferron J. Poverty experiences of young children and the quality of their home environments. *Child Dev* 1994; **65**: 331–345.

10. Sidebotham P, Heron J, Golding J, et al. Child maltreatment in the 'Children of the Nineties': deprivation, class and social networks. *Child Abuse Neglect* 2002; **26**: 1243–1259.

11. Meltzer H, Gatward R, Goodman R, et al. *The Mental Health of Children and Adolescents in Great Britain*. London: The Stationery Office, 2000.

12. Barker DJ. The developmental origins of chronic adult disease. *Acta Paediatr* 2004; **93**(Suppl): 26–33.

13. Spencer NJ, Bambang S, Logan S, et al. Socio-economic status and birth weight: comparison of an area-based measure with the Registrar General's social class. *J Epidemiol Commun Health* 1999; **53**: 495–498.

14. Wilkinson R. *Unhealthy Societies: The Afflictions of Inequality*. London: Routledge, 1996.

15. NHS Centre for Reviews and Dissemination. *Review of the Research on the Effectiveness of Health Service Interventions to Reduce Variations in Health*. CRD Report 3. University of York: CRD, 1995.

16. Roberts H. Reducing inequalities in child health. In: *What Works: Effective Care Services for Children and Families* (eds McNeish D, Newman T, Roberts H). London: Open University Press, 2002, pp. 232–251.

17. Hewlett SA. *Child Neglect in Rich Nations*. New York: Unicef, 1993.

18. Southall D, Abbasi K. Protecting children from armed conflict. *BMJ* 1998; **7144**: 1549–1551.

19. Cook J, Pcchcvis M, Waterstone A. Community participation and community diagnosis. In: *Social Paediatrics* (eds Lindstrom B, Spencer N). Oxford: Oxford University Press, 1995.

Further information

Childhealth Advocacy International: http://www.childadvocacy international.co.uk (accessed January 2007).

Children's Commissioner, England: http://www.childrenscommissioner.org (accessed January 2007).

Children's Commissioner, Northern Ireland: http://www.niccy.org (accessed January 2007).

Children's Commissioner, Scotland: http://www.scotland.gov.uk/about/ ED/CnF/00017842/Commissioner.aspx (accessed January 2007).

Children's Commissioner, Wales: http://www.childcom.org.uk (accessed January 2007).

UNCRC course for health workers available at: www.essop.org/essop-refs.html (accessed January 2007).

What Works for Children: www.whatworksforchildren.org.uk (accessed January 2007).

CHAPTER 18

References

1. Department of Health. *Getting the Right Start: National Service Framework for Children. Standard for Hospital Services*. London: DoH, April 2003, para 4.11:23. Available at: http://www.dh.gov.uk/ PolicyAndGuidance/HealthAndSocialCareTopics/ChildrenServices/ ChildrenServicesInformation/fs/en (accessed January 2007).
2. Department for Education and Skills. *Every Child Matters: Change for Children*. London: HMSO, 2003.
3. Department of Health. *Choosing Health: Making Healthy Choices Easier*. London: Stationery Office, 2004. Available at: http://www.dh.gov.uk/PublicationsAndStatistics/Publications/ PublicationsPolicyAndGuidance/PublicationsPAmpGBrowsable Document/fs/en?CONTENT_ID=4097491&chk=KPBy7H (accessed January 2007).
4. Miens E. A 'Mind-Reading' Mum – Rich or Poor – is Key to Baby's Progress, 2005. Swindon: Economic and Social Research Council, Press Release 26 May 2005. Avaiable at: http://www.esrcsocietytoday.ac.uk/ ESRCInfoCentre/PO/releases/2005/may (accessed January 2007).
5. Murray L, Cowley F, Hooper R, et al. The impact of postnatal depression and associated adversity on early mother–infant interactions and later infant outcomes. *Child Dev* 1996; **67**: 2512–2526.
6. National Research Council Institute of Medicine. *From Neurons to Neighborhoods: The Science of Early Childhood Development*. Washington, DC: National Academy Press, 2000.
7. Claus D. *Rethinking the Brain*. New York: Families and Work Institute, 1997.
8. Gerhardt S. *Why Love Matters: How Affection Shapes a Baby's Brain*. London: Routledge, 2003.
9. Patterson GR, Dishion TJ, Chamberlain P. Outcomes and methodological issues relating to treatment of antisocial children. In: *Handbook of Effective Psychotherapy* (ed. Giles TR). New York: Plenum, 1993, pp. 43–88.
10. Baumrind D. Rearing competent children. In: *Child Development Today and Tomorrow* (ed. Damon W). San Francisco, CA: Jossey-Bass, 1989, pp. 349–378.
11. Bone M, Meltzer H. *The Prevalence of Disability Among Children*. OPCS Surveys of Disability in Great Britain Report 3. London: HMSO, 1989.
12. Glazebrook C, Hollis C, Heussler H, et al. Detecting emotional and behavioural problems in paediatric clinics. *Child Care Health Dev* 2003; **29**: 141–149.
13. Gottman JM, Katz LF, Hooven C. Parental meta-emotion philosophy and the emotional life of families: theoretical models and preliminary data. *J Fam Psychol* 1996; **10**: 243–268.
14. Wickrama KAS, Lorenz FO, Conger RD. Parental support and adolescent physical health status: a latent growth curve analysis. *J Health Soc Behav* 1997; **38**: 149–163.
15. Mantymaa M, Puura K, Luopma I, et al. Infant–mother interaction as a predictor of child's chronic health problems. *Child Care Health Dev* 2003; **29**: 181–191.
16. Askildsen EC, Watten RG, Faleide AO. Are parents of asthmatic children different from other parents? Some follow up results from the Norwegian PRAD Project. *Psychother Psychosomat* 1993; **60**: 91–99.
17. Cohen D, Richardson J, Labree L. Parenting behaviours and the onset of smoking and alcohol use: a longitudinal study. *Pediatrics* 1994; **94**: 368–375.
18. Kremers SPJ, Brug J, Vries HD, et al. Parenting style and adolescent fruit consumption. *Appetite* 2003; **41**: 43–50.
19. Scaramella LV, Conger RD, Simons RL, et al. Predicting a risk for pregnancy by late adolescence: a social contextual perspective. *Dev Psychol* 1998; **34**: 1233–1245.
20. Desforges C. *The Impact of Parental Involvement, Parental Support and Family Education on Pupil Achievement and Adjustment*. London: DfES, 2003.
21. Stewart-Brown S, Fletcher L, Wadsworth M, et al. *The Roots of Social Capital II: The Impact of Parent–Child Relationships on Mental and Physical Health in Later Life: An Analysis of Data Collected in the Three British National Birth Cohort Studies*. Oxford: HSRU, 2002.
22. Conger RD, Conger K, Elder G, et al. A family process model of economic hardship and adjustment of early adolescent boys. *Child Dev* 1992; **63**: 526–541.
23. Conger RD, Patterson G, Xiaojia G. It takes two to replicate: a mediational model for the impact of parents' stress on adolescent adjustment. *Child Dev* 1995; **66**: 80–97.
24. Larzelere R, Patterson G. Parental management: mediator of the effect of socioeconomic status on early delinquency. *Criminology* 1990; **28**: 301–323.
25. Barlow J, Stewart-Brown S. Understanding parenting programmes: parents' views. *Primary Health Care Res Dev* 2001; **2**: 117–130.
26. Patterson J, Mockford C, Barlow J, et al. Need and demand for parenting programmes in a general practice setting. *Arch Dis Child* 2002; **87**: 468–471.
27. Ghate D, Ramella M. *Positive parenting: The National Evaluation of the Youth Justice Board's Parenting Programme*. London: Youth Justice Board for England and Wales, 2002.
28. Cawson P, Wattam C, Brooker S, et al. *Child Maltreatment in the United Kingdom: A Study of the Prevalence of Child Abuse and Neglect*. London: NSPCC, 2000.
29. Olds D, Eckenrode J, Henderson CR, et al. Long-term effects of home visitation on maternal life course and child abuse and neglect: fifteen-year follow-up of a randomised trial. *JAMA* 1997; **278**: 637–643.
30. Bull J, McCormick G, Swann C, et al. *Ante- and Post-Natal Home-Visiting Programmes: A Review of Reviews*. London: HAD, 2004.
31. Barlow J, Stewart-Brown S, Davis H, et al. *Working in Partnership: The Effectiveness of a Home Visiting Service for Vulnerable Families*. Warwick: University of Warwick, 2005.
32. Seeley S, Murray L, Cooper PJ. The outcome for mothers and babies of health visitor intervention. *Health Visitor* 1996; **69**: 135–138.
33. Puckering C, Roger J, Mill M, et al. Process and evaluation of a group intervention for mothers with parenting difficulties. *Child Abuse Rev* 1994; **3**: 299–310.
34. Onzawa K, Glover V, Adams D, et al. Infant massage improves mother–infant interaction for mothers with postnatal depression. *J Affect Disorder* 2001; **63**: 201–207.
35. Parr M. A new approach to parent education. *Br J Midwifery* 1998; **6**: 160–165.
36. Svanberg PO. *Sunderland Infant Programme*. OXPIP Conference: Oxford, 2005.
37. Evangelou, M, Sylva, K. *The Effects of PEEP on Children's Developmental Progress: Towards Effective Early Childhood Interventions*. London: DfES, 2002.
38. Barlow J, Stewart-Brown SL. Review article: behavior problems and parent-training programs. *J Dev Behav Pediatr* 2000; **21**: 356–370.
39. Barlow J, Coren E, Stewart-Brown S. Meta-analysis of parenting programmes in improving maternal psychosocial health. *Br J Gen Pract* 2002; **52**: 223–233.
40. Webster-Stratton C, Hancock L. Training for parents of young children with conduct problems: content methods and therapeutic processes. In: *Handbook of Parent Training*, 2nd edn (eds Briesmeister JM, Schaefer CE). New York, Wiley, 1998.
41. Hunt C. *The Parenting Puzzle: How to Get the Best Out of Family Life*. Oxford: Family Links, 2003.
42. Quinn M, Quinn T. *The 'Noughts to Sixes' Parenting Programme*. Newry: Family Caring Trust, 1995.

43. Sanders MR, Cann W, Markie-Dadds C. The Triple-P Positive Parenting Programme: a universal population-level approach to the prevention of child abuse. *Child Abuse Rev* 2003; **12**: 155–171.

44. Davis H, Day C, Bidmead C. *Working in Partnership with Parents: The Parent Advisor Approach.* London: The Psychological Corporation, 2002.

45. Window S, Richards M, Vostanis P. *Evaluation of Inter-Agency Interventions for Children with Behavioural Problems and their Families.* Leicester: University of Leicester, 2002.

46. Royal College of Paediatrics and Child Health. *Helpful Parenting.* London: RCPCH, 2002.

47. Henricson C, Katz I, Mesie J, et al. *National Mapping of Family Services in England and Wales – A Consultation Document.* London: National Family and Parenting Institute, 2001.

48. Harker L, Kendall L. *An Equal Start: Improving Support During Pregnancy and the First 12 Months.* London: IPPR, 2003.

Further reading

Anisfeld E, Casper V, Nozyce M, et al. Does infant carrying promote attachment? An experimental study of the effects of increased physical contact on the development of attachment. *Child Dev* 1990; **61**: 1617–1627.

Barlow J, Brocklehurst N, Stewart-Brown S, et al. Working in partnership: the development of a home visiting service for vulnerable families. *Child Abuse Rev* 2003; **12**: 172–189.

Department of Health. *Child Protection: Messages from Research.* HMSO: London, 1996.

Gross D, Fogg L, Tucker S. The efficacy of parent training for promoting positive parent–toddler relationships. *Res Nurs Health* 1995; **18**: 489–499.

Hall DMB, Elliman D (eds). *Health for all Children,* 4th edn. Oxford: Oxford University Press, 2003.

Henrikson C. *Government and Parenting: Is there a Case for a Policy Review and a Parents' Code?* York: Joseph Rowntree Foundation, 2003.

MacLeod J, Nelson G. Programs for the promotion of family wellness and the prevention of child maltreatment: a meta-analytic review. *Child Abuse Neglect* 2000; **24**: 1127–1149.

Puura K, Davis H, Papadopoulou K, et al. The European Early Promotion Project: a new primary health care service to promote children's mental health. *J Infant Mental Health* 2002; 23: 606–624.

CHAPTER 19

References

1. Kennedy H (Chair). *Sudden Unexpected Death In Infancy: The Report Of A Working Group Convened by the Royal College of Pathologists and the Royal College of Paediatrics and Child Health.* London: Royal College of Pathologists, 2004.

2. Dent A, Condon L, Blair P, et al. A study of bereavement care after sudden and unexpected death. *Arch Dis Child* 1996; **74**: 522–526.

3. Fleming P, Blair P, Bacon C, et al. (eds). *Sudden Unexpected Deaths in Infancy: the CESDI SUDI Studies, 1993–96.* London: The Stationery Office, 2000.

4. Meadow R. Unnatural sudden infant death. *Arch Dis Child* 1999; **80**: 7–14.

5. Wolkind S, Taylor EM, Waite AJ, et al. Recurrence of unexpected infant death. *Acta Paediatr* 1993; **82**: 873–876.

6. Lord Laming. *Inquiry into the Death of Victoria Climbié.* London: The Stationery Office, 2003.

Further information:

Foundation for the Study of Infant Deaths: http://www.sids.org.uk (accessed January 2007).

CHAPTER 20

References

1. Cook P. *Supporting Sick Children and their Families.* London: Harcourt, 1999.

2. MacCarthy D, MacKeith R. A parent's voice. *Lancet* 1965; **ii**: 1289–1291.

3. Seecharan GA, Andresen EM, Norris K, et al. Parents' assessment of the quality of care and grief following a child's death. *Arch Pediatr Adolesc Med* 2004; **158**: 515–520.

4. Li J, Precht DH, Mortensen PB, et al. Mortality in parents after death of a child in Denmark: a nationwide follow-up study. *Lancet* 2003; **361**: 363–367.

5. Oliver RC, Sturtevant JP, Scheetz JP, et al. Beneficial effects of a hospital bereavement intervention program after traumatic childhood death. *J Trauma* 2001; **50**: 440–446.

6. Yates DW, Ellison G, McGuiness S. Care of the suddenly bereaved. **BMJ** 1990; **301**: 29–31.

7. Robinson SM, Mackenzie-Ross S, Campbell Hewson GL, et al. Psychological effect of witnessed resuscitation on bereaved relatives. *Lancet* 1998; **352**: 614–617.

8. Barratt F, Wallis DN. Relatives in the resuscitation room: their point of view. *J Accid Emerg Med* 1998; **15**: 109–111.

9. Ardley C. Should relatives be denied access to the resuscitation room? *Intens Crit Care Nurs* 2003; **19**: 1–10.

10. Copnell B. Death in the pediatric ICU: caring for children and families at the end of life. *Crit Care Nurs Clin North Am* 2005; **17**: 349–360.

11. Kübler-Ross E. *On Death and Dying.* London: Tavistock/Routledge, 1969.

12. Parkes CM, Brown RJ. Health after bereavement. A controlled study of young Boston widows and widowers. *Psychosom Med* 1972; **34**: 449–461.

13. Parkes CM. Components of the reaction to loss of a limb, spouse or home. *J Psychosom Res* 1972; **16**: 343–349.

14. Worden JW. Bereavement. *Semin Oncol* 1985; **12**: 472–475.

15. Johnson LC, Rincon B, Gober C, et al. The development of a comprehensive bereavement program to assist families experiencing pediatric loss. *J Pediatr Nurs* 1993; **8**: 142–146.

16. Worden JW, Davies B, McCown D. Comparing parent loss with sibling loss. *Death Stud* 1999; **23**: 1–15.

17. American Academy of Pediatrics. Committee on Psychosocial Aspects of Child and Family Health. The pediatrician and childhood bereavement. *Pediatrics* 2000; **105**: 445–447.

18. Cook P, White DK, Ross-Russell RI. Bereavement support following sudden and unexpected death: guidelines for care. *Arch Dis Child* 2002; **87**: 36–38.

19. de Groot-Bollujt W, Mourik M. Bereavement – role of the nurse in the care of terminally ill and dying children in the pediatric intensive care unit. *Crit Care Med* 1993; **21**: S391–S392.

20. Gudmundsdottir M, Chesla CA. Building a new world: habits and practices of healing following the death of a child. *J Fam Nurs* 2006; **12**: 143–164.

21. Cox SA. Pediatric bereavement: supporting the family and each other. *J Trauma Nurs* 2004; **11**: 117–121.

22. Merlevede E, Spooren D, Henderick H, et al. Perceptions, needs and mourning reactions of bereaved relatives confronted with a sudden unexpected death. *Resuscitation* 2004; **61**: 341–348.

23. Douglas M, Pemberton S, Hewitt B. Palliative care nursing. Part 2. Addressing bereavement issues through education. *Nurs Times* 2002; **98**: 36–37.

24. Schneiderman G, Winders P, Tallett S, et al. Do child and/or parent bereavement programs work? *Can J Psychiatry* 1994; **39**: 215–217.

25. Rowa-Dewar N. Do interventions make a difference to bereaved parents? A systematic review of controlled studies. *Int J Palliat Nurs* 2002; **8**: 452–457.

26. Dent A, Condon L, Blair P, et al. A study of bereavement care after a sudden and unexpected death. *Arch Dis Child* 1996; **74**: 522–526.

CHAPTER 21

References

1. SCOPE. *Right From the Start,* 1994. Available at: http://www.scope.org.uk/earlyyears-old/prof/start.shtml (accessed January 2007).

2. Hogbin B, Fallowfield L. Getting it taped: bad news consultations with cancer patients. *Br J Hosp Med* 1989; **41**: 330–333.

3. Royal College of Paediatrics and Child Health, Royal College of Psychiatrists, Faculty for Children and Young People, British Psychological Society. *Child in Mind.* Teaching programme. Available at: http://www.rcpch.ac.uk/education/projects/child_in_mind.html (accessed January 2007).

4. Jacobson L, Owen P. Study of teenage care in one general practice. *Br J Gen Pract* 1993; **43**: 349.
5. Beresford B, Sloper P. Chronically ill adolescents' experiences of communicating with doctors: a qualitative study. *J Adolesc Health* 2003; **33**: 172–179.
6. Bluebond-Langer M. *The Private Worlds of Dying Children*. Princeton, NJ: Princeton University Press, 1978.
7. Koh THHG, Jarvis C. Promoting effective communication in NICU by audio-taping parents–neonatologists conversations. *Int J Clin Pract* 1998; **52**: 27–29.

Further reading

Hasnat MJ, Graves P. Disclosure of developmental disability: a study of paediatricians' practices. *J Pediatr Child Health* 2000; **36**: 27–31.

Hasnat MJ, Graves P. Disclosure of developmental disability: a study of parent satisfaction and the determinants of satisfaction. *J Pediatr Child Health* 2000; **36**: 32–35.

Klass D, Silverman PR, Nickman SL. *Continuing Bonds: New Understandings of Grief*. London: Taylor and Francis, 1996.

Riches G, Dawson P. *An Intimate Loneliness: Supporting Bereaved Parents and Siblings*. Buckingham: Open University Press, 2000.

Silverman P. *Never Too Young to Know: Death in Children's Lives*. Oxford: Oxford University Press, 2000.

Sloper P. Needs and responses of parents following the diagnosis of childhood cancer. *Child Care Health Dev* 1996; **22**: 187–202.

Tate P. *The Doctor's Communication Handbook*. Oxford: Radcliffe Medical, 1994.

Walker G, Bradburn J, Maher J. *Breaking Bad News*. London: King's Fund, 1997.

Further information

Child Bereavement Trust: http://www.childbereavement.org.uk (accessed January 2007).

Cruse Bereavement Care: http://www.crusebereavementcare.org.uk (accessed January 2007).

Sands – support for parents and families whose baby is stillborn or dies soon after birth, including a range of leaflets and books for adults: http://www.uk-sands.org (accessed January 2007).

SCOPE. *Sharing Concerns*, 2002. Video produced by the university of Central England, the West Birmingham Portage Service and their Parents' Group.

Winston's Wish – books and support for grieving children and their families: http://www.winstonswish.org.uk (accessed January 2007).

CHAPTER 22

References

1. Department of Health. *Together From the Start: Practical Guidance for Professionals Working with Disabled Children (Birth to Third Birthday) and their Families*. London: DoH, 2003. Available at: http://www.dh.gov.uk/PublicationsAndStatistics/LettersAndCirculars/Local AuthoritySocialServicesLetters/AllLASSLs/LocalSocialServicesLetters Article/fs/en?CONTENT_ID=4004628&chk=cTSAh5 (accessed January 2007).
2. Cunningham CC, Morgan P, McGucken RB. Down's syndrome: is dissatisfaction with disclosure of diagnosis inevitable? *Dev Med Child Neurol* 1984; **26**: 33–39.
3. Sloper P, Turner S. Determinants of parental satisfaction with disclosure of disability. *Dev Med Child Neurol* 1993; **35**: 816–825.
4. Quine L, Rutter DR. First diagnosis of severe mental and physical disability: a study of doctor–parent communication. *J Child Psychol Psychiatry* 1994; **35**: 1273–1287.
5. Baird G, Scrutton D, McConachie H. Parents' perceptions of disclosure of the diagnosis of cerebral palsy. *Arch Dis Child* 2000; **83**: 475–480.
6. Hasnat MJ, Graves P. Disclosure of developmental disability: a study of parent satisfaction and the determinants of satisfaction. *J Pediatr Child Health* 2000; **36**: 32–35.
7. Abrams EZ, Goodman JF. Diagnosing developmental problems in children: parents and professionals negotiate bad news. *J Pediatr Psychol* 1998; **23**: 87–98.
8. Bartolo PA. Communicating a diagnosis of developmental disability to parents: multiprofessional negotiation frameworks. *Child Care Health Dev* 2002; **28**: 65–71.
9. O'Sullivan P, Mahoney G, Robinson C. Perceptions of paediatricians' helpfulness: a national study of mothers of young disabled children. *Dev Med Child Neurol* 1992; **34**: 1064–1071.
10. Cottrell DJ, Summers K. Communicating an evolutionary diagnosis of disability to parents. *Child Care Health Dev* 1990; **16**: 211–218.
11. Davis H. *Counselling Parents of Children with Chronic Illness or Disability*. Leicester: BPS Books, 1993.
12. McConachie H. Breaking the news to family and friends: some ideas to help parents. *Ment Handicap* 1991; **16**: 373–381.
13. Starke M, Möller A. Parents' need for knowledge concerning the medical diagnosis of their children. *J Child Health Care* 2002; **6**: 245–257.
14. Contact a Family: http://www.cafamily.org.uk (accessed January 2007).
15. Bicknell J. The psychopathology of handicap. *Br J Med Psychol* 1983; **56**: 167–178.
16. Blacher J. *Severely Handicapped Young Children and their Families: Research in Review*. London: Academic Press, 1984.
17. Romans-Clarkson SE, Clarkson FE, Dittner ID, et al. Impact of a handicapped child on mental health of parents. *Br Med J Clin Res Educ* 1986; **293**: 1395–1397.
18. Sanders JL, Morgan SB. Family stress and adjustment as perceived by parents of children with autism or Down syndrome: implications for intervention. *Child Fam Behav Ther* 1997; **19**: 15–32.
19. Beresford B. *Expert Opinions: A National Survey of Parents Caring for a Severely Disabled Child*. Bristol: Policy Press, 1995.
20. Corden A, Sainsbury R, Sloper P. *Financial Implications of the Death of a Child*. London: Family Policy Studies Centre, 2001.
21. Beresford B. Resources and strategies: how parents cope with the care of a disabled child. *J Child Psychol Psychiatry* 1994; **35**: 171–209.
22. McConachie H. Implications of a model of stress and coping for services to families of young disabled children. *Child Care Health Dev* 1994; **20**: 37–46.
23. Hastings RP, Taunt HM. Positive perceptions in families of children with developmental disabilities. *Am J Mental Retard* 2002; **107**: 116–127.
24. Mukherjee S, Beresford B, Sloper P. *Unlocking Key Working: An Analysis and Evaluation of Key Worker Services for Families with Disabled Children*. Bristol: Policy Press, 1999.
25. Neely-Barnes S, Marcenko M. Predicting impact of childhood disability on families: results from the 1995 National Health Interview Survey. *Mental Retard* 2004; **42**(Suppl): 284–293.
26. Chamba R, Ahmad W, Hirst M, et al. *On the Edge: Minority Ethnic Families Caring for a Severely Disabled Child*. Bristol: Policy Press, 1999.
27. Kirk S, Glendinning C. Developing services to support parents caring for a technology dependent child at home. *Child Care Health Dev* 2004; **30**: 209–218.
28. Department of Health. *Getting the Right Start: National Service Framework for Children Standard for Hospital Services*. London: DoH, April 2003, para 4.11:23. Available at: http://www.dh.gov.uk/PolicyAndGuidance/HealthAndSocialCareTopics/ChildrenServices/ChildrenServicesInformation/fs/en (accessed January 2007).

Further reading

Dobson B, Middleton S, Beardsworth A. *The Impact of Childhood Disability on Family Life*. York: Joseph Rowntree Foundation, 2001.

Mitchell W, Sloper P. *User-friendly Information for Families with Disabled Children: A Guide to Good Practice*. York: York Publishing Services, 2000.

CHAPTER 23

References

1. Gortmaker SL, Sappenfield W. Chronic childhood disorders: prevalence and impact. *Pediatr Clin North Am* 1984; **31**: 3–18.
2. Wallander JL, Varni JW, Babani L, et al. Children with chronic physical disorders: maternal reports of their psychological adjustment. *J Pediatr Psychol* 1988; **2**: 197–212.
3. Gortmaker SL, Walker DK, Weitzman M, et al. Chronic conditions, socioeconomic risks, and behavioral problems in children and adolescents. *Paediatrics* 1990; **85**: 267–276.
4. Cadman D, Boyle M, Szatmari P, et al. Chronic illness, disability, and mental and social wellbeing: findings of the Ontario Child Health Study. *Pediatrics* 1987; **79**: 805–813.

5. Pless IB, Cripps HA, Davies JMC, et al. Chronic physical illness in childhood: psychological and social effects in adolescence and adult life. *Dev Med Child Neurol* 1989; **31**: 746–755.

6. Orr DP, Susan CW, Satterwhite B, et al. Psychosocial implications of chronic illness in adolescence. *J Pediatr* 1984; **104**: 152–157.

7. Goldberg S, Simmons RJ. Chronic illness and early development: the parent's perceptive. *Pediatrician* 1988; **15**: 13–20.

8. Hawkins WE, Duncan DF. Children's illnesses as risk factor for child abuse. *Psychol Rep* 1985; **56**: 638.

9. Goldberg S. Chronic illness and early development. *Pediatr Ann* 1990; **19**: 35–41.

10. Krener P. Parent salvage and parent sabotage in the care of chronically ill children. *Am J Dis Child* 1988; **142**: 945–951.

11. Sabbeth BF, Leventhal JM. Marital adjustment to chronic childhood illness: a critique of the literature. *Paediatrics* 1984; **73**: 762–768.

12. Cadman D, Rosenbaum P, Boyle M, et al. Children with chronic illness: family and parent demographic characteristics and psychosocial adjustment. *Paediatrics* 1991; **87**: 884–889.

13. Powers GM, Gaudet LM. Coping patterns of parents of chronically ill children. *Psychol Rep* 1986; **59**: 519–522.

14. Clements DB, Copeland LG, Loftus M. Critical times for families with a chronically ill child. *Pediatr Nurs* 1990; **16**: 157–161.

15. Drotar D, Crawford P. Psychological adaptation of siblings of chronically ill children: research and practice implications. *Dev Behav Pediatr* 1985; **6**: 355–362.

16. Koocher GP, O'Malley JE. *The Damocles Syndrome: Psychosocial Consequences of Surviving Childhood Cancer*. London: McGraw-Hill, 1981.

17. Seligman M. Adaptation of children to chronically ill or mentally handicapped sibling. *CMAJ* 1987; **136**: 1249–1251.

18. Kazak A. Families of chronically ill children: a systems and social-ecological model of adaptation and challenge. *J Consult Clin Psychol* 1989; **57**: 25–30.

19. Rolland JS. Anticipatory loss: a family systems developmental framework. *Fam Process* 1990; **29**: 229–243.

20. Kupst M, Schulman J, Maurer H, et al. Coping with pediatric leukemia: a two year old follow-up. *J Pediatr Psychol* 1984; **9**: 149–163.

21. Tsiantis J. Family reactions and relationships in thalassemia. *Ann NY Acad Sci* 1990; **612**: 451–461.

22. Eiser C. Psychological effects of chronic disease. *J Child Psychol Psychiatry* 1990; **31**: 85–89.

23. Sinnema G. Resilience among children with special health-care needs and among their families. *Pediatr Ann* 1991; **20**: 483–486.

24. Griffith JL, Griffith ME. Structural family therapy in chronic illness. *Psychosomatics* 1987; **28**: 202–205.

25. Williamson PS. Consequences for the family in chronic illness. *J Fam Pract* 1985; **21**: 23–32.

26. Frey J. A family/systems approach to illness-maintaining behaviors in chronically ill adolescents. *Fam Process* 1984; **23**: 251–260.

27. Collier JAH. Developmental and systems perspectives on chronic illness. *Holistic Nurs Pract* 1990; **5**: 1–9.

28. Merkens MJ, Perrin EC, Perrin JM, et al. The awareness of primary physicians of the psychosocial adjustment of children with a chronic illness. *Dev Behav Pediatr* 1989; **10**: 1–6.

29. Lau RR, Williams HS, Williams LC, et al. Psychosocial problems in chronically ill children: Physician concern, parent satisfaction, and the validity of medical records. *J Commun Health* 1982; **7**: 250–261.

CHAPTER 24

References

1. National Autistic Society for NAISA (National Initiative for Autism: Screening and Assessment) in collaboration with the Royal College of Psychiatrists, Royal College of Paediatrics and Child Health, and the All Party Parliamentary Group on Autism. *National Autism Plan for Children*, 2003. Available at: http://www.nas.org.uk/nas/jsp/polopoly.jsp?d=368&a=2178 (accessed January 2007).

2. Gillberg C, Coleman M. *The Biology of the Autistic Syndromes*, 3rd edn. Cambridge: MacKeith Press, 2000.

3. Melville CA, Cameron J. Autism. In: *Seminars in the Psychiatry of Learning Disabilities*, 2nd edn (eds Fraser W, Kerr M). London: Gaskell Press, 2003.

4. Hall DH, Elliman D. *Health for All Children*. Oxford: Oxford University Press, 2003.

5. Lloyd Evans A, Knight-Jones E, Nicholson J. *Standards for Child Development Services*. London: British Association of Community Child Health (BACCH), Child Development and Disability Group, 1999.

6. National Autistic Society, EarlyBird Programme. Available at: http://www.nas.org.uk/nas/jsp/polopoly.jsp?d=142 (accessed January 2007).

7. Treatment and Education of Autistic and related Communication-handicapped Children (TEACCH). Available at: http://www.teacch.com (accessed January 2007).

8. Picture Exchange Communication System (PECS). Available at: http://www.childrenwithspecialneeds.com/pecs.html (accessed January 2007).

9. Kuoch H, Mirenda P. Social story interventions for children with autism spectrum disorders. *Focus on Autism and Other Developmental Disabilities* 2003; **18**: 73–79.

CHAPTER 25

Further reading

Aitken S, Millar S. *Listening to Children with Communication Support Needs*, Books 1 and 2. Glasgow: Sense Scotland, CALL Centre and Scottish Executive Education Department, 2002.

Aitken S, Millar S. *Listening to Children 2004*. Glasgow: Sense Scotland, CALL Centre and Scottish Executive Education Department, 2004.

Cockerill H, Carroll-Few L (eds). *Communicating without Speech: Practical Augmentative and Alternative Communication*. London: MacKeith, 2001.

Gompertz J. Developing communication: early intervention and augmentative signing. In: *Children with Learning Difficulties: A Collaborative Approach to their Education and Management* (ed. Fawcus M). London: Whurr, 1997, pp. 64–96.

Howlin P. *Children with Autism and Asperger Syndrome: A Guide for Practitioners and Carers*. Chichester: Wiley, 1998.

NSPCC, Joseph Rowntree Foundation, Triangle. *Two-Way Street: Communicating with Disabled Children and Young People* (video and handbook). Leicester: NSPCC, 2001.

Von Tetzchner S, Martinsen H. *Introduction to Augmentative and Alternative Communication*, 2nd edn. London: Whurr, 2000.

CHAPTER 26

References

1. Department of Health. *Assessing Children in Need and their Families: Practice Guidance*. London: Stationery Office, 2000.

2. Disability Alliance. *Disability Rights Handbook. A Guide to Benefits and Services for all Disabled People, Their Families, Carers and Advisers*, 31st edn. London: Disability Alliance, 2006.

3. Department for Work and Pensions. *DLA1 Child April 2001. Notes about Claiming Under the Special Rules for a Child under 16*. London: DWP, 2001.

4. Department for Work and Pensions. Topic areas. In: *DLA1 Child April 2001. Section 2, Application Form – How the Child's Illness or Disability Affects Them*. London: DWP, 2001.

5. Department for Work and Pensions. *DLA1 Child April 2001. Notes About Claiming Disability Living Allowance for a Child Under 16*. London: DWP, 2001.

6. Family Fund Trust. *Are You Caring for a Severely Disabled Child?* York: Family Fund Trust, 2002.

Further reading

Disability Alliance. *Disability Rights Handbook. A Guide to Benefits and Services for all Disabled People, Their Families, Carers and Advisers*, 31st edn. London: Disability Alliance, 2006.

Further information

Benefits Enquiry Line: Tel. 0800 882200.

Citizens Advice Bureau (National): Myddelton House, 115–123 Pentonville Road, London N1 9LZ; Tel. 020 7833 2181; http://www.nacab.org.uk (accessed January 2007).

Central London Congestion Charging Office: Tel. 0845 900 1234.

Contact a Family: 209–211 City Road, London EC1V 1JN; Tel. 020 7608 8700; freephone for parents and families 0808 808 3555; http://www.cafamily.org.uk (accessed January 2007).

Department for Work and Pensions, online application for benefits: http://www.direct.gov.uk (accessed January 2007).

Disability Alliance: Universal House, 88–94 Wentworth Street, London E1 7SA; Tel: 020 7247 8776; http://www.disabilityalliance.org (accessed January 2007).

Family Fund Trust: Unit 4, Alpha Court, Monks Cross Drive, Huntington, York YO32 9WN Tel. 0845 130 4542; http://www.familyfund.org.uk (accessed January 2007).

Motability: Warwick House, Roydon Road, Harlow, Essex CM19 5PX; Tel. 01279 635666; http://www.motability.co.uk (accessed January 2007).

CHAPTER 27

References

1. HM Treasury. *Securing our Future Health: Taking a Long Term View*. Wanless Report. London: HMSO, 2002.
2. Department of Health. *Choosing Health: Making Healthy Choices Easier*. London: Stationery Office, 2004. Available at: http://www.dh.gov.uk/PublicationsAndStatistics/Publications/PublicationsPolicyAndGuidance/PublicationsPAmpGBrowsableDocument/fs/en?CONTENT_ID=4097491&chk=KPBy7H (accessed January 2007).
3. Sure Start: http://www.surestart.gov.uk (accessed January 2007).
4. Department of Health. *Getting the Right Start: National Service Framework for Children. Standard for Hospital Services*. London: DoH, April 2003, para 4.11:23. Available at: http://www.dh.gov.uk/PolicyAndGuidance/HealthAndSocialCareTopics/ChildrenServices/ChildrenServicesInformation/fs/en (accessed January 2007).
5. Department of Education and Skills. *National Healthy Schools Status 2005: A Guide for Schools*. Available at: http://www.wiredforhealth.gov.uk/PDF/NHSS_A_Guide_for_Schools_10_05.pdf (accessed January 2007).
6. Welsh Assembly Government. *National Service Framework for Children, Young People and Maternity*, 2006. Available at: http://new.wales.gov.uk/consultations/closed/childrenyoungpeople/cons-child-nsf-disabled/?lang=en (accessed March 2007).
7. Breast Feeding etc. (Scotland) Act 2005. Available at: http://www.opsi.gov.uk/legislation/scotland/acts2005/20050001.htm (accessed January 2007).
8. Healthcare Commission: http://www.healthcarecommission.org.uk (accessed January 2007).
9. National Institute for Health and Clinical Excellence (NICE): http://www.nice.org.uk (accessed January 2007).
10. Ham C, Pickard S. *Tragic Choices in Health Care – The Case of Child B*. London: King's Fund, 1998.
11. Griffiths S, Hill A, Gillam S. *Public Health and Primary Care*. Oxford: Oxford University Press, 2007, Chap. 1 (in press).
12. Department of Health. *Shifting the Balance of Power in England*. London: HMSO, 2001.
13. New B. *A Good Enough Service – Values, Trade Offs and the NHS*. London: King's Fund, 1999.
14. Moynihan R, Smith R. Too much medicine? *BMJ* 2002; **324**: 859–860.
15. Griffiths S, Jewell T, Hope T. *Developing Health System Strategy*. Oxford: Oxford University Press, 2006, pp. 404–410.
16. Hope T, Hicks N, Reynolds DJM, et al. Rationing and the health authority. *BMJ* 1998; **317**: 1067–1069.

CHAPTER 28

References

1. Report of the Independent Inquiries into Paediatric Cardiac Services at the Royal Brompton Hospital and Harefield Hospital (the Brompton Report). Available at: http://www.rbh.nthames.nhs.uk (accessed January 2007).
2. Rawls J. *A Theory of Justice*. Oxford: Oxford University Press, 1972.
3. Daniels N. *Just Health Care: Studies in Philosophy and Health Policy*. Cambridge: Cambridge University Press, 1985.
4. Harris J. What is the good of health care? *Bioethics* 1996; **10**: 269–291.
5. Williams A. Economics of coronary artery bypass grafting. *BMJ* 1985; **291**: 326–329.
6. Airedale NHS Trust v Bland [1993] 1 All ER 821; Re John Storar (1981) 420 NE 2d 64 (NY CA); Re the Treatment and Care of Infant Doe, No GU 8204-004A (Ind Cir Ct, April 12, 1982); Re C (A Minor) (Wardship: Medical Treatment) [1989] 2 All ER 782, CA; Re J (A Minor) (Wardship: Medical Treatment) [1990] 3 All ER 930 [1991] Fam 33 (CA); Re R (Adult: Medical Treatment) [1996] 2 FLR 99.
7. R v. Cambridge Health Authority, ex p. B [1995] 2 All ER 129, 133 (CA).
8. General Medical Council. *Priorities and Choices: Guidance from the General Medical Council*. London: GMC, 2000. Available at: http://www.gmc-uk.org/guidance/archive/Priorities_and_choices_2000.pdf (accessed January 2007).
9. Harris J. QALYfying the value of human life. *J Med Ethics* 1987; **13**: 117–123.
10. Harris J. More and better justice. In: *Philosophy and Medical Welfare* (eds Bell JM, Mendus SM). Cambridge: Cambridge University Press, 1988.
11. Harris J. Double jeopardy and the veil of ignorance – a reply. *J Med Ethics* 1995; **21**: 151–157.
12. Savulescu J. Warning: smoking harms your chances. *Aust Med* 2001; **13**: 10–11.
13. Savulescu J. Resources, Down's syndrome and cardiac surgery. Do we really want 'equality of access'? *BMJ* 2001; **322**: 875–876.
14. Neville B. Response to: Resources, Down's syndrome and cardiac surgery. *BMJ* 2001; **322**: 875–876. Available at: http://www.bmj.com/cgi/eletters/322/7291/875#14548 (accessed January 2007).

Further reading

Battin M, Rhodes R, Silvers A (eds). *Medicine and Social Justice*. New York: Oxford University Press, 2002.

Daniels N. Accountability for reasonableness in private and public health insurance. In: *The Global Challenge of Health Care Rationing* (eds Coulter A, Ham C). Buckingham: Pen University Press, 2000. pp. 89–106.

Daniels N, Sabin J. Limits to health care: fair procedures, democratic deliberation and the legitimacy problem for insurers. *Philos Public Affairs* 1997; **26**: 303–350.

Edgar A, Salek S, Shickle D, et al. *The Ethical QALY: Ethical Issues in Healthcare Resource Allocations*. Haslemere: Euromed Communications, 1998.

McKie J. *The Allocation of Health Care Resources: An Ethical Evaluation of the 'QALY' Approach*. Dartmouth: Ashgate, 1998.

New B. Defining a package of health care services the NHS is responsible for. In: *Rationing, Talk and Action in Health Care* (ed. New B). London: King's Fund/BMJ Books, 1997, pp. 79–84.

Nord E. *Cost–Value Analysis in Health Care: Making Sense of QALYs*. Cambridge: Cambridge University Press, 1999.

CHAPTER 29

References

1. Wood NS, Costeloe K, Gibson AT, et al. The EPICure Study: associations and antecedents of neurological and developmental disability at 30 months of age following extremely preterm birth. *Arch Dis Child Fetal Neonatal Edn* 2005; **90**: F134–F140.
2. Roy R, Aladangady N, Costeloe K, et al. Decision making and modes of death in a tertiary neonatal unit. *Arch Dis Child Fetal Neonatal Edn* 2004; **89**: F527–F530.
3. Royal College of Paediatrics and Child Health. *Withholding or Withdrawing Life Saving Treatment in Children: A Framework for Practice*. London: RCPCH, 2004.
4. British Medical Association. *Withholding and Withdrawing Life-Prolonging Medical Treatment*. London: BMJ, 1999.
5. Doyal L, Larcher V. Drafting guidelines for the withholding or withdrawing of life-sustaining treatment in critically ill children and neonates. *Arch Dis Child Fetal Neonatal Edn* 2000; **83**: F60–F63.
6. Airedale NHS Trust v Bland [1993] 1 All ER 821.
7. Chantler C, Doyal L. Medical Ethics; the duties of care in principle and practice. In: *Clinical Negligence* (eds Powers M, Harris N). London: Butterworths, 2000.
8. Mr Justice Hedley (2004) EWHC 2247 (Fam).
9. Kennedy I, Grubb A. *Medical Law: Text and Materials*. London: Butterworth, 2000.

10. Elbourne D, Snowdon D, Garcia J. Informed consent. Subjects may not understand concept of clinical trials. *BMJ* 1997; **315**: 248–249.
11. Children Act 1989. Available at: http://www.opsi.gov.uk/acts/acts1989/Ukpga_19890041_en_1.htm (accessed January 2007).
12. Re B [1981] 1 WLR 1421.
13. Re C [1989] 2 All ER 782.
14. Re J [1990] 6 BMLR 25.
15. Re J [1992] 9 BMLR 10.
16. Elias-Jones AC, Samanta J. The implications of the David Glass case for future clinical practice in the UK. *Arch Dis Child* 2005; **90**: 822–825.
17. Stevenson RC, Cooke RWI. Economics and ethics in neonatology. *Semin Neonatol* 1998; **3**: 315–321.
18. Chiswick ML. Withdrawal of life support in babies: deceptive signals. *Arch Dis Child* 1990; **65**: 1096–1097.
19. Royal College of Physicians. *Ethics in Clinical Practice: Background and Recommendations for Enhanced Support.* Report of a Working Party. London: RCP, 2005.
20. Wood NS, Marlow N, Costeloe K, et al. Neurologic and developmental disability after extremely preterm birth. *N Engl J Med* 2000; **343**: 378–384.
21. Hawdon JM, Williams S, Weindling AM. Withdrawal of neonatal intensive care in the home. *Arch Dis Child* 1994; **71**: F142–F144.
22. McHaffie HE, Lyon AJ, Fowlie PW. Lingering death after treatment withdrawal in the neonatal intensive care unit. *Arch Dis Child Fetal Neonatal Edn* 2001; **85**: F8–F12.
23. McHaffie HE, Fowlie PW, Hume R, et al. Consent to autopsy for neonates. *Arch Dis Child Fetal Neonatal Edn* 2001; **85**: F4–F7.
24. McHaffie HE, Laing IA, Lloyd DJ. Follow up care of bereaved parents after treatment withdrawal from newborns. *Arch Dis Child Fetal Neonatal Edn* 2001; **84**: F125–F128.

CHAPTER 30

References

1. Gillon R. *Philosophical Medical Ethics.* New York: Wiley, 1996.
2. Royal College of Paediatrics and Child Health. *Withholding or Withdrawing Life Saving Treatment in Children: A Framework for Practice.* London: RCPCH, 1997.
3. Slowther AM, Hope T. Clinical ethics committees. *BMJ* 2000; **321**: 649–650.
4. Slowther A, Bunch C, Woolnough B, et al. Clinical ethics support services in the UK: an investigation of the current provision of ethics support to health professionals in the UK. *J Med Ethics* 2001; **27**(Suppl I): i2–i8.
5. Szeremeta M, Dawson J, Manning D, et al. Snapshots of five clinical ethics committees in the UK. *J Med Ethics* 2001; **27**(Suppl I): i9–ii17.
6. Watson AR. An ethics of clinical practice committee: should every hospital have one? *Proc R Coll Phys Edinburgh* 1999; **29**: 335–337.
7. Rudd PT. The clinical ethical committee at the Royal United Hospital, Bath, England. *HEC Forum* 2002;**14**: 37–44.
8. Campbell AV. Clinical governance - watchword or buzzword? *J Med Ethics* 2001; **27**(Suppl I): i54–i56.
9. Jonsen AR, Siegler M, Winslade WJ. *Clinical Ethics. A Practical Approach to Ethical Decisions in Clinical Medicine,* 4th edn. New York: McGraw-Hill, 1998.
10. Gillon R. Medical ethics: four principles plus attention to scope. *BMJ* 1994; **309**: 184–188.
11. Association of Anaesthetists of Great Britain and Ireland. *Management of Anaesthesia for Jehovah's Witnesses.* Available at: http://www.aagbi.org (accessed January 2007).
12. British Medical Association the Resuscitation Council (UK) and The Royal College of Nursing. *Decisions Relating to Cardiopulmonary Resuscitation,* 2002. Available at: http://www.bma.org.uk/ap.nsf/Content/cardioresus (accessed January 2007).
13. Law Society/British Medical Association. *Assessment of Mental Capacity: Guidance for Doctors and Lawyers.* London: BMA, 1995.
14. Gillick vs West Norfolk and Wisbech. AHA 1985; I A II: ER533.
15. Who decides for the child? *Bull Med Ethics* 1999;**149**: 3–4.
16. Re W. (A minor) medical treatment court's jurisdiction. 1992; 4 AII: ER 627.
17. Royal College of Physicians. *Ethics in Practice: Background and Recommendations for Enhanced Support.* London: RCP, 2005. Available

at: http://www.rcplondon.ac.uk/pubs/books/ethics/index.asp (accessed January 2007).
18. UK Clinical Ethics Network: http://www.ethics-network.org.uk (accessed January 2007).
19. Larcher VF, Lask B, McCarthy JM. Paediatrics at the cutting edge: do we need clinical ethics committees? *J Med Ethics* 1997; **23**: 245–249.
20. DuVal G, Sartouis L, Clarridge BM, et al. What triggers requests for ethics consultations? *J Med Ethics* 2001; **27**(Suppl 1): i24–i29.

Further reading

British Medical Association. *Consent, Rights and Choices in Health Care for Children and Young People.* London: BMJ Books, 2001.
Watson AR. Ethics support in clinical practice. *Arch Dis Child* 2005; **90**: 943–946.

CHAPTER 31

References

1. Rudd PT. The role of clinical ethics committees. *Curr Paediatr* 2001; **11**: 381–385, 493–497.
2. Lincoln JA. Quoted In: Sherrin N (ed.), *The Oxford Dictionary of Humorous Quotations.* Oxford: Oxford University Press, 1995.
3. Beauchamp TL, Childress JF. *Principles of Biomedical Ethics,* 5th edn. Oxford: Oxford University Press, 2001.
4. Sweeney KG, Edwards K, Stead J, et al. A comparison of professionals' and patients' understanding of asthma: evidence of emerging dualities? *Med Humanities* 2001; **27**: 20–25.

CHAPTER 32

References

1. Baum D, Curtis H, Elston S, et al. *A Guide to the Development of Children's Palliative Care Services,* 1st edn. Bristol: ACT/RCPCH, 1997.
2. Davies R, Harding Y. The first Diana Team in Wales: an update. *Paediatr Nurs* 2002; **14**: 24–25.
3. Hain RDW, Hughes E. Children referred for specialist palliative care: first 25 patients. *Arch Dis Child* 2001; **84**: A56–A57.
4. Lenton S, Stallard P, Lewis M, et al. Prevalence and morbidity associated with non-malignant, life-threatening conditions in childhood. *Child Care Health Dev* 2001; **27**: 389–398.
5. Association for Children's Palliative Care (ACT): http://www.act.org.uk (accessed January 2007).
6. Horrocks S, Somerset M, Salisbury C. Determining the need for terminal care for children. *Eur J Palliat Care* 2002; **9**: 78–79.
7. Joint Working Party on Palliative Care for Adolescents and Young Adults. *Palliative Care for Young People Aged 13–24 Years.* Bristol: ACT, 2001.
8. Friedrichsdorf S, Zernikow B. Die Versorgung sterbender Kinder in Deutschland – Status Quo der pädiatrischen Palliativmedizin. *Prakt Pädiatr* 2004; **10**: 68-72.
9. Kane B. Children's concepts of death. *J Genet Psychol* 1979; **134**: 141–153.
10. Piaget J. *Dreams and Imitations in Childhood.* New York: Norton, 1962.
11. Nagy M. The child's theories concerning death. *J Genet Psychol* 1948; **73**: 3–27.
12. World Health Organization. Guidelines for analgesic drug therapy. In: *Cancer Pain Relief and Palliative Care in Children.* Geneva: WHO/IASP, 1998, pp. 24–28.
13. Hain R, Hardcastle A, Pinkerton C, et al. Morphine metabolism and morphine-6-glucuronide in the plasma and cerebrospinal fluid of children. *J Pharmacol* 1999; **48**: 37–42.
14. Hunt A, Joel S, Dick G, et al. Population pharmacokinetics of oral morphine and its glucuronides in children receiving morphine as immediate release liquid or sustained release tablets for cancer pain. *J Pediatr* 1999; **135**: 47–55.
15. Kart T, Christrup L, Rasmussen M. Recommended use of morphine in neonates, infants and children. *Paediatr Anaesth* 1997; **7**: 93–101.
16. Vermeire A, Remon JP. Compatibility and stability of ternary admixtures of morphine with haloperidol or midazolam and dexamethasone or methylprednisolone. *Int J Pharm* 1999; **177**: 53–67.

17. Schrijvers D, Tai-Apin C, De Smet MC, et al. Determination of compatibility and stability of drugs used in palliative care. *J Clin Pharm Ther* 1998; **23**: 311–314.

18. Grassby PF, Hutchings L. Drug combinations in syringe drivers: the compatibility and stability of diamorphine with cyclizine and haloperidol. *Palliat Med* 1997; **11**: 217–224.

19. Back I. Syringe driver drug compatibility database, patient information leaflets on the Internet. *Palliat Med* 2001; **15**: 77.

20. Neuberger J. *Caring for Dying People of Different Faiths*. London: Mosby, 1994.

21. Goldman A, Beardsmore S, Hunt J. Palliative care for children with cancer – home, hospital, or hospice? *Arch Dis Child* 1990; **65**: 641–643.

22. Ashby M, Kosky RJ, Laver HT, et al. An enquiry into death and dying at Adelaide Children's Hospital: a useful model. *Med J Aust* 1991; **154**: 165–170.

23. Hain RDW. The view from a bridge. *Eur J Palliat Care* 2002; **9**: 75–77.

24. Initiative for Pediatric Palliative Care (IPPC): http://www.ippcweb.org (accessed January 2007).

25. Goldman A, Hain RDW, Liben S (eds). *Oxford Textbook of Palliative Care for Children*, 1st edn. Oxford, Oxford University Press, 2006.

CHAPTER 33

References

1. Pappworth MH. *Human Guinea Pigs: Experimentation on Man*. London: Routledge, 1967.

2. Ticktin HE, Zimmerman HJ. Hepatic dysfunction and jaundice in patients receiving triacetyloleandomycin. *N Engl J Med* 1962; **267**: 964–968.

3. Youngson RM, Schott I. *Medical Blunders – Amazing True Stories of Mad, Bad and Dangerous Doctors*. London: Robinson, 1996.

4. Lock S. Lessons from the Pearce affair: handling scientific fraud. *BMJ* 1995; **310**: 1547–1548.

5. Department of Health Research Governance Framework. Available at: http://www.dh.gov.uk/PolicyAndGuidance/ResearchAndDevelopment/ResearchAndDevelopmentAZ/ResearchGovernance/ResearchGovernanceArticle/fs/en?CONTENT_ID=4002112&chk=PJlaGg (accessed January 2007).

6. *Inquiry into the Management of Care of Children Receiving Complex Heart Surgery at the Bristol Royal Infirmary*. Central Office of Information, May 2000. BRRO JOO-5418/1K. Available at: http://www.bristol-inquiry.org.uk (accessed January 2007).

7. *The Royal Liverpool Children's Enquiry Report* (The Redfern Report). London: Stationery Office, 2002. Available at: http://www.rlcinquiry.org.uk (accessed January 2007).

8. Smith R. Cheating in medical school. *BMJ* 2000; **321**: 398.

9. Glick SM. Cheating at medical school. *BMJ* 2001; **322**: 250–251.

10. Gale E, Clarke A. A drug on the market? *Lancet* 2000; **355**: 61–63.

11. Stephenson TJ, Barbor P. Ethical dilemmas of diagnosis and intervention. In: *Fetal and Neonatal Neurology and Neurosurgery*, 2nd edn (eds Levene MI, Lilford RJ, Bennett MJ, et al.). London: Churchill Livingstone, 1995, pp. 709–718.

12. Stephenson TJ, Walker DA. Ethics of randomised controlled trials. *BMJ* 1996; **313**: 362–363.

13. Lennon R, Quinn M, Collard K. Support for studies in paediatric medicine is needed. *BMJ* 2000; **321**: 1228.

14. Stephenson T. Worst outcome of Griffiths report would be that research becomes increasingly difficult. *BMJ* 2000; **321**: 1345.

15. Turner S, Longworth A, Nunn AJ, et al. Unlicensed and off label drug use in paediatric wards: prospective study. *BMJ* 1998; **316**: 343–345.

16. McIntyre J, Conroy S, Avery A, et al. Unlicensed and off label drug use in general practice. *Arch Dis Child* 2000; **83**: 498–501.

17. Chalumeau M, Treluyer JM, Salanave B, et al. Off label and unlicensed drug use among French office based paediatricians. *Arch Dis Child* 2000; **83**: 502–505.

18. Regulations requiring manufacturers to assess the safety and effectiveness of new drugs and biological products in paediatric patients. Pages 66631–66674 [FR doc 98-31902] OC 98412. Docket No. 97M-0165 [REFT] [PDF].

19. Royal College of Paediatrics and Child Health, Ethics Advisory Committee. *Guidelines for the Ethical Conduct of Medical Research Involving Children*. London: RCPCH, 2000.

20. Medical Research Council. *The Ethical Conduct of Research on Children*. London: MRC, 1991.

21. Campbell H, Surry S, Royle E. A review of randomised controlled trials published in *Archives of Disease in Childhood* from 1982–1996. *Arch Dis Child* 1997; **79**: 192–197.

22. Rudolf M, Lyth N, Bundle A, et al. A search for the evidence supporting community paediatric practice. *Arch Dis Child* 1999; 80: 257–261.

23. Department of Health. Report of the Ad Hoc Advisory Group on the Operation of NHS Research Ethics Committees. London: Stationery Office, 2005. Available at: http://www.dh.gov.uk/PublicationsAndStatistics/Publications/PublicationsPolicyAndGuidance/PublicationsPolicyAndGuidanceArticle/fs/en?CONTENT_ID=4112410&chk=kw5gAf (accessed January 2007).

24. NHS Executive West Midlands Regional Office. *Report of a Review of the Research Framework in North Staffordshire Hospital NHS Trust* (Griffiths Report). Leeds: NHS Executive, 2000.

25. Murray GD. Commentary: research governance must focus on research training. *BMJ* 2001; **322**: 1461–1462.

26. Faulder C. *Whose Body Is It? The Troubling Issue of Informed Consent*. London: Virago, 1985, p. 158.

27. Gillick v West Norfolk and Wisbech Area Health Authority [1985] 3 All ER 402.

28. British Medical Association. *Withholding and Withdrawing Life-prolonging Medical Treatment*. London: BMJ Books, 2001, p. 94.

29. Calvert S, on behalf of the UKOS trial. *Autumn Newsletter*. London: St George's Hospital Medical School, 2000.

30. Somerville A. Informed consent and human rights in medical research. In: *Informed Consent in Medical Research* (eds Doyal L, Tobias JS). London: BMJ Books, 2000, pp. 249–256.

31. Edwards SJ, Lilford RJ, Braunholtz DA, et al. Ethical issues in the design and conduct of randomised controlled trials. *Health Technol Assess* 1998; **2**: 1–6.

32. Galloway J. Game plan for cancer care. *Lancet* 2000; **355**: 150.

33. Lantos J. The inclusion benefit in clinical trials. *J Pediatr* 1999; **134**: 130–131.

34. Djulbegovic B, Lacavic M, Cantor A, et al. The uncertainty principle and industry-sponsored research. *Lancet* 2000; **356**: 635–638.

35. Kemmeren JM, Algra A, Grobbee DE. Third generation oral contraceptives and risk of venous thrombosis: meta-analysis. *BMJ* 2001; **323**: 131–134.

36. Stelfox HT, Chua G, O'Rourke K, et al. Conflict of interest in the debate over calcium-channel antagonists. *N Engl J Med* 1998; 338: 101–106.

37. Rochon PA, Gurwitz JH, Simms RW, et al. A study of manufacturer-supported trials of nonsteroidal anti-inflammatory drugs in the treatment of arthritis. *Arch Intern Med* 1994; **154**: 157–163.

38. Smyth R. Research with children. *BMJ* 2001; **322**: 1377–1378.

39. Stephenson TJ. Medicines for children – the last century and the next. *Arch Dis Child* 2001; **85**: 177–179.

40. Smithells R. Iatrogenic hazards and their effects. *Postgrad Med J* 1975; **15**: 39–52.

41. Royal College of Paediatrics and Child Health, Neonatal and Paediatric Pharmacists Group. *Medicines for Children*. London: RCPCH, 1999, p. 667.

42. Bolam v Friern Hospital Management Committee [1957] 2 All ER 118, [1957] 1 WLR 582.

43. Royal College of Paediatrics and Child Health. *Safer and Better Medicines for Children*. London: RCPCH, 2004.

CHAPTER 34

Further reading

British Medical Association. *Consent, Rights and Choices in Healthcare for Children and Young People*. London: BMJ Books, 2001.

Derbyshire P. *Living with a Sick Child in Hospital. The Experiences of Parents and Nurses*. London: Chapman and Hall, 1994.

Macnab A, Macrae D, Henning R (eds). *Care of the Critically Ill Child*. London: Churchill Livingstone, 1999.

Pillitteri A. *Child Health Nursing. Care of the Child and Family*. Philadelphia, PA: Lippincott, 1999. (Comprehensive review with many practical nursing suggestions.)

Royal College of Paediatricians and Child Health. *Bridging the Gaps: Healthcare for Adolescents. Report of the Joint Working Party on*

Adolescent Health of the Royal Medical and Nursing Colleges of the UK. London: RCPCH, 2003.

Scal P, Ireland M. Addressing transition to adult healthcare for adolescents with special health care needs. *Paediatrics* 2005; **115**: 1607–1612. (An overview and reference list for a therapeutic success but new source of conflict.)

Shooter M. The ethics of withholding and withdrawing therapy in infants and young children. In: *CAPD/CCPD in Children*, 2nd edn (eds Fine R, Alexander S, Warady B). Boston, MA: Kluwer Academic, 1998. (The most critical of issues for staff and parents.)

Shooter MS. Children and adolescents who have chronic physical illness. In: *Strategic Approaches to Planning and Delivery of Child and Adolescent Mental Health Services* (eds Williams R, Kerfoot M). Oxford: Oxford University Press, 2005.

Sloper P. Predictors of distress in parents of children with cancer. A prospective study. *J Paediatr Psychol* 2005: **25**: 79–91. (What to watch out for.)

Viner R. (ed.). ABC of Adolescence. Series of 12 articles. *BMJ* 2005; **330**(Feb–Apr). (Good review of many adolescent, family and health issues.)

CHAPTER 35

References

1. Department of Health. *The New NHS: Modern. Dependable.* Cmnd Paper 3807. London: DoH, 1997.
2. Department of Health. *Complaints: Listening ... Acting ... Improving. Guidance on Implementation of the NHS Complaints Procedure.* London: DoH, 1996.
3. NHS Scotland. *Can I Help You? Learning from Comments, Concerns and Complaints.* Available at: http://www.show.scot.nhs.uk/publications/me/complaints/docs/1guidance010405.pdf (accessed January 2007).
4. Scottish Executive Health Department. *The NHS Complaints Procedure: Revised Guidance for Family Health Service, Hospital and Health Board Complaints.* NHS MEL(1999)49. Edinburgh: Scottish Executive Health Department, 1999.
5. Commission for Patient and Public Involvement in Health. Independent Complaints Advocacy Service (ICAS). Available at: http://www.cppih.org/icas.html (accessed January 2007).
6. Healthcare Commission. Available at: http://www.healthcarecommission.org.uk/ContactUs/ComplainAboutNHS/fs/en (accessed January 2007).
7. Health Service Ombudsman. Available at: http://www.ombudsman.org.uk (accessed January 2007).
8. General Medical Council. *Good Medical Practice.* London: GMC, 2006. Available at: http://www.gmc-uk.org/guidance/good_medical_practice/GMC_GMP_V41.pdf (accessed January 2007).
9. General Medical Council. *A Guide for Doctors Referred to the GMC.* London: GMC, 2005. Available at: http://www.gmc-uk.org/concerns/doctors_under_investigation/guide_for_doctors.pdf (accessed January 2007).
10. General Medical Council. How to Make a Complaint about a Doctor: A Guide for Doctors, Medical Directors and Clinical Governance Managers. London: GMC, 2005. Available at: http://www.gmc-uk.org/concerns/making_a_complaint/guide_for_directors.pdf (accessed January 2007).
11. BBC News UK edition. *Profile: Professor David Southall.* Available at: http://news.bbc.co.uk/1/hi/health/3542880.stm (accessed January 2007).
12. BBC News UK edition. *Profile: Sir Roy Meadow.* Available at: http://news.bbc.co.uk/2/hi/health/3307427.stm (accessed January 2007).
13. Koralage N. Rising child abuse complaints and paediatrics. *BMJ Career Focus* 2004; **328**: 159. Available at: http://careerfocus.bmjjournals.com/cgi/reprint/328/7445/159.pdf (accessed January 2007).
14. Royal College of Paediatrics and Child Health. The RCPCH *Child Protection (CP) Survey.* Available at: http://www.rcpch.ac.uk/publications/recent_publications/Latest%20news/CP%20report.pdf (accessed January 2007).

Further information

Action Against Medical Accidents. Available at: http://www.avma.org.uk (accessed January 2007).

British Medical Association. *Consultant Handbook – The NHS Complaints Procedure.* BMA: London, 2005.

Citizens Advice Bureau. Advice guide. Available at: http://www.adviceguide.org.uk (accessed January 2007).

Commission for Patient and Public Involvement in Health. Available at: http://www.cppih.org (accessed January 2007).

NHS Complaints Procedure. Available at: http://www.dh.gov.uk/PolicyAndGuidance/OrganisationPolicy/ComplaintsPolicy/NHSComplaintsProcedure/fs/en (accessed January 2007).

NHS Complaints Procedure (Scotland). Available at: http://www.show.scot.nhs.uk/publications/me/complaints (accessed January 2007).

Quick Guide to the NHS Complaints Procedure. Available at: http://www.icasresources.com/images/QuickGuide.pdf (accessed January 2007).

CHAPTER 36

References

1. Burton JL, Wells M. The Alder Hey affair: implications for pathology practice. *J Clin Pathol* 2001; **54**: 820–823.
2. Bristol Royal Infirmary Inquiry. *The Inquiry into the Management of Care of Children receiving Complex Heart Surgery at The Bristol Royal Infirmary. Interim Report: Removal and Retention of Human Material.* July 2001. Available at: http://www.bristol-inquiry.org.uk/interim_report/index.htm (accessed January 2007).
3. The Royal Liverpool Children's Hospital Inquiry. Report (Alder Hey). London: The Stationery Office, 2001. Available at: http://www.rlcinquiry.org.uk (accessed January 2007).
4. NHS Scotland. *Review Group on Retention of Organs at Post Mortem.* November 2001. Chairman, Professor Sheila McLean. Available at: http://www.show.scot.nhs.uk/scotorgrev (accessed January 2007).
5. Royal College of Pathologists. *Guidelines for the Retention of Tissues and Organs at Post-mortem Examination.* London: Royal College of Pathologists, 2000.
6. British Medical Association. *Interim BMA Guidelines on Retention of Human Tissue at Post-mortem Examination for the Purposes of Medical Education and Research.* London: BMA, 2000.
7. Department of Health. *Families and Post Mortems: A Code of Practice.* London: DoH, 2003.
8. Bove KE, Autopsy Committee of the College of American Pathologists. Practice guidelines for autopsy pathology. *Arch Pathol Lab Med* 1997; **121**: 368–376.
9. Human Tissues Authority. Codes of Practice. July 2006. Available at: http://www.hta.gov.uk/guidance/codes_of_practice.cfm (accessed February 2007).
10. Evans HM. What's wrong with 'retained organs'? Some personal reflections in the afterglow of 'Alder Hey'. *J Clin Pathol* 2001; **54**: 824–826.
11. Confidential Enquiry into Maternal and Child Health. (CEMACH). Stillbirth, Neonatal and Post-neonatal Mortality 2000–2002. CEMACH, 2005. Available at: http://www.cemach.org.uk/publications/CEMACHPerinatalMortalityReportApril2005.pdf (accessed January 2007).
12. Stocker JT, Macpherson TA. The pediatric autopsy. In: *Pediatric Pathology*, Vol. 1 (eds Stocker JT, Dehner LP). Philadelphia, PA: Lippincott Williams & Wilkins, 2001, pp. 5–17.
13. Brodlie M, Laing IA, Keeling JW, et al. Ten years of neonatal autopsies in tertiary referral centre: retrospective study. *BMJ* 2005; **324**: 761–763.
14. Sutton L, Bajuk B, New South Wales Intensive Care Unit Study Group. Post-mortem examinations in a statewide audit of neonatal intensive care unit admissions in Australia in 1992. *Acta Paediatr* 1996; **85**: 865–869.
15. Kumar P, Angst DB, Taxy J, et al. Neonatal autopsies: a ten year experience. *Arch Pediatr Adolesc Med* 2000; **154**: 38–42.
16. Royal College of Obstetricians and Gynaecologists, Royal College of Pathologists. Joint Working Party. *Fetal and Perinatal Pathology.* London: RCOG/RCP, 2001.
17. General Medical Council. *Making and Using Visual and Audio Recordings of Patients.* London: GMC, 2002. Available at: http://www.gmc-uk.org/guidance/current/library/making_audiovisual.asp (accessed January 2007).
18. Department of Health. *What is the Human Tissue Act 2004?* London: DoH, 2005. Available at: http://www.opsi.gov.uk/acts/acts2004/20040030.htm (accessed February 2007).

19. Many of the points in this section were outlined by Professor Margot Brazier, former Chairman of the Retained Organs Commission at Royal College of Pathologists' seminar on *The Human Tissue Act 2004: What does it mean for you?* 4 May 2005.
20. Nationwide Organ Group Litigation. Medical Litigation. April 2004, pp. 2–5.
21. Becher JC, Bell JE, Keeling JW, et al. The Scottish perinatal neuropathology study: clinicopathological correlation in early neonatal deaths. *Arch Dis Child Fetal Neonatal Ed* 2004; 89: F399–F407.

CHAPTER 37

References

1. Baumer JH. International randomised trial of patient trigger ventilation in respiratory distress syndrome. *Arch Dis Child Fetal Neonatal Ed* 2000; 82: F5–F10.
2. Ventriculomegaly Trial Group. Randomised trial of early tapping in neonatal post-haemorrhagic ventricular dilatation. *Arch Dis Child* 1994; 65: F3–F10.
3. Anon. UK collaborative randomised trial of neonatal extracorporeal membrane oxygenation. *Lancet* 1996; 348: 75–82.
4. Kennedy I, Grubb A. *Medical Law: Text with Materials*, 2nd edn. London: Butterworths, 1994, p. 1052.
5. McLean S. Commentary: no consent means not treating the patient with respect. *BMJ* 1997; 314: 1076.
6. Mason S, Allmark PJ, Euricon Study Group. Obtaining informed consent to neonatal randomised controlled trials: interviews with parents and clinicians in the Euricon study. *Lancet* 2000; 356: 2045–2051.
7. Samuels MP, Raine J, Wright T, et al. Continuous negative extrathoracic pressure in neonatal respiratory failure. *Pediatrics* 1996; 98: 1154–1601.
8. NHS Executive West Midlands Regional Office. *Report of a Review of the Research Framework in North Staffordshire Hospital NHS Trust* (Griffiths Report). Leeds: NHS Executive, 2000.
9. Hey E. Chalmers I. Investigating allegations of research misconduct: the vital need for due process. *BMJ* 2000; 321: 752–755.
10. Neuberger J. *The Role of Research Ethics Committees in the United Kingdom. Ethics and Health Care*. London: King's Fund, 1992.
11. Beauchamp T, Childress J. *Principles of Biomedical Ethics*, 4th edn. New York: Oxford University Press, 1994, pp. 142–146.
12. Dalla-Vorgia P, Mason S, Megone C, et al. Overview of European legislation on informed consent for neonatal research. *Arch Dis Child Fetal Neonatal Ed* 2001; 84: F70–F73.
13. Megone C, Mason S, Allmark P, et al. The attitudes of RECs in 11 European countries to informed consent in neonatal research. In: *European Neonatal Research. Consent, Ethics Committees and Law* (eds Mason S, Megone C). Dartmouth: Ashgate, 2001, pp. 43–62.
14. Department of Health. *Research Governance Framework for Health and Social Care*, 2d edn. London: DoH, 2005. Available at: http://www.dh.gov.uk/assetRoot/04/12/24/27/04122427.pdf (accessed January 2007).
15. Modi N. Is parental 'informed consent' always necessary for research involving newborn infants? In: *European Neonatal Research. Consent, Ethics Committees and Law* (eds Mason S, Megone C). Dartmouth: Ashgate, 2001, pp. 237–247.
16. International PHVD Drug Trial Group. International randomised controlled trial of acetazolamide and furosemide in posthaemorrhagic ventricular dilatation in infancy. *Lancet* 1998; 352: 433–440.
17. Halliday H. The effect of post-natal steroids on growth and development. *J Perinatal Med* 2001: 29: 281–285.

Further reading

Mason S, Megone C. *European Neonatal Research. Consent, Ethics Committees and Law*. Dartmouth: Ashgate, 2001.

CHAPTER 38

References

1. Department of Health. *Seeking Consent: Working with Children*. London: DoH, 2001, p. 6.

2. Children Act 1989. Section 3(5). Available at: http://www.opsi.gov.uk/acts/acts1989/Ukpga_19890041_en_1.htm (accessed January 2007).
3. General Medical Council. *Seeking Patients' Consent: The Ethical Considerations*. London: GMC, 1998, pp. 3–4.
4. Thornton H. Clinical trials – a brave new partnership? *J Med Ethics* 1994; 20: 19–22.
5. McCabe MA. Involving children and adolescents in medical decision-making: developmental and clinical considerations. *J Pediatr Psychol* 1996; 21: 505–516.
6. British Medical Association. *Report of Consent Working Party*. London: BMA, 2001, p. 30.
7. Family Law Reform Act 1969 s8(1).
8. Re W [1992] 4 All ER 627 at 639.
9. BMA. *Consent, Rights and Choices in Health Care for Children and Young People*. London: BMJ Books, 2001, p. 40.
10. Gillick v West Norfolk and Wisbech Area Health Authority [1985] 3 All ER 402.
11. BBC News. *Mother Angry at Secret Abortion*. Available at: http://news.bbc.co.uk/1/hi/england/nottinghamshire/3709681.stm (accessed January 2007).
12. Daily Mail. *Sent for Abortion by 21-Year-Old*. Available at: http://www.dailymail.co.uk/pages/live/articles/health/womenfamily.html?in_article_id=302780&in_page_id=1799 (accessed January 2007).
13. NHS Health Advisory Service. *Children and Young People: Substance Misuse Services: The Substance of Young Needs: Commissioning and Providing Services for Children and Young People Who Use and Misuse Substances*. London: HMSO, 1996.
14. R (on the application of Axon) v Secretary of State for Health [2006] Q.B.539.
15. Children Act 1989. Section 38(6). Available at: http://www.opsi.gov.uk/acts/acts1989/Ukpga_19890041_en_1.htm (accessed January 2007).
16. British Medical Association. *Consent, Rights and Choices in Health Care for Children and Young People*. London: BMJ Books, 2001, p. 4.
17. Ginsberg KR, Slap GB, Cnaan A, et al. Adolescents' perceptions of factors affecting their decisions to seek health care. *JAMA* 1995; 273: 1913–1918.
18. Ford CA, Millstein SG, Halpern-Felsher BL, et al. Influence of physician confidentiality assurances on adolescents' willingness to disclose information and seek future health care. *JAMA* 1997; 278: 1029–1034.
19. Thrall JS, McCloskey L, Ettner SL, et al. Confidentiality and adolescents' use of providers for health information and for pelvic examinations. *Arch Pediatr Adolesc Med* 2000; 154: 885–892.
20. American Academy of Pediatrics Committee on Adolescence. Suicide and suicide attempts in adolescence. *Pediatrics* 2000; 105: 871–874.
21. Re M (Child: Refusal of Treatment) [1999] 2 FLR 810.
22. Royal College of Paediatrics and Child Health. *Withholding or Withdrawing Life Saving Treatment in Children: A Framework for Practice*. RCPCH: London, 1997.
23. Traugott I, Alpers A. In their own hands: adolescents' refusals of medical treatment. *Arch Pediatr Adolesc Med* 1997; 151: 922–927.
24. General Medical Council. http://www.gmc-uk.org/news/index.asp#young_people (accessed March 2007).

CHAPTER 39

Further information

Children Act 1989. Available at: http://www.opsi.gov.uk/acts/acts1989/Ukpga_19890041_en_1.htm (accessed January 2007).
Gillick v West Norfolk and Wisbech Area Health Authority [1986] AC112.
Human Rights Act 1998. Available at: http://www.opsi.gov.uk/ACTS/acts1998/19980042.htm (accessed January 2007).
United Nations (UN) Convention on the Rights of the Child. Available at: http://www.ohchr.org/english/law/pdf/crc.pdf (accessed January 2007).

CHAPTER 40

References

1. Wilson JMG, Jungner G. *Principles and Practices of Screening for Disease*. Geneva: World Health Organisation, 1968.

2. Parsonnet J, Axon ATR. Principles of screening and surveillance. *Am J Gastroenterol* 1996; **91**: 847–849.

3. National Screening Committee. *First Report of the National Screening Committee.* London: Health Departments of the United Kingdom, 1998.

4. Clarke A. The process of genetic counselling. Beyond nondirectiveness. In: *Genetics, Society and Clinical Practice* (eds Harper PS, Clarke A). Oxford: Bios Scientific, 1997, pp. 179–200.

5. Elwyn G, Gray J, Clarke A. Shared decision-making and nondirectiveness in genetic counselling. *J Med Genet* 2000; **37**: 135–138.

6. Gekas J, Gondry J, Mazur S, et al. Informed consent to serum screening for Down syndrome: are women given adequate information? *Prenat Diagn* 1999; **19**: 1–7.

7. Freda MC, DeVore N, Valentine-Adams N, et al. Informed consent for maternal serum alpha-fetoprotein screening in an inner city population: how informed is it? *J Obstet Gynecol Neonatal Nurs* 1998; **27**: 99–106.

8. Press NA, Browner CH. Why women say yes to prenatal diagnosis. *Soc Sci Med* 1997; **45**: 979–989.

9. Sadler M. Serum screening for Down's syndrome: how much do health professionals know? *Br J Obstet Gynaecol* 1997; **104**: 176–179.

10. Asch DA, Hershey JC, Pauly MV, et al. Genetic screening for reproductive planning. methodological and conceptual issues in policy analysis. *Am J Public Health* 1996; **86**: 684–690.

11. Koch L, Stemerding D. The sociology of entrenchment: a cystic fibrosis test for everyone? *Soc Sci Med* 1994; **39**: 1211–1220.

12. Nelkin D. The social dynamics of genetic testing: the case of fragile-X. *Med Anthropol Quar* 1996; **10**: 537–550.

13. Wilcken B, Travert G. Neonatal screening for cystic fibrosis: present and future. *Acta Paediatr* 1999; **88**(Suppl): 33–35.

14. Clarke A, Parsons EP. Screening, ethics and the law. *BMJ* 1993; **306**: 209.

15. Parsons EP, Clarke AJ, Bradley DM. Newborn screening for Duchenne muscular dystrophy: a psychosocial study. *Arch Dis Child* 2002; **86**: F91–F95.

16. Parsons EP, Clarke AJ, Hood K, et al. Feasibility of a change in service delivery: the case of optimal newborn screening for Duchenne muscular dystrophy. *Commun Genet* 2000; **3**: 17–23.

17. Parsons EP, Bradley D, Clarke A. Disclosure of Duchenne muscular dystrophy after newborn screening. *Arch Dis Child* 1996; **74**: 550–553.

18. Goddard P. Newborn screening for medium chain acyl-CoA dehydrogenase deficiency (MCADD) in the UK. *J Fam Health Care* 2004; **14**: 90–92

19. Wilcken B. Ethical issues in newborn screening and the impact of new technologies. *Eur J Pediatr* 2003; **162**(Suppl 1): S62–S66.

20. Chamberlain JM. Which prescriptive screening programmes are worthwhile? *J Epidemiol Commun Health* 1984; **38**: 270–277.

21. Atkin K, Ahmad WIU. Genetic screening and haemoglobinopathies: ethics, politics and practice. *Soc Sci Med* 1998; **46**: 445–458.

22. Clarke A. Population screening for genetic susceptibility to disease. *BMJ* 1995; **311**: 35–38.

CHAPTER 41

References

1. McClean SAM. Mapping the human genome – friend or foe? *Soc Sci Med* 1994; **39**: 1221-1227.

2. Clarke A (ed.). *The Genetic Testing of Children.* Oxford: BIOS Scientific, 1998, Chap. 1.

3. Marteau TM, Croyle RT. Psychological responses to genetic testing. *BMJ* 1998; **316**: 693–696.

4. Craufurd D, Harris R. Ethics of predictive testing for Huntington's chorea: the need for more information. *BMJ* 1986; **293**: 249–251.

5. Harper PS, Clarke A. Should we test children for 'adult' genetic diseases? *Lancet* 1990; **335**: 1205–1206.

6. Ross LF. Predictive genetic testing for conditions that present in childhood. *Kennedy Inst Ethics J* 2002, **12**: 225–244.

7. Michie S, Marteau TM. Predictive genetic testing in children: the need for psychological research. *Br J Health Psychol* 1996; **1**: 3 16.

8. Michie S, McDonald V, Bobrow M, et al. Parents' responses to predictive genetic testing in their children: report of a single case study. *J Med Genet* 1996; **33**: 313–318.

9. Michie S, Bobrow M, Marteau TM. Predictive genetic testing in children and adults: a study of emotional impact. *J Med Genet* 2001; **38**: 519–526.

10. Grosfeld FJM, Lips CJM, Beemer FA, et al. Psychological risks of genetically testing children for a hereditary cancer syndrome. *Patient Educ Couns* 1997; **32**: 63–67.

11. Cohen CB. Moving away from the Huntington's disease paradigm in the predictive genetic testing of children. In: *The Genetic Testing of Children* (ed. Clarke A). Oxford: Bios Scientific, 1998, Chap. 12.

12. Broadstock M, Michie S, Marteau TM. The psychological consequences of predictive genetic testing: a systematic review. *Eur J Hum Genet* 2000; **8**: 731–738.

13. Codori A-M, Petersen GM, Boyd PA, et al. Genetic testing for cancer in children. *Arch Pediatr Adolesc Med* 1996; **150**: 1131–1138.

14. Geller G. Commentary. Weighing burdens and benefits rather than competence. *BMJ* 1999; **318**: 1066.

15. McConkie-Rosell A, Spiridigliozzi GA. 'Family matters': a conceptual framework for genetic testing in children. *J Genet Couns* 2004; **13**: 9–29.

16. Codori AM, Zawacki KL, Petersen GM, et al. Genetic testing for hereditary colorectal cancer in children: long-term psychological effects. *Am J Med Genet* 2003; **116**: 117–128.

17. Sarangi S, Clarke A. Constructing an account by contrast in counselling for childhood genetic testing. *Soc Sci Med* 2002; **54**: 295–308.

18. Clinical Genetics Society. Report of the Working Party on the Genetic Testing of Children. *J Med Genet* 1994; **31**: 785–797.

19. Reder P, Fitzpatrick G. What is sufficient understanding? *Clinical Child Psychol Psychiatry* 1998; **3**: 103–113.

20. Dickenson DL. Can children and young people consent to be tested for adult onset genetic disorders? *BMJ* 1999; **318**: 1063–1065.

21. Alderson P. In the genes or in the stars? Children's competence to consent. *J Med Ethics* 1992; **18**: 119–124.

22. Alderson P. *Children's Consent to Surgery.* Milton Keynes: Open University Press, 1993.

23. Binedell J. Adolescent requests for predictive genetic tests. In: *The Genetic Testing of Children* (ed. Clarke A). Oxford: BIOS Scientific, 1998, pp. 123–132.

24. Binedell J, Soldan JR, Scourfield J, et al. Huntington's disease predictive testing: the case for an assessment approach to requests from adolescents. *J Med Genet* 1996; **33**: 912–918.

25. Procter AM, Clarke A, Harper PS. *Survey of Genetic Testing in Childhood.* Poster presentation, British Human Genetics Conference, University of York, 27–29 September 1999.

26. Brunger JW, Murray GS, O'Riordan M, et al. Parental attitudes toward genetic testing for pediatric deafness. *Am J Hum Genet* 2000; **67**: 1621–1625.

27. Rosen A, Wallenstein S, McGovern MM. Attitudes of pediatric residents toward ethical issues with genetic testing in children. *Pediatrics* 2002; **110**: 360–363.

28. Parker M, Lucassen A. Working towards ethical management of genetic testing. *Lancet* 2002; **360**: 1685–1658.

Further reading

American Society of Human Genetics, American College of Medical Genetics. ASHG/ACMG Report. Points to consider: ethical, legal and psychosocial implications of genetic testing in children and adolescents. *Am J Hum Genet* 1995; **57**: 1233–1241.

Dalby S. Genetics Interest Group response to the UK Clinical Genetics Society Report. The genetic testing of children. *J Med Genet* 1995; **32**: 490–491.

Davis DS. Discovery of children's carrier status for recessive genetic disease: some ethical issues. *Genet Test* 1998; **2**: 323–327.

Hoffmann DE, Wulfsberg EA. Testing children for genetic predispositions: is it in their best interest? *J Law Med Ethics* 1995; **23**: 331–344.

Welkenhuysen M, Evers-Kiebooms G, Decruyenaere M, et al. Adolescents' attitude towards carrier testing for cystic fibrosis and its relative stability over time. *Eur J Hum Genet* 1996; **4**: 52–62.

Wertz DC, Reilly PR. Laboratory policies and practices for the genetic testing of children: a survey of the Helix network. *Am J Hum Genet* 1997; **61**: 1163–1168.

CHAPTER 42

References

1. General Medical Council, Education Committee. *Recommendations on Basic Medical Education.* Rochester: Stanhope Press, 1980.

2. British Medical Association. Annual Representatives Meeting, London. British Medical Association 1986, Minutes 335 and 33.

3. Pond K (ed.). *Report of a Working Party on the Teaching of Medical Ethics* (Pond Report). London: Institute of Medical Ethics, 1987.

4. Teaching medical ethics and law within medical education: a model for the UK core curriculum. *J Med Ethics* 1998; **24**: 188–192.

5. General Medical Council, Education Committee. *Tomorrow's Doctors*. London: General Medical Council, 1993.

6. Davies DP. The changing face of undergraduate medical education. Consensus statement by teachers of medical ethics and law in UK medical schools. *Curr Paediatr* 2001; **11**: 212–217.

7. General Medical Council. *Good Medical Practice*. London: GMC, 1998.

8. Herbert PC, Meslin EM, Dunn EV. Measuring the ethical sensitivity of medical students: a study at the University of Toronto. *J Med Ethics* 1992; **18**: 142–147.

9. Kohlberg L. *Essays on Moral Development*: Vol. II. *The Psychology of Moral Development*. San Francisco, CA: Harper & Row, 1976.

10. Davies DP, Evans I, Lloyd-Richards R, et al. Improving awareness of ethical issues. *Arch Dis Child* 1996; **74**: 172–175.

11. Sritharan K, Russel G, Fritz Z, et al. Medical oaths and declarations. *BMJ* 2001; **323**: 1440–1441.

CHAPTER 43

References

1. McIntosh N. On behalf of the Ethics Advisory Committee of the Royal College of Paediatrics and Child Health. Guidelines for the ethical conduct of medical research involving children. *Arch Dis Child* 2000; **82**: 177–182.

2. Stiller CA. Centralised treatment, entry to trials and survival. *Br J Cancer* 1994; **70**: 352–362.

3. Schmidt B, Gillie P, Caco C, et al. Do sick newborn infants benefit from participation in a randomised clinical trial? *J Pediatr* 1999; **134**: 151–155.

4. Shuster E. The Nuremberg Code: hippocratic ethics and human rights. *Lancet* 1998; **351**: 974–977.

5. The World Medical Assembly. The Declaration of Helsinki. *N Engl J Med* 1964; **271**: 473–474.

6. Riis P. Perspectives of the Fifth Revision of the Declaration of Helsinki. *JAMA* 2000; **284**: 3045–3046.

7. Biros MH, Lewis RJ, Olson CM, et al. Informed consent in emergency research. Consensus statement from the coalition conference on acute resuscitation and critical care researchers. *JAMA* 1995; **273**: 1283–1287.

8. Smithells R. Iatrogenic hazards and their effects. *Postgrad Med J* 1975; **51**(Suppl 2): 39–52.

9. Modi N. Ethical and legal issues in neonatal research. *Semin Neonatol* 1999; **3**: 303–314.

10. McIntosh N. Strengthen ethical committees' role. *BMJ* 1993; **307**: 1496.

11. Zupancic JAF, Gillie P, Streiner DL, et al. Determinants of parental authorisation for involvement of newborn infants in clinical trials. *Pediatrics* 1997; **99**: e6.

12. Harth S, Thong Y. Parental perceptions and attitudes about informed consent in research involving children. *Soc Sci Med* 1995; **40**: 1537–1577.

13. Stenson BJ, Becher J-C, McIntosh N. Neonatal research – the parental perspective. *Arch Dis Child* 2004; 89: F321–F324.

14. Zelen M. A new design for randomised controlled trials. *N Engl J Med* 1979; **300**: 1242–1245.

15. Mason S. Obtaining informed consent for neonatal randomised controlled trials – an elaborate ritual? *Arch Dis Child* 1997; **76**: F143–F144.

16. Rogers GC, Tyson JE, Kennedy KA, et al. Conventional consent with opting in versus simplified consent with opting out: an explanatory trial for studies that do not increase patient risk. *J Pediatr* 1998; **132**: 606–611.

17. Doyal L. Journals should not publish research to which patients have not given fully informed consent – with three exceptions. *BMJ* 1997; **314**: 1107–1111.

Index